AF838812

AGE RELATED MACULAR DEGENERATION – THE RECENT ADVANCES IN BASIC RESEARCH AND CLINICAL CARE

Edited by **Gui-Shuang Ying**

Age Related Macular Degeneration – The Recent Advances in Basic Research and Clinical Care
Edited by Gui-Shuang Ying

Published by InTech
Janeza Trdine 9, 51000 Rijeka, Croatia

Copyright © 2011 InTech
All chapters are distributed under the Creative Commons Attribution 3.0 license, which allows users to download, copy and build upon published articles even for commercial purposes, as long as the author and publisher are properly credited, which ensures maximum dissemination and a wider impact of our publications. After this work has been published by InTech, authors have the right to republish it, in whole or part, in any publication of which they are the author, and to make other personal use of the work. Any republication, referencing or personal use of the work must explicitly identify the original source.

As for readers, this license allows users to download, copy and build upon published chapters even for commercial purposes, as long as the author and publisher are properly credited, which ensures maximum dissemination and a wider impact of our publications.

Notice
Statements and opinions expressed in the chapters are these of the individual contributors and not necessarily those of the editors or publisher. No responsibility is accepted for the accuracy of information contained in the published chapters. The publisher assumes no responsibility for any damage or injury to persons or property arising out of the use of any materials, instructions, methods or ideas contained in the book.

Publishing Process Manager Iva Simcic

Technical Editor Teodora Smiljanic

Cover Designer InTech Design Team

Additional hard copies can be obtained from orders@intechopen.com

Age Related Macular Degeneration –
The Recent Advances in Basic Research and Clinical Care, Edited by Gui-Shuang Ying
p. cm.
ISBN 978-953-307-864-9

We are IntechOpen, the world's leading publisher of Open Access books

Built by scientists, for scientists

4,100+
Open access books available

116,000+
International authors and editors

120M+
Downloads

151
Countries delivered to

Our authors are among the
Top 1%
most cited scientists

12.2%
Contributors from top 500 universities

CLARIVATE ANALYTICS
BOOK CITATION INDEX
INDEXED

WEB OF SCIENCE™

Selection of our books indexed in the Book Citation Index
in Web of Science™ Core Collection (BKCI)

Interested in publishing with us?
Contact book.department@intechopen.com

Numbers displayed above are based on latest data collected.
For more information visit www.intechopen.com

For EU product safety concerns:
IN TECH d.o.o., Prolaz Marije Krucifikse Kozulić 3, 51000 Rijeka, Croatia,
info@intechopen.com or visit our website at intechopen.com.

Meet the editor

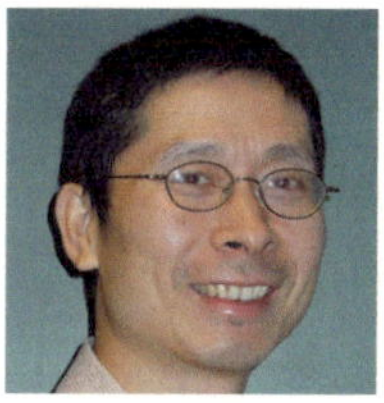

Dr Ying is an Assistant Professor of Ophthalmology, a faculty biostatistician in the Center of Preventive Ophthalmology and Biostatistics at the Department of Ophthalmology, and an Associate Scholar at the Department of Biostatistics, Perelman School of Medicine, University of Pennsylvania. He has more than 10 years of research experience in Age-related Macular Degeneration (AMD) and is the senior biostatistician for several multi-center AMD clinical trials, including the Complications of AMD Prevention Trial (CAPT), and the Comparison of AMD Treatment Trials (CATT). He collaborates with ophthalmologists and vision scientists and has authored or co-authored more than 80 papers in peer-reviewed journals. Dr Ying received a MD in Preventive Medicine and a MPH in Toxicology, both from ZheJiang University in China, and a PhD in Biostatistics from the University of Pennsylvania in the United States.

Contents

Preface

In the past decade, great progress has been made in understanding the pathobiology and genetics of Age-Related Macular Degeneration (AMD), and the effective therapies for this blinding disease have become available. These advancements have lead to the substantial change in the management of AMD patients. The online book *Age Related Macular Degeneration – The Recent Advances in Basic Research and Clinical Care* presents the most recent advances in basic research and clinical care of AMD. Different from other AMD books, this book aims to cover the new findings from basic and translational research on the biological and genetic mechanism of AMD, and the new interventions to prevent and treat this disease.

The book has a total of 15 chapters, grouped into two sections. Section one includes six chapters covering the basic and translational research of AMD. Section two includes nine chapters describing the clinical research and management of AMD. Each chapter has been contributed to by outstanding researchers or clinicians in the area of AMD. They present a very detailed review of new research and findings in the topic-specific AMD area, and also provide direction for future research. The book is targeted at researchers and clinicians who are interested in learning about new advances in the understanding and treatment of AMD, and insights into future research of AMD.

We hope that this AMD book will provide the latest information to its readers. The large amount of information presented in this book will help clinicians to take best care of their AMD patients. Additionally, it will assist researchers in conducting further AMD research and, eventually, achieve the goal of finding effective and safe ways to prevent or treat AMD.

Gui-Shuang Ying, PhD
Assistant Professor of Ophthalmology
University of Pennsylvania, Perelman School of Medicine
Philadelphia, PA
USA

Part 1

Basic and Translational Research

1

Wet Age Related Macular Degeneration

Fardad Afshari, Chris Jacobs, James Fawcett and Keith Martin
University of Cambridge,
UK

1. Introduction

Age related macular degeneration (AMD) is the leading cause of blindness in the developed countries. Approximately 8 million people in America have AMD and the number of advanced AMD is likely to rise by 50% by year 2020 due to the projected increase in the number of elderly people (Friedman et al., 2004). AMD is a condition of significant morbidity in terms of both physical and mental health (Hassell et al 2006). The burden of this disease is multifaceted as both the individual and society bear a cost. The individual has a loss of independence and ability of self care, with a pressure on society to fulfil the need for community and vision related support.

In this review of AMD, we will explore the epidemiology of AMD, the criteria for diagnosis with particular focus on the pathophysiology and treatments of wet AMD.

1.1 Epidemiology

AMD affects a large proportion of the elderly population. By applying the criteria of presence of macular drusen greater than 63 micrometres in diameter on fundus photography, up to 61% of adults over 60 years have some degree of AMD (Piermarocchi et al 2011). With a high estimated prevalence, it is important to understand the potential risk factors for this condition.

A meta analysis of published data suggests that increasing age, current cigarette smoking, previous cataract surgery, and a family history of AMD show strong and consistent associations with late AMD. Risk factors with moderate and consistent associations were higher body mass index, history of cardiovascular disease, hypertension, and higher plasma fibrinogen. Risk factors with weaker and inconsistent associations were gender, ethnicity, diabetes, iris colour, history of cerebrovascular disease, and serum total and HDL cholesterol and triglyceride levels (Chakravarthy et al 2010).

Direct associations between AMD and age, cataract, family history, alcohol consumption, the apolipoproteins A1 and B were also found in a 14 year follow up amongst a city populations (Buch et al 2005). In addition, recent data on human genome project have linked a complement H polymorphism Try402His on chromosome 1 to increased risk of AMD (Klein et al.,2005). Ala69ser polymorphism in the ARMS2 gene on chromosome 10 is yet another instance where genetic susceptibility for this condition has been established (Rivera et al., 2005). It has also been shown that ARMS2 polymorphism together with smoking, can synergistically increase the risk of developing AMD (Schmidt et al., 2006). Therefore it is evident that AMD is a result of interplay of genetic and environmental factors leading to the final pathology.

Better understanding of risk factors can help to identify individuals at high risk for wet AMD who may benefit from early intervention with existing or novel therapies. Using visual acuity as an outcome measure, visual prognosis is more favourable in patients with early intervention (Wong et al 2008).

1.2 Classification of AMD and diagnosis

AMD is characterized by the deposition of polymorphous material between the retinal pigmented epithelium and Bruch's membrane (Jager et al., 2008). These depositions are named Drusen. Drusen are categorised by sizes as, small(<63µm), medium (63-124 µm) and large (>124µm) (Bird et al., 1995). They are also considered as hard or soft depending on the appearance of their margins on opthalmological examination. While hard drusens have clearly defined margins, soft ones have less defined and fluid margins (Bird et al., 1995).

Classically the condition is divided in to two main subtypes; dry/non exudative and wet/exudative. The Age-related Eye Disease Study (AREDS) fundus photographic severity scale is one of the main classification systems used for this condition (Sallo et al 2009):

No AMD (AREDS category 1)

No or a few small (<63 micrometres in diameter) drusen.

Early AMD (AREDS category 2)

Many small drusen or a few intermediate-sized (63-124 micrometres in diameter) drusen, or macular pigmentary changes.

Intermediate AMD (AREDS category 3)

Extensive intermediate drusen or at least one large (≥125 micrometres) drusen, or geographic atrophy not involving the foveal centre.

Advanced AMD (AREDS category 4)

Geographic atrophy involving the foveal centre (atrophic, or dry AMD)

Choroidal neovascularisation (wet AMD) or evidence for neovascular maculopathy (subretinal haemorrhage, serous retinal or retinal pigment epithelium detachments, lipid exudates, or fibrovascular scar).

Wet AMD results from the abnormal growth of blood vessels from the choriocapillaris (choroidal neovascularisation), through Bruch's membrane. The fragility of the blood vessels and inflammatory processes lead to subretinal haemorrhages and fibrovascular scarring. This process can occur de novo or as a progression of dry AMD.

As with many classification systems, there is variability in AMD grading between clinicians. Therefore although such scales are important for accurate follow up of AMD progression, care is needed in their interpretation.

To classify AMD, multiple ophthalmological tools have proven to be useful including dilated indirect ophthalmoscopy, stereoscopic fundus photography, amsler grid testing, fundus fluorescein angiography (FFA) and optical coherence tomography (OCT). Of the mentioned techniques available, FFA is of great importance as it allows differentiation between neovascularisation attributable to AMD and that caused by other conditions. The use of FFA has enabled sub-classification of wet AMD according to the appearance of the lesions and the location of choroidal neovascularisation in relation to the fovea. The appearance can be described as classic or occult, which is according to the defined features of the membrane at early and late phases. The location can be extrafoveal (choroidal neovascularisation greater than 200um from the foveal avascular zone), juxtafoveal (choriodal neovascularisation is closer than 200um from the fovealavascualr zone) and sub-foveal (originating or extension of choroidal neovascularisation to the centre of the avascular zone). OCT provides a cross sectional image of the macula and identifies retinal pigment detachment, fluid accumulation and vitero-macular attachments. OCT has become an important tool in the monitoring progression of wet AMD especially in light of new therapeutic possibilities.

2. Pathophysiology of wet AMD

In this section we will explore the clinical presentation and the current pathophysiological mechanism underlying the development of AMD.

2.1 Clinical presentation of wet AMD

Clinically, AMD presents with visual loss of varying severity. Early in the course of disease, patients can present with very mild symptoms or be completely asymptomatic. Some patients, however, do experience a loss of contrast sensitivity, blurred vision and scotomas as the disease progresses to the intermediate stage (Jager et al., 2008). Other visual abnormalities associated with AMD include metamophopsia(distortion of straight lines), disparity of image size, macropisa and micropsia, hyperopic refractive shift with associated anisometriopia, light glare, floaters, photopsia (Schmidt-Erfurth et al 2004). However, neovascular or wet AMD, unlike the dry subtype, can have a sudden onset of presentation due to subretinal haemorrhages and exudates leading to retinal detachment and a acute visual loss (Jager et al., 2008). Although wet AMD is only responsible for 15% of the total AMD, it is responsible for more than 80% of AMD-related severe visual loss and blindness (Fine et al., 1986).

2.2 Pathophysiological models for AMD development

Various theories and models have been proposed to explain the pathophysiology of AMD with multiple factors contributing to the final outcome. Most models proposed focus either on the Bruch's membrane or on the retinal pigmented cells overlying this membrane.

Retinal pigment epithelial (RPE) cells, form a single layer of cells overlying Bruch's membrane with photoreceptors located anterior to RPE layer. RPE cells play a very complex role in preserving photoreceptors and their function. One of their major functions is to remove the shed outer segments of the photoreceptors by phagocytosis (Chang and Finnemann, 2007;Finnemann and Silverstein, 2001). It has been shown that failure of this process will result in build up of debris between the retinal layer and the Bruch's membrane leading to retinal degeneration (Nandrot et al., 2004).

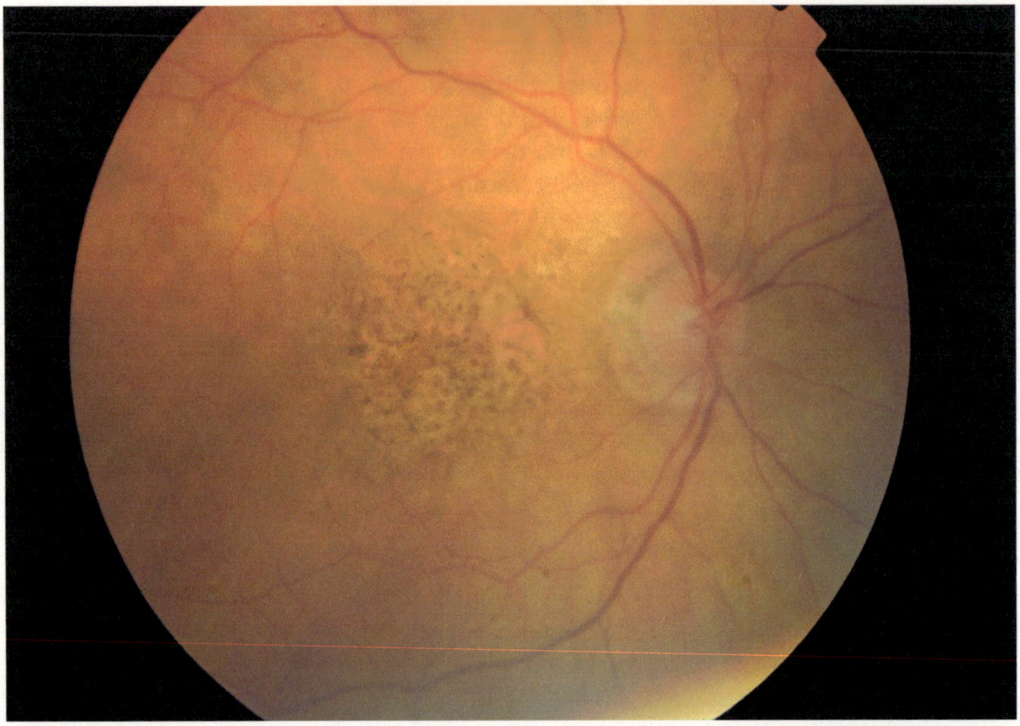

Fig. 1. Fundoscopic view- dry AMD. Note there is no neovascularisation evident.

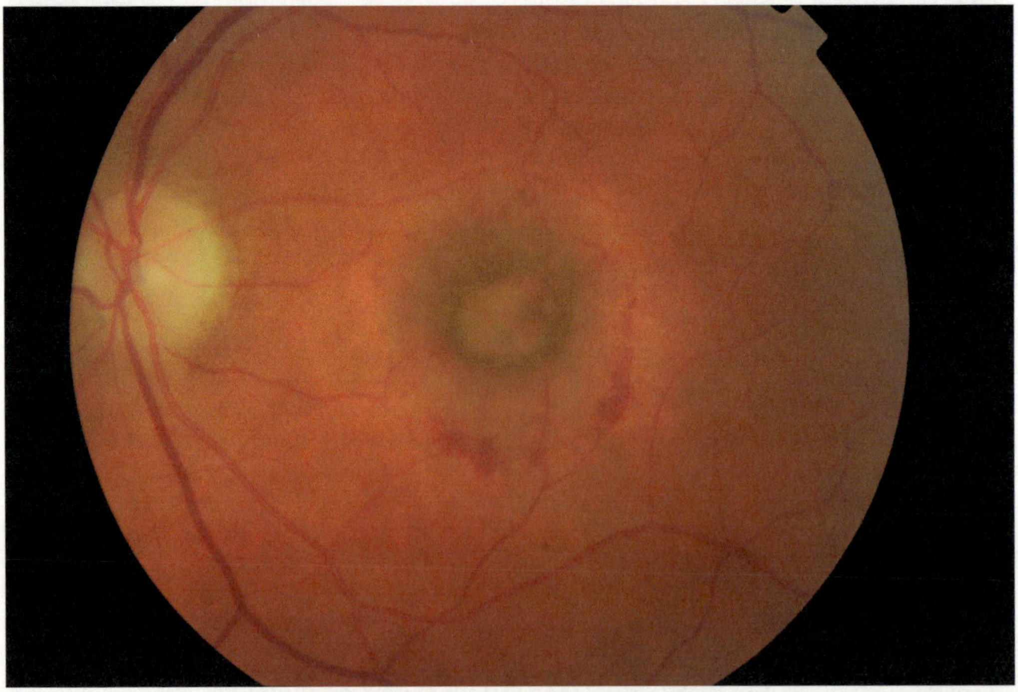

Fig. 2. Fundoscopic view of wet AMD. Excessive neovascularisation in macular region.

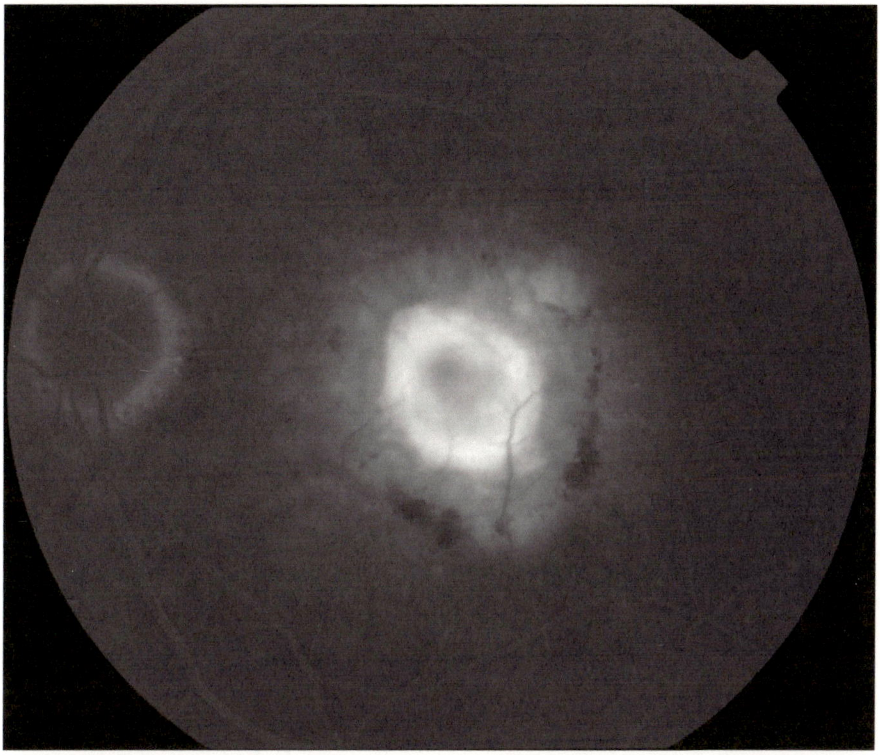

Fig. 3. Fundus fluorescein angiography (FFA) image of corresponding eye affected by wet AMD.

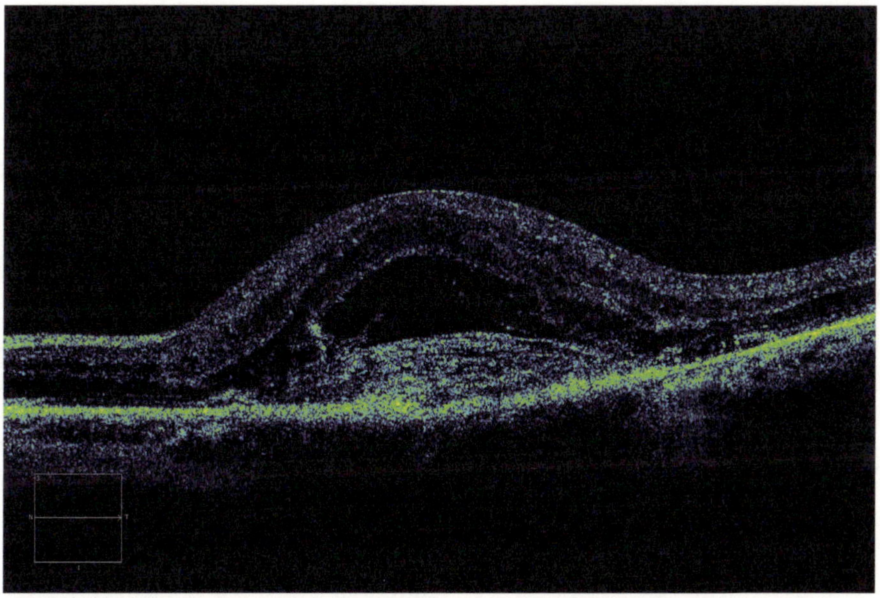

Fig. 4. Optical coherence tomography (OCT) image of corresponding eye. Significant macular oedema is evident.

In AMD, various abnormalities in the Bruch's membrane have been shown to lead to the disruption of RPE function (Sun et al., 2007), and this in turn can lead to the disruption of photoreceptor function and their loss. Therefore, Bruch's membrane has been the focus of great deal of AMD research.

To understand the pathophysiology of AMD, it is necessary to understand the basic normal structure of Bruch's membrane. Bruch's membrane is a penta-laminar structure, composed of RPE basement membrane, inner collagenous layer, elastin lamina, outer collagenous layer and choriocapillary basement membrane (Zarbin et al 2003). Each layer has a different composition of extracellular ligands, capable of interacting with integrins on the RPE cells. The top layer of Bruch's membrane (the RPE basement membrane) is of great importance as it contains an important extracellular matrix called laminin (Das et al., 1990; Zarbin,2003; Pauleikhoff et al., 1990) necessary for RPE adhesion and attachment.

Over the years, molecular analysis of Bruch's membrane has lead to the identification of composition of each layer as summarized in the table below (Das et al., 1990; Zarbin, 2003; Pauleikhoff et al., 1990).

Layer 1. Basement membrane (Immediately underneath RPE layer)	Collagen IV, Collagen V, laminin, Heparan sulphate
Layer 2. Inner collagenous layer	Collagen I, Collagen III, Collagen V, fibronectin, Chondroitin sulphate, dermatan sulphate
Layer 3. Elastic lamina	Elastin, Collagen I, Fibronectin
Layer 4. Outer collagenous layer	Collagen I, Collagen III, Collagen V, fibronectin, Chondroitin sulphate, Dermatan sulphate
Layer 5. Choriocapillaries basement membrane	Collagen IV, Collagen V, Collagen VI, laminin, heparan sulphate

Table 1. Matrix components of different layers of Bruch's membrane.

Each layer of Bruch's membrane is composed of mixture of proteoglycans and adhesive ligands. Adhesive ligands interact with integrins on the surface of RPE cells. Different subunits of integrins interact with different class of ligands. RPE cells attachment to Bruch's membrane is largely dependent on integrin's ability to anchor the cell to the membrane firmly. Pathological states affecting the membrane or RPE cells therefore, may disrupt this important interaction leading to loss of adhesion and death of RPE cells.

A large number of hypotheses have existed regarding pathological processes involved in AMD. Overall, the pathological mechanisms proposed in AMD can be divided into 4 categories of inflammation, oxidative stress, abnormal ECM production, formation of CNVs and neovascularisation (Zarbin, 2004). These various components can happen either sequentially or they can occur simultaneously, leading to the final outcome seen in AMD (Zarbin, 2004).

2.2.1 The inflammation component

Although drusen formation is one of the hallmarks of AMD, controversy exists as to whether they are directly involved in the pathology of AMD. Drusen can be found in non-AMD patient eyes incidentally associated with aging (Zarbin, 2004). However, others have suggested that the accumulation of large numbers of macular drusen is a necessity for the development of geographic atrophy and choroidal neovascularization characteristic of advanced AMD (Harman, 1956; Wallace, 1999).

Biochemical and immunohistological studies suggest drusen consist of immunoglobulins and components of the complement pathway (such as the C5b-C9 complex), acute phase response proteins raised in inflammation (CRP, amyloid P component and alpha1-antitrypsin), proteins that modulate the immune response (such as vitronectin, clusterin, apolipoprotein E, membrane cofactor protein and complement receptor1), major histocompatibility complex class 2 antigens, and HLA-DR and cluster differentiation antigens (Hageman et al., 1999; Johnson et al., 2000; Mullins et al.,2000; Sakaguchi et al., 2002; Zarbin, 2004). In addition, there are cellular components in drusen including RPE membrane debris, lipofuscin, melanin and choroidal dendritic cells (Ishibashi et al., 1986; Killingsworth, 1987; Mullins et al., 2000).

In support of this inflammatory theory, intravitreal injections of corticosteroids reduce the incidence of laser-induced CNVs in non human primates, possibly by reducing inflammation (Ishibashi et al., 1985).

2.2.2 Oxidative stress

It has been shown that with increasing age, oxidative damage in RPE cells also increases (Wallace et al., 1998). This is associated with a decrease in levels of antioxidant protective agents such as plasma glutathione, while oxidized glutathione levels increase. Also antioxidant vitamins, such as vitamin C and E, show a decline with increasing age (Rikans and Moore, 1988; Vandewoude and Vandewoude, 1987).

In support of oxidation stress as one of the factors involved, accumulation of lipofuscin has been observed in aging eyes. Lipofuscins are derivatives of vitamin A metabolites (Katz et al., 1994). It has been shown that in the first decade of life, they only constitute 1% of the cytoplasmic volume of RPE cells where as this is increased to 19% of cytoplasmic volume in the elderly (De La Paz and Anderson, 1992; Feeney-Burns et al., 1984).

In vitro studies suggest that RPE lipofuscin is a photo-inducible generator of reactive oxygen species. Lipofuscin granules are continuously exposed to visible light and to high oxygen tension, which causes the production of reactive oxygen species and oxidative damage to RPE cells (Wassell et al., 1999; Winkler et al.,1999; Zarbin, 2004).

RPE lipofuscin accumulation can ultimately lead to the disruption of lysosomal integrity, induce lipid peroxidation, reduce the phagocytic capacity of RPE cells and ultimately lead to loss of RPE cells (Boulton et al., 1993; De La Paz and Anderson, 1992; Sundelin and Nilsson, 2001; Zarbin, 2004).

Consistent with the oxidative stress model, clinical studies on the use of antioxidants has shown that in patients with extensive intermediate drusen, supplementation with antioxidant vitamins and minerals reduces the risk of developing advanced AMD from 28% to 20% (Age related eye disease study research group, 2001).

2.2.3 Abnormal ECM production

With aging, various changes can happen to the extracellular matrix deposited within the Bruch's membrane. It has been shown that there is a decline of laminin, fibronectin and type

IV collagen in the aging RPE basement membrane, particularly over the drusen (Pauleikhoff et al., 1999).

There is an age dependent increase in type I collagen within the Bruch's membrane, with an increase in the thickness of the membrane from 2 micrometres at birth, to up to 6 micrometres in the elderly ages (Ramrattan et al., 1994). During aging , the membrane glycosaminglycans in Bruch's membrane increase in size, and there is an increase in the heparan sulphate proteoglycan content of the membrane (Hewitt et al., 1989). Furthermore, glycation end products can accumulate within the Bruch's membrane with aging, trapping other macromolecules (King and Brownlee, 1996; Schmidt et al., 2000).

RPE cells themselves are the source of many of these ECM molecules. Histologically, abnormal extracellular matrix can be found between the RPE cells and the basement membrane (basal laminar deposits) and external to the basement membrane within the collagenous layers of the membrane (basal linear deposits) (Bressler et al., 1994; Green and Enger, 2005). Drusen therefore can be a localized accentuation of these deposits in AMD (Bressler et al., 1994).

The increase in thickness and change in composition of the Bruch's membrane in AMD can lead to a disruption of the exchange of molecules between choriocapillaris and the subretinal space (Starita et al., 1997).

In support of this model, it has been shown that the hydraulic conductivity of the Bruch's membrane falls exponentially with age. Measurements have shown that most of the resistance to water flow lies in the inner collagenous layer of the Bruch's membrane which is possibly due to accumulation of abnormal entrapped material within this plane (Starita et al., 1997). Therefore, the thickened Bruch's membrane in AMD may lead to a diffusion barrier, leading to RPE and retinal dysfunction (Pauleikhoff et al., 1999; Remulla et al., 1995).

2.2.4 CNV formation

Multiple factors have been proposed as promoters of new blood vessels formation in wet AMD. Changes in the ECM is one of the abnormalities seen in AMD which can lead to the formation of new blood vessels. The mechanism by which this phenomenon occurs is not completely understood but is likely to be a multifactorial. The risk of CNV in AMD increases with the increase in Drusen. Some drusen components and advanced glycation end products stimulate the production of angiogenic factors (Lu et al., 1998; Mousa et al., 1999). The increased thickness of Bruch's membrane can also lead to reductions in choriocapillary blood flow and hypoxia (Remulla et al., 1995). Hypoxia in turn can upregulate genes Ang-1 and Ang-2, with Ang-1 promoting maturation and stabilization of blood vessels, and Ang-2 conferring endothelial cell responsiveness to angiogenic factors (Hanahan, 1997; Maisonpierre et al.,1997). In addition, RPE cells are themselves known to produce angiogenic factors, such as VEGF, (Kim et al., 1999) which can lead to neovascularisation. High concentrations of VEGF and its receptors are found in CNV and RPE cells (Kliffen et al., 1997; Kvanta et al., 1996). Furthermore, anti-VEGF treatments prevent laser induced CNV formation in primate models of AMD (Krzystolik et al., 2002).

It has been shown that overexpression of VEGF in transgenic mice leads to the formation of aberrant choriocapillaries. However, these vessels are not capable of penetrating the intact Bruch's membrane (Schwesinger et al., 2001). Therefore, damage to Bruch's membrane due to various factors in combination with the upregulation of VEGF, can synergistically lead to the choriocapillary CNVs penetrating the membrane and reaching the subretinal space (Schwesinger et al.,2001; Zarbin ,2004).

One of the molecules that has been studied extensively in our lab is a glycoprotein called tenascin C, known to be overexpressed in angiogenesis (Zagzag and Capo, 2002; Zagzaget al., 1996), neovascularisation and wound healing (Maseruka et al., 1997). Tenascin C deposition can occur in the Bruch's membrane in wet AMD on the basal side of RPE cells (Fasler-Kan et al., 2005) and in association with CNVs in the pathological Bruch's membrane (Nicolo et al., 2000). Tenascin C has been shown to prevent adhesion of RPE cells to extracellular matrix (Afshari et al 2010). Therefore accumulation of this molecule associated with CNV formation may play an important role in RPE loss from the Bruch's membrane seen in AMD (Afshari et al 2010).

In summary, different pathological processes during aging and in AMD can lead to modifications in the Bruch's membrane which ultimately becomes a less supportive environment for the RPE adhesion and function.

3. Experimental models available for studying wet AMD

3.1 *In vitro* and *ex vivo* models - Advantages vs disadvantages

In vitro models have allowed development of simplified systems to study processes involved in wet AMD. Most *in vitro* models have focused on the role of angiogenesis and isolation of Bruch's membrane to assess adhesion and survival of RPE cells.

Tezel and Del priore first described methodology for accessing different layers of Bruch's membrane to allow *in vitro* assessment of RPE adhesion at different levels of Bruch's membrane. A combination of enzymatic treatment and mechanical techniques were used to expose each layer sequentially starting from the top basal lamina and moving to deeper structures. Using this technique, it was shown that deeper layers of Bruch's membrane are less supportive of RPE attachment (Del priore et al 1998; Tezel TH 1999 FEB; Tezel TH 1999 March). RPE cell adhesion to Bruch's membrane may play a detrimental role both in AMD and following RPE transplantation.

An alternative way of accessing Bruch's membrane used in our lab is the water lysis technique (Afshari et al 2010). In this method, eye globes are dissected out and separated from their muscle attachments. The anterior chamber is then dissected away leaving the posterior chamber and retina and Bruch's-choroid-sclera. Retinal layer is then carefully removed leaving the Bruch's-choroid-sclera trilaminar structure which can be subsequently exposed to water. Exposure to water leads to lysis of endogenous RPE cells. Lysed RPE cells are then flushed away from the surface of Bruch's membrane using a mini water jet. This procedure therefore results in formation of a denuded Bruch's membrane which can allow further experiments such as transplanting exogenous RPE cells to assess adhesion and migration of the transplanted cells (Afshari et al 2010). The advantages of this technique is that minimal treatment of the tissue is required with preservation of natural Bruch's membrane. In addition the preparation of the Bruch's membrane for adhesion and migration assay is a short procedure. Immunostaining of both frozen sections and electron microscopy of the membranes following water treatment have confirmed complete removal of endogenous RPE layer therefore creating a suitable environment for transplanting exogenous cells (Afshari et al 2010). However for assessment of adhesion on different layers such as deeper collagen layers of Bruch's membrane, methodology by Tezel and Del priore et al can be used (Del priore et al 1998; Tezel TH 1999 FEB; Tezel TH 1999 March).

Although much has been learned from the use of eyes derived from experimental animals such as rats and rabbits, a major problem faced is the unique human age related changes and AMD related pathological processes that have been hard to recapitulate in animal models. Therefore recent attention has been on use of human derived Bruch's membrane and *ex vivo* models whereby pathological or normal samples can be used from donors. A great advantage of this technique is that good methodology exists for isolation of layers of Bruch's membrane, and eyes from various stages of the disease can be studied. A disadvantage of using human samples is the difficulty in obtaining high quality tissue before post mortem deterioration occurs.

3.2 *In vivo* models - Advantages vs disadvantages

In vivo animal models have been used widely in studying AMD. Creating animal models specific for AMD has been a difficult task to achieve. One of the older animal models used in AMD research is Royal College of Surgeons rats (RCS rats) where RPE cells are gradually lost over time along with photoreceptors. RCS rats have been used in RPE transplantation experiments widely to assess efficiency of transplanted cells in replacing the lost endogenous RPE cells and preventing photoreceptor loss (Li and Turner 1988). However these rats are a better model for studying retinitis pigmentosa and therefore may differ considerably with regards to pathology from AMD.

Another used animal model comprises of mechanically scratching the RPE layer. This allows creation of focal areas devoid of RPE cells allowing studying various transplantation or pharmacological treatments. Rabbits are used generally in this model (Philips 2003) due to bigger size of the eye globes allowing easier access.

None of the models above recapitulate the neovascularisation seen in wet AMD. However recently more models have emerged which reproduce the neovascularisation process. Some of these models use growth factors such as b-fibroblast growth factor (FGF) or vascular endothelial growth factor (VEGF) to induce the endothelial cells proliferation and migration to promote CNV formation in rats, rabbits and monkeys (Montezumas.R 2009, Edwards A. 2007, Lassota N 2008, Baba T 2010). Over the years different techniques have been used to deliver growth factors ranging from direct injections, lentiviral vectors, cells secreting growth factors or transgenic animals secreting the VEGF (Spilsbury 2000; julien 2008; Okamoto et al1997; Cui et al 2000) .

Newer techniques which can stimulate CNV formation include injection of matrigel subretinally which allows a suitable environment for blood vessels to grow into (Cao J 2010). An alternative to this has been use of polyethylene glycol injections subretinally which leads to activation of complement cascade and generation of VEGF leading to CNV formation in mouse (Lyzogubov et al 2011).

Multiple transgenic mice lines also have been created which produce CNV through different methods. One of such animal models is use of transgenic mice producing mitogen prokineticin 1 (Hpk1) which specifically stimulates fenestrated endothelial cells.

Introduction of this mitogen can lead to CNV formation from choriocapillaries (Tanaka N 2006). By generating transgenic mice expressing Hpk1 in retina, Tanaka et al were able to show that Hpk1 promotes development of CNV with no effect on retinal vasculature. Interestingly, these mice also show increased levels of lipofuscin which is also seen in AMD (Tanaka N 2006).

One of the most interesting examples of transgenic mice used in studying wet AMD is the ccr2/ccl2 transgenic mice which are unable to recruit macrophages to RPE layer and Bruch's membrane. This leads to accumulation of C5a and Immunoglobulin G which in turn leads to stimulation of VEGF production (Ambati 2003; Takeda et al. 2009).

An alternative method of CNV formation is application of laser to generate a focal area of burn within the Bruch's membrane which in turn leads to CNV formation. This technique over the years has become one of the most standard and widely used techniques in studying wet AMD. Various laser treatments using krypton, argon and diode have all been able to induce CNV formation in mice, rats, pigs and monkeys (Dobi et al 1989; Frank et al 1989;Ryan et al. 1979; Saishin et al 2003). To initiate CNV formation using laser, it is necessary for RPE layer, Bruch's membrane and the underlying choroid to be damaged by the laser to allow penetration and initiation of new blood vessel formation. The laser induced CNV formation is VEGF mediated, as different methods of blocking VEGF using peptides and antibodies in mice, rats and monkeys are all able to block the neovascularisation process (Hua J 2010; Goody RJ 2011).

4. Treatments available for AMD and their mode of action

4.1 Surgical and cellular transplantation/replacement

Since defects in Bruch's membrane in age related macular degeneration leads to RPE loss, replacement of RPE cells by transplantation has been proposed as a technique to prevent secondary photoreceptor death. In the past two decades, studies in various animal models of retinal degeneration and RPE loss have shown that RPE cell replacement may be a feasible technique to prevent a secondary photoreceptor loss due to RPE damage (Lund et al., 2001).

Li et al in 1988 demonstrated that RPE transplantation in young neonatal and adult rats allows a repopulation of denuded areas on the Bruch's membrane and prevent the photoreceptor degeneration in dystrophic RCS rat models of AMD (Liand Turner, 1988a, b). In separate studies, Castillo et al have shown that transplantation of adult young human RPE cells derived from cadaveric eye samples, into the dystrophic RCS rats can salvage the photoreceptor loss in this model (Castillo et al., 1997).

Furthermore, subretinal transplantation of the RPE cell line ARPE-19, the most widely used adult human RPE cell line, in dystrophic RCS rats can rescue the photoreceptors (Wang et al., 2005). Other animal models, such as rabbit models of RPE damage, showed that mechanical debridement of the Bruch's membrane followed by autologous RPE transplantation leads to the repopulation of debrided Bruch's membrane with preservation of photoreceptors (Phillips et al., 2003).

In humans patients with AMD, the formation of choroidal new vessels is part of the pathology of advanced wet AMD. The removal of CNVs has also been carried out in human patients with AMD. This can be followed by autologous transplantation of RPE cells, either harvested from the periphery of the Bruch's membrane which is not affected by the disease process (Binder et al., 2007), or from RPE cells from other donors (Algvere et al.,1994).

Algevere et al at in 1994 assessed the effect of human fetal RPE transplantation in 5 patients with AMD after the removal of CNVs. Human fetal RPE cells survived up to 3 months and covered the denuded areas of the Bruch's membrane (Algvere et al., 1994).

Other studies have also assessed the effect of adult autologous transplantation of RPE cells in AMD. It has been shown that autolgous transplantation following the removal of CNVs is a feasible technique and associated with some visual acuity improvement (Binder et al., 2004).

In 2007 Maclaren et al carried out autologous transplantation of the RPE cells, following submacular CNV excision, and reported viable grafts at 6 months time point and some level of visual function improvement in some patients. However, the complications associated with the surgery remained high (MacLaren et al., 2007).

RPE transplantation has traditionally been carried out as cell suspension but, due to problems with RPE attachment to Bruch's membrane, more recently RPE-choroid sheets have been tried as a means of delivering RPE cells (Treumer et al 2007). In 2011, Falkner-Radler et al, carried out a study comparing RPE cell suspension with that of RPE-choroid sheet transplantation. This study showed that anatomical and functional outcome in both cases were comparable with no significant difference between the two techniques in humans (Falkner-RadlerCl 2011).

Despite some improvements gained in the visual function, the results from the CNV removal combined with RPE transplantation, have not been as successful as those observed with animal models. This may be due to age related changes specific to human AMD which are absent in the animal models used in studying AMD and RPE transplantation.

RPE transplantation as a therapeutic technique faces major limitations, including poor adhesion of RPE cells when transplanted subretinally. Studies have shown that RPE cells require rapid adhesion to avoid apoptosis (Tezel and Del Priore, 1997,1999). Therefore, there is a limited time period after subretinal injection during which RPE cells need to reattach before undergoing cell death.

The lack of adhesion following transplantation is likely to be multifactorial due to the molecular changes resulting from pathological age related changes in the membrane, and other changes contributed by the disturbance of normal architecture of the membrane from the surgery.

Various studies using *ex vivo* models have demonstrated major differences between RPE and Bruch's membrane in patients from different ages, emphasizing the important role of aging in the pathological process. Studies by Gullapalli et al have shown that aged submacular human Bruch's membrane does not support adhesion, survival and differentiation of fetal RPE cells effectively (Gullapalli et al., 2005). Multiple studies have shown that RPE cell adhesion to the Bruch's membrane is reduced on aged membranes, when compared to the membrane derived from younger donors (Del Priore and Tezel,1998; Tezel et al., 1999).

In addition to changes in adhesion, survival and differentiation, it has been shown that the capacity of RPE cells to phagocytose the shed outer segment of rod photoreceptors is reduced when RPE cells are seeded on aged membranes than the young membranes (Sun, et al., 2007).

These functional differences are further backed up by the changes in gene expression between RPE cells cultured on aged and young membranes. It has been shown that the RPE cells seeded on aged membranes up-regulate 12 genes and downregulate 8 genes compared to RPE cells cultured on membranes derived from young donors suggesting the differences between ages are also reflected at gene level (Cai and Del Priore, 2006).

Therefore, it is evident that there is a significant age-dependent decline in the Bruch's membrane's ability to support the RPE cell adhesion and function, and therefore RPE loss and dysfunction in AMD can be at least partially reflective of changes within the membrane. These changes in Bruch's membrane therefore pose an obstacle for the transplanted RPE cells, which require fast attachment and adhesion, to survive post-transplantation.

In addition, data from our lab and others have shown that in wet AMD, there is increased deposition of a glycoprotein associated with neovascularisation. This glycoprotein named tenascin C is deposited on the upper layer of Bruch's membrane. Using purified tenascin C, we were able to show that human RPE cells lack the necessary integrins to attach to surfaces coated with this glycoprotein and therefore deposition of this molecule in pathological AMD Bruch's membrane further reduces the chance of adhesion. Using *in vitro* assays we were able to show that if RPE cells are engineered to express a necessary receptor called alpha9beta1 integrin for tenascin C, they are able to attach following transplantation to the wet AMD derived Bruch's membrane where as in the absence of this receptor, control RPE cells were unable to attach to the membrane effectively (Afshari et al 2010).

In addition to changes mentioned above, surgical techniques used in removal of CNVs have been shown to damage the normal architecture of Bruch's membrane. It is well established that surgical removal of CNVs in the wet AMD generally leads to excision of the basement membrane of the Bruch's membrane (Grossniklaus et al., 1994). Tsukahara et al using *ex vivo* models of aged Bruch's membrane have shown that the resurfacing of the Bruch's membrane is highly dependent on whether the basement membrane is intact or removed. The adhesion of RPE cells was much higher on aged Bruch's membrane if the basement membrane was not damaged and removed (Tsukahara et al., 2002). Therefore, one of the limitations of the CNV removal procedure is the iatrogenic removal of the laminin rich basement membrane, which reduces the chance of adhesion of RPE cells transplanted subsequently into the subretinal space.

In addition to the removal of the laminin rich basement membrane of Bruch'smembrane, the surgical procedures also lead to the exposure of deeper layers of the Bruch's membrane. Various studies have assessed the adhesion rate and the survival of RPE cells on different layers of the Bruch's membrane. They have revealed that RPE cell reattachment is the highest on the uppermost layers of the Bruch's membrane which include basement membrane. As deeper layers are exposed, this adhesion rate decreases (Del Priore and Tezel, 1998). Thus, following CNV removal, depending on which layer of the Bruch's membrane is exposed , the outcome of adhesion will differ which diminishes the chances of fast and efficient adhesion of the RPE cells following transplantation (Del Priore and Tezel, 1998).

RPE cells are known to attach to the human Bruch's membrane through beta1 integrin-mediated interaction, with extracellular ligands such as laminin, fibronectin, vitronectin and collagen IV (Ho and DelPriore, 1997). Tezel et al have demonstrated that laminin and fibronectin supported the adhesion of RPE cells best and prevented cellular apoptosis (Tezel and Del Priore,1997). Since the upper most layers of the Bruch's membrane are rich in laminin and fibronectin, removal of basement membrane combined with the exposure of deeper less adhesive substrates, limits adhesion following transplantation.

Therefore, there is a great need for promoting cell adhesion post transplantation to allow resurfacing and seeding of the pathologically and surgically altered membranes. Multiple problems faced with transplantation therefore haves lead to more attention on pharmacological and less invasive techniques to halt the CNV formation.

4.2 Photodynamic therapy and laser treatment

Laser photocoagulation is one of the techniques that was developed to treated neovascularisation problem in wet AMD. Since this technique leads to full thickness retinal burns, this can lead to loss of visual acuity if carried out in foveal region and therefore it is reserved for extrafoveal CNVs. In addition, there is a high rate of recurrence of CNVs following treatment with this method (Vedula SS and Krzystolik M 2011). However this technique is effective in reducing the progression of non-subfoveal CNVs compared to observation alone (Virgil 2007; Verdula SS and Krzystolik M 2011).

Photodynamic therapy on the other hand is a technique that works by injecting a photosensitive dye intravenously which preferentially binds to CNVs. On exposure of the eye to laser light, the dye can be activated leading to obliteration of the CNVs. This technique has the advantage of causing minimal trauma to normal choroid and membrane and the overlying retina. It therefore can be used for subfoveal lesions. The disadvantage with this technique is the necessity to repeat this procedure at least multiple times due to high rate of recurrence (TAP 1999;Verdula SS 2011).

4.3 Anti-VEGF monoclonal antibodies

One of the most recent approaches in battling wet AMD is the use of anti-VEGF monoclonal antibodies. Vascular endothelial growth factor has been shown to be involved in promoting formation of new blood vessels. The source of VEGF in AMD is believed to be the RPE cells themselves. Multiple studies have demonstrated presence of VEGF in RPE cells and its association with CNVs (Kim et al. 1999; Klifen 1997; Kvanata 1996). Although VEGF is necessary for neovascularisation, animal research shows that in the presence of intact normal Bruch's membrane, blood vessels will not invade the subretinal area and therefore a pathological process must render the membrane permeable to invading growing new blood vessels in AMD setting (Schwesinger 2001). Regardless of this finding, use of blocking agents against VEGF or its receptor holds promise in halting neovascularisation.

Animal studies have shown that blocking VEGF using different approaches can halt the neovascularisation process. Multiple clinical trials have assessed efficacy and safety of anti-VEGF monoclonal antibodies which include Bevacizumab, ranibizumab, pegabtanib (Vendula SS and KrzystolikM 2011). A recent systematic review of randomised controlled trials compared recent trials using anti-VEGF in wet AMD. Pegabtanib and Ranibizumab were shown to be both effective in reducing the neovascularisation with improvements in visual acuity and quality of life (Vendula SS and Krzystolik M 2011). There are currently no trials comparing these two drugs directly together. Bevacizumab, which also blocks VEGF and is considerably cheaper than its counterparts, has also been used off licence for treating wet AMD although originally it was licensed for colorectal carcinoma (Avery 2006, Emerson 2007). Although multiple studies have shown efficacy of this monoclonal antibody in reducing neovascularisation, the safety profile of this antibody is not as clear as other two (Mitchell P 2011).

5. Problems and challenges for future

With increasing aging population, the number of patients with AMD is likely to rise sharply. The projected number of advanced AMD cases is likely to rise by 50% by year 2020 (Friedman et al 2004). Therefore with increasing incidence of this condition, screening programs may be of value to allow early detection and treatment of this condition. This is of paramount importance as early detection has been shown to be associated with a better outcome and prognosis (Wong et al 2008).

With recent advances in cell transplantation and knowledge of stem cells, it may be possible that stem cell derived RPE cells can be used in the treatment of AMD (Lee and Maclaren 2011). Use of these cells may be of benefit as they have the potential to replace the lost cells and may not be hindered by the obstacles such as poor adhesion faced with cadaveric or donor derived RPE cells. For dry AMD, cell transplantation strategies are also undergoing clinical trials in several centres worldwide . Strategies to compare improve the survival and adhesion of transplanted cells to damaged Bruch's membrane are a key focus of our ongoing work.

Manipulation of integrins on RPE cells or genetic engineering of transplanted cells is a new field that holds promise in overcoming the obstacles faced in cell transplantation. Activating integrins by enhancing their function or introduction of new subunits of integrins into RPE cells have been shown to overcome the poor attachment and integration of RPE cells over Bruch's membrane (Afshari et al 2010; Fang et al 2009). It is therefore possible that with better understanding of RPE biology, adhesion and survival of cells following transplantation could be improved.

With the advent of the new therapies such as monoclonal anti-VEGF treatments, major advances have occurred in the treatment of wet AMD. At this point the challenges reside in wide access and affordable costs to allow early recognition and prevention of loss of vision at an early stage. Currently repeated injections of monoclonal antibodies limit their use in areas where access to such therapies is limited. With better understanding and experience of using such therapies, it is hoped that treatments with longer half lives and more affordable prices can be available to increasing aging population.

6. References

Afshari FT, Kwok JC, Andrews MR, Blits B, Martin KR, Faissner A, Ffrench-Constant C, Fawcett JW. Integrin activation or alpha 9 expression allows retinal pigmented epithelial cell adhesion on Bruch's membrane in wet age-related macular degeneration. Brain. 2010 Feb;133(Pt 2):448-64.

Age related eye disease study research group (2001). A randomized, placebocontrolled, clinical trial of high-dose supplementation with vitamins C and E, beta carotene, and zinc for age-related macular degeneration and vision loss: AREDS report no. 8. Arch Ophthalmol *119*, 1417-1436.

Algvere, P.V., Berglin, L., Gouras, P., and Sheng, Y. (1994). Transplantation of fetal retinal pigment epithelium in age-related macular degeneration with subfoveal neovascularization. Graefes Arch Clin Exp Ophthalmol *232*, 707-716.

Ambati J, Anand A, Fernandez S, Sakurai E, Lynn BC, Kuziel WA, Rollins BJ, Ambati BK. An animal model of age-related macular degeneration in senescent Ccl-2- or Ccr-2-deficient mice. Nat Med. 2003 Nov;9(11):1390-7.

Avery RL, Pieramici DJ, Rabena MD, Castellarin AA, Nasir MA, Giust MJ. Intravitreal bevacizumab (Avastin) for neovascular age-related macular degeneration. Ophthalmology. 2006 Mar;113(3):363-372.e5.

Baba T, Bhutto IA, Merges C, Grebe R, Emmert D, McLeod DS, Armstrong D, Lutty GA. A rat model for choroidal neovascularization using subretinal lipid hydroperoxide injection. Am J Pathol. 2010 Jun;176(6):3085-97.

Binder, S., Krebs, I., Hilgers, R.D., Abri, A., Stolba, U., Assadoulina, A., Kellner, L., Stanzel, B.V., Jahn, C., and Feichtinger, H. (2004). Outcome of transplantation of autologous retinal pigment epithelium in age-related macular degeneration: a prospective trial. Invest Ophthalmol Vis Sci *45*, 4151-4160.

Bird, A.C., Bressler, N.M., Bressler, S.B., Chisholm, I.H., Coscas, G., Davis, M.D.,de Jong, P.T., Klaver, C.C., Klein, B.E., Klein, R., and et al. (1995). An international classification and grading system for age-related maculopathy and age-related macular degeneration. The International ARM Epidemiological Study Group. Surv Ophthalmol *39*, 367-374.

Boulton, M., Dontsov, A., Jarvis-Evans, J., Ostrovsky, M., and Svistunenko, D. (1993). Lipofuscin is a photoinducible free radical generator. J Photochem Photobiol B *19*, 201-204.

Bressler, N.M., Silva, J.C., Bressler, S.B., Fine, S.L., and Green, W.R. (1994).Clinicopathologic correlation of drusen and retinal pigment epithelial abnormalities in age-related macular degeneration. Retina *14*, 130-142.

Buch H, Vinding T, la Cour M, Jensen GB, Prause JU, Nielsen NV. Risk factors for age-related maculopathy in a 14-year follow-up study: the Copenhagen City Eye Study. Acta Ophthalmol Scand. 2005 Aug;83(4):409-18.

Cai, H., and Del Priore, L.V. (2006). Gene expression profile of cultured adult compared to immortalized human RPE. Mol Vis *12*, 1-14.

Cao J, Zhao L, Li Y, Liu Y, Xiao W, Song Y, Luo L, Huang D, Yancopoulos GD, Wiegand SJ, Wen R. A subretinal matrigel rat choroidal neovascularization (CNV) model and inhibition of CNV and associated inflammation and fibrosis by VEGF trap.Invest Ophthalmol Vis Sci. 2010 Nov;51(11):6009-17.

Castillo, B.V., Jr., del Cerro, M., White, R.M., Cox, C., Wyatt, J., Nadiga, G., and del Cerro, C. (1997). Efficacy of nonfetal human RPE for photoreceptor rescue: a study in dystrophic RCS rats. Exp Neurol *146*, 1-9.

Chakravarthy U, Wong TY, Fletcher A, Piault E, Evans C, Zlateva G, Buggage R, Pleil A, Mitchell P. Clinical risk factors for age-related macular degeneration: a systematic review and meta-analysis. BMC Ophthalmol. 2010 Dec 13;10:31.

Chang, Y., and Finnemann, S.C. (2007). Tetraspanin CD81 is required for the alpha v beta5-integrin-dependent particle-binding step of RPE phagocytosis. J Cell Sci *120*, 3053-3063.

Cui JZ, Kimura H, Spee C, Thumann G, Hinton DR, Ryan SJ. Natural history of choroidal neovascularization induced by vascular endothelial growth factor in the primate. Graefes Arch Clin Exp Ophthalmol. 2000 Apr;238(4):326-33.

Das, A., Frank, R.N., Zhang, N.L., and Turczyn, T.J. (1990). Ultrastructural localization of extracellular matrix components in human retinal vessels and Bruch's membrane. Arch Ophthalmol *108*, 421-429.

De La Paz, M., and Anderson, R.E. (1992). Region and age-dependent variation in susceptibility of the human retina to lipid peroxidation. Invest Ophthalmol Vis Sci *33*, 3497-3499.

Del Priore, L.V., and Tezel, T.H. (1998). Reattachment rate of human retinal pigment epithelium to layers of human Bruch's membrane. Arch Ophthalmol *116*, 335-341

Dobi ET, Puliafito CA, Destro M. A new model of experimental choroidal neovascularization in the rat. Arch Ophthalmol. 1989 Feb;107(2):264-9.

Edwards AO, Malek G. Molecular genetics of AMD and current animal models. Angiogenesis. 2007;10(2):119-32.

Emerson MV, Lauer AK, Flaxel CJ, Wilson DJ, Francis PJ, Stout JT, Emerson GG, Schlesinger TK, Nolte SK, Klein ML. Intravitreal bevacizumab (Avastin) treatment of neovascular age-related macular degeneration.Retina. 2007 Apr-May;27(4):439-44.

Falkner-Radler CI, Krebs I, Glittenberg C, Povazay B, Drexler W, Graf A, Binder S. Human retinal pigment epithelium (RPE) transplantation: outcome after autologous RPE-choroid sheet and RPE cell-suspension in a randomised clinical study. Br J Ophthalmol. 2011 Mar;95(3):370-5.

Fang, I.M., Yang, C.H., Yang, C.M., and Chen, M.S. (2008). Overexpression of integrin alpha(6) and beta(4) enhances adhesion and proliferation of human retinal pigment epithelial cells on layers of porcine Bruch's membrane. Exp Eye Res. 2009 Jan;88(1):12-21.

Fasler-Kan, E., Wunderlich, K., Hildebrand, P., Flammer, J., and Meyer, P. (2005). Activated STAT 3 in choroidal neovascular membranes of patients with agerelated macular degeneration. Ophthalmologica *219*, 214-221.

Feeney-Burns, L., Hilderbrand, E.S., and Eldridge, S. (1984). Aging human RPE: morphometric analysis of macular, equatorial, and peripheral cells. Invest Ophthalmol Vis Sci *25*, 195-200.

Fine, A.M., Elman, M.J., Ebert, J.E., Prestia, P.A., Starr, J.S., and Fine, S.L. (1986). Earliest symptoms caused by neovascular membranes in the macula.Arch Ophthalmol *104*, 513-514.

Finnemann, S.C., and Silverstein, R.L. (2001). Differential roles of CD36 and alphavbeta5 integrin in photoreceptor phagocytosis by the retinal pigment epithelium. J Exp Med *194*, 1289-1298.

Frank RN, Das A, Weber ML. Curr Eye Res. A model of subretinal neovascularization in the pigmented rat. 1989 Mar;8(3):239-47.

Friedman, D.S., O'Colmain, B.J., Munoz, B., Tomany, S.C., McCarty, C., de Jong, P.T., Nemesure, B., Mitchell, P., and Kempen, J. (2004). Prevalence of agerelated macular degeneration in the United States. Arch Ophthalmol *122*, 564-572.

Goody RJ, Hu W, Shafiee A, Struharik M, Bartels S, López FJ, Lawrence MS. Optimization of laser-induced choroidal neovascularization in African green monkeys. Exp Eye Res. 2011 Jun;92(6):464-72.

Green, W.R., and Enger, C. (2005). Age-related macular degeneration histopathologic studies: the 1992 Lorenz E. Zimmerman Lecture. 1992. Retina *25*, 1519-1535.

Grossniklaus, H.E., Hutchinson, A.K., Capone, A., Jr., Woolfson, J., and Lambert, H.M. (1994). Clinicopathologic features of surgically excised choroidal neovascular membranes. Ophthalmology *101*, 1099-1111.

Hageman, G.S., Mullins, R.F., Russell, S.R., Johnson, L.V., and Anderson, D.H. (1999). Vitronectin is a constituent of ocular drusen and the vitronectin gene is expressed in human retinal pigmented epithelial cells. FASEB J *13*, 477-484.

Hanahan, D. (1997). Signaling vascular morphogenesis and maintenance. Science *277*, 48-50.

Hassell JB, Lamoureux EL, Keeffe JE. Impact of age related macular degeneration on quality of life. Br J Ophthalmol. 2006 May;90(5):593-6.

Hewitt, A.T., Nakazawa, K., and Newsome, D.A. (1989). Analysis of newly synthesized Bruch's membrane proteoglycans. Invest Ophthalmol Vis Sci *30*,478-486.

Ho, T.C., and Del Priore, L.V. (1997). Reattachment of cultured human retinal pigment epithelium to extracellular matrix and human Bruch's membrane. Invest Ophthalmol Vis Sci *38*, 1110-1118.

Hua J, Spee C, Kase S, Rennel ES, Magnussen AL, Qiu Y, Varey A, Dhayade S, Churchill AJ, Harper SJ, Bates DO, Hinton DR. Recombinant human VEGF165b inhibits experimental choroidal neovascularization. Invest Ophthalmol Vis Sci. 2010 Aug;51(8):4282-8.

Ishibashi, T., Miki, K., Sorgente, N., Patterson, R., and Ryan, S.J. (1985). Effects of intravitreal administration of steroids on experimental subretinal neovascularization in the subhuman primate. Arch Ophthalmol *103*, 708-711.

Ishibashi, T., Patterson, R., Ohnishi, Y., Inomata, H., and Ryan, S.J. (1986). Formation of drusen in the human eye. Am J Ophthalmol *101*, 342-353.

Jager, R.D., Mieler, W.F., and Miller, J.W. (2008). Age-related macular degeneration. N Engl J Med *358*, 2606-2617.

Johnson, L.V., Ozaki, S., Staples, M.K., Erickson, P.A., and Anderson, D.H. (2000). A potential role for immune complex pathogenesis in drusen formation. Exp Eye Res *70*, 441-449.

Julien S, Kreppel F, Beck S, Heiduschka P, Brito V, Schnichels S, Kochanek S, Schraermeyer U. A reproducible and quantifiable model of choroidal neovascularization induced by VEGF A165 after subretinal adenoviral gene transfer in the rabbit. Mol Vis. 2008 Jul 30;14:1358-72.

Katz, M.L., Christianson, J.S., Gao, C.L., and Handelman, G.J. (1994). Iron induced fluorescence in the retina: dependence on vitamin A. Invest Ophthalmol Vis Sci *35*, 3613-3624.

Killingsworth, M.C. (1987). Age-related components of Bruch's membrane in the human eye. Graefes Arch Clin Exp Ophthalmol *225*, 406-412.

Kim, I., Ryan, A.M., Rohan, R., Amano, S., Agular, S., Miller, J.W., and Adamis,A.P. (1999). Constitutive expression of VEGF, VEGFR-1, and VEGFR-2 in normal eyes. Invest Ophthalmol Vis Sci *40*, 2115-2121.

King, G.L., and Brownlee, M. (1996). The cellular and molecular mechanisms of diabetic complications. Endocrinol Metab Clin North Am *25*, 255-270.

Klein, R.J., Zeiss, C., Chew, E.Y., Tsai, J.Y., Sackler, R.S., Haynes, C., Henning, A.K., SanGiovanni, J.P., Mane, S.M., Mayne, S.T., *et al.* (2005). Complement factor H polymorphism in age-related macular degeneration. Science *308*, 385-389.

Kliffen, M., Sharma, H.S., Mooy, C.M., Kerkvliet, S., and de Jong, P.T. (1997). Increased expression of angiogenic growth factors in age-related maculopathy. Br J Ophthalmol *81*, 154-162.

Krzystolik, M.G., Afshari, M.A., Adamis, A.P., Gaudreault, J., Gragoudas, E.S., Michaud, N.A., Li, W., Connolly, E., O'Neill, C.A., and Miller, J.W. (2002). Prevention of experimental choroidal neovascularization with intravitreal antivascular endothelial growth factor antibody fragment. Arch Ophthalmol *120*,338-346.

Kvanta, A., Algvere, P.V., Berglin, L., and Seregard, S. (1996). Subfoveal fibrovascular membranes in age-related macular degeneration express vascular endothelial growth factor. Invest Ophthalmol Vis Sci *37*, 1929-1934.

Lassota N. Clinical and histological aspects of CNV formation: studies in an animal model. Acta Ophthalmol. 2008 Sep;86 Thesis 2:1-24.

Lee E, Maclaren RE. Sources of retinal pigment epithelium (RPE) for replacement therapy. Br J Ophthalmol. 2011 Apr;95(4):445-9.

Li, L.X., and Turner, J.E. (1988a). Inherited retinal dystrophy in the RCS rat: prevention of photoreceptor degeneration by pigment epithelial cell transplantation. Exp Eye Res *47*, 911-917. 313

Li, L.X., and Turner, J.E. (1988b). Transplantation of retinal pigment epithelial cells to immature and adult rat hosts: short- and long-term survival characteristics. Exp Eye Res *47*, 771-785.

Lu, M., Kuroki, M., Amano, S., Tolentino, M., Keough, K., Kim, I., Bucala, R.,and Adamis, A.P. (1998). Advanced glycation end products increase retinal vascular endothelial growth factor expression. J Clin Invest *101*, 1219-1224.

Lund, R.D., Kwan, A.S., Keegan, D.J., Sauve, Y., Coffey, P.J., and Lawrence, J.M. (2001). Cell transplantation as a treatment for retinal disease. Prog Retin Eye Res *20*, 415-449

Lyzogubov VV, Tytarenko RG, Liu J, Bora NS, Bora PS. Polyethylene glycol (PEG)-induced mouse model of choroidal neovascularization. J Biol Chem. 2011 May 6;286(18):16229-37.

MacLaren, R.E., Uppal, G.S., Balaggan, K.S., Tufail, A., Munro, P.M., Milliken, A.B., Ali, R.R., Rubin, G.S., Aylward, G.W., and da Cruz, L. (2007).

Maisonpierre, P.C., Suri, C., Jones, P.F., Bartunkova, S., Wiegand, S.J., Radziejewski, C., Compton, D., McClain, J., Aldrich, T.H., Papadopoulos, N.,*et al.* (1997). Angiopoietin-2, a natural antagonist for Tie2 that disrupts in vivo angiogenesis. Science *277*, 55-60.

Maseruka, H., Bonshek, R.E., and Tullo, A.B. (1997). Tenascin-C expression in normal, inflamed, and scarred human corneas. Br J Ophthalmol *81*, 677-682.

Mitchell P. A systematic review of the efficacy and safety outcomes of anti-VEGF agents used for treating neovascular age-related macular degeneration: comparison of ranibizumab and bevacizumab. Curr Med Res Opin. 2011 Jul;27(7):1465-75.

Montezuma SR, Vavvas D, Miller JW. Review of the ocular angiogenesis animal models. Semin Ophthalmol. 2009 Mar-Apr;24(2):52-61.

Mousa, S.A., Lorelli, W., and Campochiaro, P.A. (1999). Role of hypoxia and extracellular matrix-integrin binding in the modulation of angiogenic growth factors secretion by retinal pigmented epithelial cells. J Cell Biochem *74*, 135-143.

Mullins, R.F., Russell, S.R., Anderson, D.H., and Hageman, G.S. (2000). Drusen associated with aging and age-related macular degeneration contain proteins common to extracellular deposits associated with atherosclerosis, elastosis, amyloidosis, and dense deposit disease. FASEB J *14*, 835-846.

Nandrot, E.F., Kim, Y., Brodie, S.E., Huang, X., Sheppard, D., and Finnemann, S.C. (2004). Loss of synchronized retinal phagocytosis and age-related blindness in mice lacking alphavbeta5 integrin. J Exp Med *200*, 1539-1545.

Nicolo, M., Piccolino, F.C., Zardi, L., Giovannini, A., and Mariotti, C. (2000). Detection of tenascin-C in surgically excised choroidal neovascular membranes. Graefes Arch Clin Exp Ophthalmol *238*, 107-111.

Okamoto N, Tobe T, Hackett SF, Ozaki H, Vinores MA, LaRochelle W, Zack DJ, Campochiaro PA. Transgenic mice with increased expression of vascular endothelial growth factor in the retina: a new model of intraretinal and subretinal neovascularization. Am J Pathol. 1997 Jul;151(1):281-91.

Pauleikhoff, D., Harper, C.A., Marshall, J., and Bird, A.C. (1990). Aging changes in Bruch's membrane. A histochemical and morphologic study. Ophthalmology *97*, 171-178.

Pauleikhoff, D., Spital, G., Radermacher, M., Brumm, G.A., Lommatzsch, A., and Bird, A.C. (1999). A fluorescein and indocyanine green angiographic study of choriocapillaris in age-related macular disease. Arch Ophthalmol *117*, 1353-1358.

Phillips, S.J., Sadda, S.R., Tso, M.O., Humayan, M.S., de Juan, E., Jr., and Binder,S. (2003). Autologous transplantation of retinal pigment epithelium after mechanical debridement of Bruch's membrane. Curr Eye Res *26*, 81-88.

Piermarocchi S, Varano M, Parravano M, Oddone F, Sartore M, Ferrara R, Sera F, Virgili G. Quality of Vision Index: a new method to appraise visual function changes in age-related macular degeneration. Eur J Ophthalmol. 2011 Jan-Feb;21(1):55-66.

Ramrattan, R.S., van der Schaft, T.L., Mooy, C.M., de Bruijn, W.C., Mulder, P.G., and de Jong, P.T. (1994). Morphometric analysis of Bruch's membrane, the choriocapillaris, and the choroid in aging. Invest Ophthalmol Vis Sci *35*, 2857-2864.

Remulla, J.F., Gaudio, A.R., Miller, S., and Sandberg, M.A. (1995). Foveal electroretinograms and choroidal perfusion characteristics in fellow eyes of patients with unilateral neovascular age-related macular degeneration. Br J Ophthalmol *79*, 558-561.

Rikans, L.E., and Moore, D.R. (1988). Effect of aging on aqueous-phase antioxidants in tissues of male Fischer rats. Biochim Biophys Acta *966*, 269-275.

Rivera, A., Fisher, S.A., Fritsche, L.G., Keilhauer, C.N., Lichtner, P., Meitinger, T., and Weber, B.H. (2005). Hypothetical LOC387715 is a second major susceptibility gene for age-related macular degeneration, contributing independently of complement factor H to disease risk. Hum Mol Genet *14*,3227-3236.

Ryan SJ. The development of an experimental model of subretinal neovascularization in disciform macular degeneration. Trans Am Ophthalmol Soc. 1979;77:707-45.

Saishin Y, Saishin Y, Takahashi K, Lima e Silva R, Hylton D, Rudge JS, Wiegand SJ, Campochiaro PA. VEGF-TRAP(R1R2) suppresses choroidal neovascularization and VEGF-induced breakdown of the blood-retinal barrier. J Cell Physiol. 2003 May;195(2):241-8.

Sakaguchi, H., Miyagi, M., Shadrach, K.G., Rayborn, M.E., Crabb, J.W., and Hollyfield, J.G. (2002). Clusterin is present in drusen in age-related macular degeneration. Exp Eye Res *74*, 547-549.

Sallo FB, Peto T, Leung I, Xing W, Bunce C, Bird AC. The International Classification system and the progression of age-related macular degeneration. Curr Eye Res. 2009 Mar;34(3):238-40.

Schmidt, A.M., Yan, S.D., Yan, S.F., and Stern, D.M. (2000). The biology of the receptor for advanced glycation end products and its ligands. Biochim Biophys Acta *1498*, 99-111.

Schmidt, S., Hauser, M.A., Scott, W.K., Postel, E.A., Agarwal, A., Gallins, P.,Wong, F., Chen, Y.S., Spencer, K., Schnetz-Boutaud, N., *et al.* (2006). Cigarette smoking strongly modifies the association of LOC387715 and age related macular degeneration. Am J Hum Genet *78*, 852-864.

Schmidt-Erfurth UM, Elsner H, Terai N, Benecke A, Dahmen G, Michels SM. Effects of verteporfin therapy on central visual field function. Ophthalmology. 2004 May;111(5):931-9.

Schwesinger, C., Yee, C., Rohan, R.M., Joussen, A.M., Fernandez, A., Meyer, T.N., Poulaki, V., Ma, J.J., Redmond, T.M., Liu, S., *et al.* (2001). Intrachoroidal neovascularization in transgenic mice overexpressing vascular endothelial growth factor in the retinal pigment epithelium. Am J Pathol *158*, 1161-1172.

Spilsbury K, Garrett KL, Shen WY, Constable IJ, Rakoczy PE. Overexpression of vascular endothelial growth factor (VEGF) in the retinal pigment epithelium leads to the development of choroidal neovascularization. Am J Pathol. 2000 Jul;157(1):135-44.

Starita, C., Hussain, A.A., Patmore, A., and Marshall, J. (1997). Localization of the site of major resistance to fluid transport in Bruch's membrane. Invest Ophthalmol Vis Sci 38, 762-767.

Sun, K., Cai, H., Tezel, T.H., Paik, D., Gaillard, E.R., and Del Priore, L.V. (2007). Bruch's membrane aging decreases phagocytosis of outer segments by retinal pigment epithelium. Mol Vis *13*, 2310-2319.

Sundelin, S.P., and Nilsson, S.E. (2001). Lipofuscin-formation in retinal pigment epithelial cells is reduced by antioxidants. Free Radic Biol Med *31*, 217-225.

Tanaka N, Ikawa M, Mata NL, Verma IM. Choroidal neovascularization in transgenic mice expressing prokineticin 1: an animal model for age-related macular degeneration. Mol Ther. 2006 Mar;13(3):609-16. Epub 2005 Nov 2.

Treatment of Age-related macular degeneration with Photodynamic therapy (TAP) Study Group. Photodynamic therapy of subfoveal choroidal neovascularization in age-related macular degeneration with verteporfin: one-year results of 2 randomized clinical trials--TAP report. *Archives of Ophthalmology* 1999;117(10):1329–45.

Tezel, T.H., and Del Priore, L.V. (1997). Reattachment to a substrate prevents apoptosis of human retinal pigment epithelium. Graefes Arch Clin Exp Ophthalmol *235*, 41-47.

Tezel, T.H., and Del Priore, L.V. (1999). Repopulation of different layers of host human Bruch's membrane by retinal pigment epithelial cell grafts. Invest Ophthalmol Vis Sci *40*, 767-774.

Tezel, T.H., Kaplan, H.J., and Del Priore, L.V. (1999). Fate of human retinal pigment epithelial cells seeded onto layers of human Bruch's membrane. Invest Ophthalmol Vis Sci *40*, 467-476

Treumer F, Bunse A, Klatt C, Roider J. Autologous retinal pigment epithelium-choroid sheet transplantation in age related macular degeneration: morphological and functional results.Br J Ophthalmol. 2007 Mar;91(3):349-53.

Tsukahara, I., Ninomiya, S., Castellarin, A., Yagi, F., Sugino, I.K., and Zarbin, M.A. (2002). Early attachment of uncultured retinal pigment epithelium from aged donors onto Bruch's membrane explants. Exp Eye Res *74*, 255-266.

Vandewoude, M.F., and Vandewoude, M.G. (1987). Vitamin E status in a normal population: the influence of age. J Am Coll Nutr *6*, 307-311.

Vedula S.S, Krzystolik M.G.(2008). Antiangiogenic therapy with anti-vascular endothelial growth factor modalities for neovascular age-related macular degeneration. Cochrane Database Syst Rev. 2008 Apr 16;(2):CD005139.

Virgili G, Bini A. Laser photocoagulation for neovascular agerelated macular degeneration. *Cochrane Database of Systematic Reviews* 2007, Issue 3.

Wallace, D.C., Brown, M.D., Melov, S., Graham, B., and Lott, M. (1998). Mitochondrial biology, degenerative diseases and aging. Biofactors *7*, 187-190.

Wallace, D.C. (1999). Mitochondrial diseases in man and mouse. Science *283*, 1482-1488. Harman, D. (1956). Aging: a theory based on free radical and radiation chemistry. J Gerontol *11*, 298-300.

Wang, S., Lu, B., Wood, P., and Lund, R.D. (2005). Grafting of ARPE-19 and Schwann cells to the subretinal space in RCS rats. Invest Ophthalmol Vis Sci *46*, 2552-2560.

Wassell, J., Davies, S., Bardsley, W., and Boulton, M. (1999). The photoreactivity of the retinal age pigment lipofuscin. J Biol Chem *274*, 23828-23832.

Winkler, B.S., Boulton, M.E., Gottsch, J.D., and Sternberg, P. (1999). Oxidative damage and age-related macular degeneration. Mol Vis *5*, 32.

Wong TY, Hyman L. Population-based studies in ophthalmology. Am J Ophthalmol. 2008 Nov;146(5):656-63.

Zagzag, D., and Capo, V. (2002). Angiogenesis in the central nervous system: a role for vascular endothelial growth factor/vascular permeability factor and tenascin-C. Common molecular effectors in cerebral neoplastic and nonneoplastic "angiogenic diseases". Histol Histopathol *17*, 301-321.

Zagzag, D., Friedlander, D.R., Dosik, J., Chikramane, S., Chan, W., Greco, M.A.,Allen, J.C., Dorovini-Zis, K., and Grumet, M. (1996). Tenascin-C expression by angiogenic vessels in human astrocytomas and by human brain endothelial cells *in vitro*. Cancer Res *56*, 182-189.

Zarbin, M.A. (2003). Analysis of retinal pigment epithelium integrin expression and adhesion to aged submacular human Bruch's membrane. Trans Am Ophthalmol Soc *101*, 499-520.

Zarbin, M.A. (2004). Current concepts in the pathogenesis of age-related macular degeneration. Arch Ophthalmol *122*, 598-614.

2

Pathogenic Roles of Sterile Inflammation in Etiology of Age-Related Macular Degeneration

Suofu Qin
Retinal Disease Research, Department of Biological Sciences, Allergan, Inc., Irvine, CA USA

1. Introduction

Inflammation is vital for host defense against invasive pathogens via the recruitment of innate inflammatory cells, which in turn phagocytose infectious agents and produce additional cytokines that then activate adaptive immune responses. Inflammation is also crucial to protect cells and facilitate wound healing as a result of mechanic or chemical injury. Because of the absence of infection, the inflammation induced by metabolic or chemical injury has been termed as 'sterile inflammation' to distinguish from that induced by pathogens. Similar to microbially induced inflammation, the immune system has evolved mechanisms to sense necrotic cell death by responding with innate and adaptive immune response, which is marked by the recruitment of macrophages and the production of inflammatory cytokines. However, unresolved and persistent inflammation due to un-removal or un-containment of the offending agents would turn it into a destructive process that is detrimental to the host. The production of reactive oxygen species (ROS), proteases and inflammatory cytokines causes tissue destruction and fibrosis. Thus, sterile inflammation has been demonstrated to be associated with human diseases such as cardiac ischaemia–reperfusion injury, the restoration of blood flow causes tissue destruction as a result of enhanced production of ROS and inflammatory responses to necrotic cells (Camara et al., 2011).

Sterile inflammation in the etiology of age-related macular degeneration (AMD) has been highlighted by the observations that individuals with genetic mutation in complement factor H confer a significantly higher risky for AMD (Montezuma et al., 2007), an idiopathic retinal degenerative disease that leads to irreversible, profound vision loss in people over 60 year old in developed countries (Evans & Wormald, 1996). AMD occurs in two major forms: atrophic (dry) AMD and exudative (wet) AMD. The atrophic AMD is characterized by RPE atrophy and subjacent photoreceptor degeneration and accounts for approximately 25% of cases with severe central vision loss (Klein et al., 1997). Exudative AMD, which accounts for approximately 75% of cases with severe central vision loss (Klein et al., 1997), is characterized by choroidal neovascularization (CNV) and retinal hemorrhage. These two forms of AMD are both part of the same disease process and share similar risk factors for their development. Although the vision loss results from photoreceptor damage in the central retina, the initial pathogenesis of AMD has been proposed to involve the degeneration of retinal pigment epithelial (RPE) cells (Hageman et al., 2001). The RPE cells *in vivo* has limited regenerating capability upon damage as they are in general post-mitotic and their mitochondria are very susceptible to oxidative damage (Qin & Rodrigues, 2010b). The specific genetic and biochemical mechanisms responsible for RPE degeneration in AMD have not been determined. However, cumulative oxidative stress and chronic inflammation have been recently appreciated to play important roles in the biogenesis of drusen, the extracellular lipid-containing deposits that are the hallmark of early AMD and may therefore be central to the etiology of this disease (Hageman et al., 2001; Rodrigues, 2007). The eye with its intense exposure to light, robust metabolic activity and high oxygen tension in the macular region, is particularly susceptible to oxidative damage. Thus, there is considerable interest in elucidating the mechanisms responsible for oxidative stress- and sterile inflammation-associated RPE injury, which would provide the basis for designing new strategies to treat or prevent AMD.

Chronic sterile inflammation in the retina might cause RPE cell dysfunction and death that subsequently contribute to retinal degeneration, however, the underlining molecular mechanisms remain elusive. Recently, the damage-associated molecular pattern (DAMP) molecules, a structurally-diverse family of endogenous molecules either released from necrotic cells or breakdown products of the extracellular matrix during cellular injury, are demonstrated to alert host cells for the coming danger by inciting inflammatory responses. Persistent stimulation by the DAMP molecules leads to cell dysfunction and eventually cell death. Some of the DAMP molecules are recognized by pattern recognition receptors, which normally sense pathogen-associated molecular patterns. The role of oxidative stress in the etiology of AMD has been reviewed elsewhere (Qin & Rodrigues, 2010b). In this review, discussed are the nature of the DAMPs, DAMP-initiated inflammatory signaling and the therapeutic potentials of anti-DAMP therapy for AMD intervention.

2. Damage-associated molecular patterns

The danger hypothesis was first proposed by Matzinger in 1994 to explain how both infectious and non-infectious agents can stimulate adaptive immune responses (Matzinger, 1994). It is postulated that the adaptive immune system has evolved to respond not only to infection but also to non-physiological cell death due to damage or environmental stress. Necrotic cell death is considered as a sign of danger to the organism. According to this danger model, dying cells will release endogenous DAMPs, using similar nomenclature to pathogen-associated molecular patterns (PAMPs). A candidate molecule as a *bona fide* DAMP should meet at least the following three criteria as proposed by Kono and Rock (Kono & Rock, 2008). First, a DAMP should be active as a highly purified molecule rather than owing to endotoxin contamination. Second, the DAMPs should be active at concentrations that are actually present in pathophysiological conditions. Finally, selectively eliminating or inactivating DAMPs will ideally block the biological activity of necrotic cells in *in vitro* and *in vivo* assays (Kono & Rock, 2008). DAMPs are normally sequestered intracellularly and are hidden from recognition by the innate immune system by the plasma membrane under physiological conditions. However, these molecules, when cells undergo injury or necrosis, are released into the extracellular milieu and then trigger inflammation under sterile conditions. Based on their origin, DAMPs are classified into two categories: intracellular and extracellular DAMPs.

2.1 Intracellular DAMPs

Intracellular DAMPs are bioactive mediators of intracellular origin that directly stimulate cells of the innate system. They are pre-existed within the cells and released into extracellular environment after cell injury or death. The DAMPs associated with retinal pathogenesis are summarized in Figure 1.

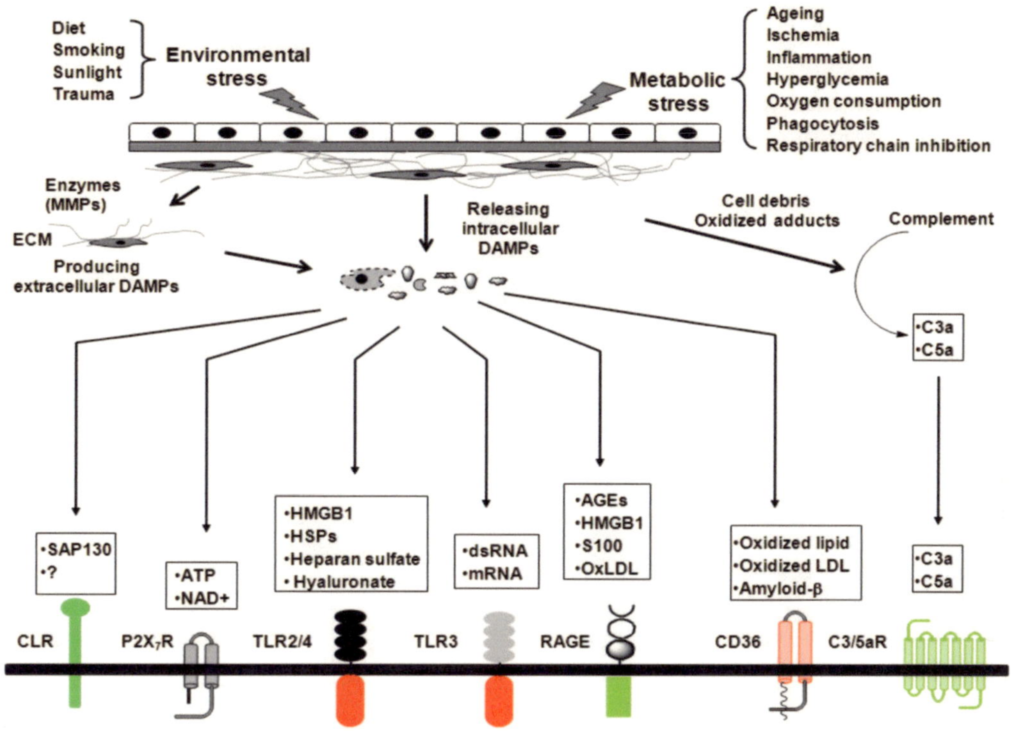

Fig. 1. Cell-surface DAMP receptors that detect a variety of DAMP molecules.

Necrotic cells due to environmental and metabolic stress release intracellular damage-associated molecular patterns (DAMPs) or hydrolytic enzymes that degrade extracellular components to generate extracellular DAMPs. Necrotic cells also activate the complement system to generate C3a and C5a. Additionally, oxidized products or oxidized adducts that are strong inflammatory stimuli are also appreciated as DAMP molecules. These DAMPs are sensed by DAMP receptors on host cells, thereby triggering host defense via sterile inflammation. AGEs, advanced glycation-end products; CLRs, c-type lectin receptors; HMGB1, high mobility group box 1; HSPs, heat-shock proteins; oxLDL, oxidized low density proteins; $P2X_7R$, purinergic receptor P2X, ligand-gated ion channel, 7; RAGE, receptor for AGEs; SAP130, spliceosome-associated protein 130; TLRs, toll-like receptors.

2.1.1 Nucleic acids

Upon releasing from dying or necrotic cells, nucleic acids such as RNA and fragments of genomic DNA can activate innate and adaptive immune systems. Necrotic synovial fluid cells from the patients with rheumatoid arthritis activated fibroblast cells with production of inflammatory cytokines in a toll-like receptor-3 (TLR-3)-dependent manner (Brentano et al., 2005), indicating that the RNA released from necrotic cells is involved in fibroblast cell activation. Heterologous RNA from necrotic cells or *in vitro* transcribed mRNA can activate dendritic cells, which is abolished by RNase pretreatment (Kariko et al., 2004). Moreover, genomic DNA released into cytosol upon cell injury has been found to activate thyroid cells in concert with histone H2B with cytokine production (Kawashima et al., 2011). Mitochondrial DNA released from injured mitochondria can activate neutrophils *in vitro* and *in vivo*, eliciting neutrophil-mediated tissue injury (Zhang et al., 2010). Intriguingly, *Alu* RNA, a double-stranded RNA (dsRNA) isolated from drusen of the patients with geographic atrophy can cause RPE cell death *in vitro* and RPE layer degeneration *in vivo* (Kaneko et al., 2011). Knockout of TLR3, the receptor for RNA, protects necrosis-induced retinal degeneration in mouse (Shiose et al., 2011). These results implicate that released nucleic acids from necrotic cells might have a role in etiology of AMD.

2.1.2 Interlukin-1α (IL-1α)

IL-1α is synthesized as a biologically active cytokine but is retained in cytosol and nucleus under physiological conditions (Cohen et al., 2010). However, IL-1α is released with its cellular contents when cells undergo necrosis and released IL-1α activates its cognate receptor, leading to rapid recruitment of inflammatory cells into the surrounding injured tissue (Cohen et al., 2010). IL-1α in dying cells and functional IL-1R are required for neutrophilic response to dead cells and tissue injury *in vivo* while this pathway is not essential for the neutrophil response to a microbial stimulus (Chen et al., 2007). Role of IL-1α in sterile inflammation appears to be dependent on its sources. IL-1α released from necrotic cells primarily triggers initial neutrohphil response and primes resident macrophage that produces IL-1α, required for necrosis-induced sterile inflammation (Kono et al., 2010b). Interestingly, IL-1α from necrotic dendritic cells primes mesothelial cells that generate chemokine (C-X-C motif) ligand 1, then recruiting neutrophils into sterile inflammation sites (Eigenbrod et al., 2008).

2.1.3 ATP and uric acid

The cytoplasm of each cell contains high concentrations of ATP, however, extracellular levels are quite low as ATP is quickly degraded by ecto-ATPases in normal tissues (Di Virgilio, 2007). Upon cell damage due to chemical or mechanical injury, ATP levels in extracellular environment is increased rapidly. High levels of ATP in extracellular space have been observed during airway inflammation *in vivo* (Idzko et al., 2007). The increase in extracellular ATP concentrations subsequently triggers inflammatory responses since lowering ATP levels by apyrase abolishes cardinal features of asthma such as cytokine production (Idzko et al., 2007). Addition of ATP to cell culture results in significant release/production of inflammatory mediators and causes cell death if under persistent stimulation (Surprenant et al., 1996). Stimulation of RPE cells with ATP enhances cytokine production (Relvas et al., 2009) and then RPE cell death (Yang et al., 2010). Uric acid, a ubiquitous metabolite of purine-degradation pathway, can be produced in high quantities upon cellular injury (Kono et al., 2010a). Uric acid, presented as monosodium urate (MSU) crystals in salt-rich fluids, promotes acute inflammatory responses *in vivo* which is substantially inhibited by uric acid depletion (Kono et al., 2010a).

2.1.4 High-mobility group box 1 protein (HMGB1)

HMGB1 is a chromatin-binding protein with key role in nuclear homeostasis. HMGB1 in extracellular mellitus behaves as a cytokine, promoting inflammation and disease pathogenesis. HMGB1 was first identified to mediate endotoxin-induced lethality in mouse (Wang et al., 1999). Addition of purified recombinant HMGB1 stimulates production of inflammatory cytokines in human monocytes (Andersson et al., 2000) and knockout of HMGB1 significantly inhibits the capability of necrotic cells to promote inflammation

(Scaffidi et al., 2002). HMGB1 release has been detected from retinal cell death by oxidative stress *in vitro* and retinal detachment *in vivo* (Arimura et al., 2009). The increase in the vitreous HMGB1 level is correlated with that of monocyte chemotactic protein-1 (MCP-1) in human eyes with retinal degeneration.

2.1.5 Heat-shock proteins (HSPs)

HSPs are a highly conserved group of intracellular proteins classified into HSP110, HSP90, HSP70, HSP60, and small molecular HSPs based on their molecular weights, and function as molecular chaperones to promote the refolding of damaged proteins and inhibit protein aggregation under stress conditions (Georgopoulos & Welch, 1993). Purified HSP70 stimulates activation of NF-*k*B in monocytes with production of inflammatory cytokines (Asea et al., 2000) and transgenic expression of HSP70 enhances the extent of *in vivo* sterile inflammation upon β-cell damage (Alam et al., 2009). HSPs also can function as a chaperone to target the antigenic peptides to antigen-presenting cells, thereby initiating immune responses (Binder et al., 2007). Dying cells express higher levels of HSPs (Decanini et al., 2007), thereby providing danger signals to alert the neighboring cells for upcoming danger. However, caution should be exercised as it is still controversial whether extracellular HSPs function as cytokines.

2.1.6 S100 proteins

The S100 proteins are a family of about 20 related small, acidic calcium-binding proteins that modulate an array of intracellular functions, like calcium homeostasis, cell cycle and cytoskeletal organization (Heizmann et al., 2002). S100 proteins are higher in extracellular milieu at inflammation site. S100A8 and/or S100A9 stimulate migration of neutrophils and monocytes in gouty arthritis, which is inhibited by anti-S100 antibodies (Ryckman et al., 2003). Additionally, S100B induces cell death in cultured RPE cells (Howes et al., 2004). Whether S100 proteins contribute to disease pathogenesis remains to be confirmed.

2.2 Extracellular DAMPs

Extracellular DAMPs, such as hyaluronan, heparan sulphate and biglycan, are generated as a result of proteolysis by enzymes released from dying cells or by proteases activated to promote tissue repair and remodeling (Babelova et al., 2009). Extracellular DAMPs can also be generated from activation of complement system by the degraded or released molecules from necrotic cells (Garg et al., 2010).

2.2.1 Breakdown products of extracellular matrix

Extracellular matrix components, which are thought to function as structural elements, are now gaining recognition as signaling molecules triggering or enhancing sterile inflammation once cleaved by released proteolytic enzymes during tissue injury. Hyaluronan fragments generated upon cell injury activate endothelial cells *in vitro* and *in vivo* with significant production of chemokine interleukin-8 (IL-8) (Taylor et al., 2004) and induce maturation of dendritic cells (Termeer et al., 2002). In addition, biglycan has been shown to activate macrophages accompanied with NF-κB-dependent cytokine production (Schaefer et al., 2005). Activated macrophages also release biglycan, further amplifying inflammatory responses (Schaefer et al., 2005). Biglycan can stimulate synthesis of immature

IL-1β via toll-like receptor signaling and in the mean time promote the processing of immature IL-1β to its mature form through P2X receptor signaling (Babelova et al., 2009). Importantly, elevation of hyaluronan contributes to the development of laser-induced choroidal neovascularization with recruitment of macrophages to the lesion sites (Mochimaru et al., 2009), shedding light on understanding the roles of extracellular components in etiology of AMD.

2.2.2 C3a and C5a

In the retina, photooxidation causes oxidative stress and complement activation, leading to cell death *in vitro* and *in vivo* (Radu et al., 2011; Zhou et al., 2006). Thus, the chance of RPE/photoreceptor cells being attacked by activated complement systems is increased. During the process of complement cascade activation, the cleaved complement components C3a, C4a and C5a, known as anaphylotoxins, stimulate inflammation. In cultured RPE cells, treatment with C5a stimulates production of IL-8 (Fukuoka et al., 2003) and MCP-1 (Ambati et al., 2003). Furthermore, C3a and C5a have been shown to be present in drusen (Ambati et al., 2003) and are generated early in the course of laser-induced CNV where activation of C3aR or C5aR is required for CNV formation (Nozaki et al., 2006), supporting the idea that RPE cells are constantly stimulated by C3a and C5a and complement-driven sterile inflammation is involved in the etiology and progression of AMD.

2.3 Oxidized adducts

With its unusually abundance in poly-unsaturated fatty acids (PUFAs), glucose-enriched and oxidative environment, the retina is an ideal place to form free radicals and bioactive small molecules, then oxidizing proteins, lipids and DNA. Many oxidized adducts of proteins with lipid or glucose accumulate within and around RPE/photoreceptor cells as a function of ageing. Accumulation of these oxidized adducts triggers transcriptional alterations in genes related to cell death and inflammatory response, perturbs the lysosomal function of the RPE via delayed processing of photoreceptor outer segments (POS), thereby resulting in the disease pathogenesis. Although they are not necessarily associated with necrosis, oxidized adducts also generate pattern recognition sites such as oxidized phospholipids, oxidized lipoproteins and long-chain fatty acids that are strong sterile stimuli. These oxidized adducts play important roles in sterile inflammation and potentially in the etiology of human diseases so that they should be recognized as DAMP molecules. Discussed here are four examples of oxidized adducts, advanced glycation endproducts (AGEs), carboxyethyl pyrole (CEP)-protein adducts, oxidized low-density lipoproteins (oxLDL) and oxidized bis-retinoid pyridinium (A2E) with relevance to AMD etiology.

2.3.1 Advanced glycation end-products (AGEs)

AGEs are heterogeneous non-enzymatic glycation products of proteins, lipids and DNA on free amino groups by aldehyde groups on sugars. AGEs accumulate during normal ageing with their formation being accelerated in a setting of oxidative stress and inflammation (Schleicher et al., 1997). There is little or no AGE products detected in normal retina, but expression of AGE products increases concomitantly with drusen formation and development of early AMD (Howes et al., 2004). AGE products are also present in RPE lipofuscin, an enzymatically undegradable heterogeneous mixture of numerous biomolecules (Schutt et al.,

2003). With the accumulation of AGEs, receptor for AGEs (RAGE) is simultaneously induced (Yamada et al., 2006), further amplifying cellular activation. Induction of AGE formation *in vivo* leads to the increased transcription of inflammatory genes, resulting in ageing of the RPE/choroid (Tian et al., 2005). In cultured human RPE cells, activation of AGE-RAGE pathway stimulates expression of VEGF (Ma et al., 2007), and production of IL-8 and MCP-1 (Bian et al., 2001). Moreover, activation of RAGE can trigger RPE cell death *in vitro* (Howes et al., 2004), demonstrating that AGEs are toxic to retinal cells.

2.3.2 Carboxyethyl pyrole (CEP) adducts

Lipid peroxidation, triggered by direct photobleaching of PUFAs or indirect excitation of photosensitizers contained in RPE lipofuscin, generates a number of reactive dicarbonyl compounds (aldehydes) such as acrolein, 4-hydroxy-2-nonenal (4-HNE), malondialdehyde (MDA) and CEP (Glenn & Stitt, 2009). These aldehydes can deplete cellular thiols, resulting in cell death. Direct exposure of RPE cells to 4-HNE causes dysregulation of chemokine production, increase in cell permeability, and finally cell death (Qin & Rodrigues, 2010a). Moreover, these aldehydes can alter cell functions via formation of lipid adducts on free amino groups of proteins. Among them, CEP adducts, uniquely generated by the oxidation of the most oxidizable fatty acid docosahexaenoate in human retina (Gu et al., 2003), are the most abundant class of oxidized proteins found in drusen. CEP adducts are higher in photoreceptors from AMD patients than healthy retinas (Gu et al., 2003). Mice immunized with mouse serum albumin (MSA) adducted with CEP (CEP-MSA) develop an atrophic AMD-like phenotype including RPE loss and drusen formation with accumulation of macrophages in the interphotoreceptor matrix and C3 fragments in Bruch's membrane (Hollyfield et al., 2008). CEP-MSA also stimulates angiogenesis in ex-vivo models and subretinal injection of CEP-MSA exacerbates laser-induced CNV in mice (Ebrahem et al., 2006). These observations definitely implicate oxidized lipid adducts in the perturbation of RPE cell function, leading RPE cell death both *in vitro* and *in vivo*.

2.3.3 Oxidized low-density lipoproteins (oxLDL)

Low-density lipoproteins (LDL) are complex particles containing cholesterol, phosphlipids, and triglycerides. The PUFAs in those molecules are susceptible to free radical-initiated oxidation, generating chemically-reactive such as MDA and 4-HNE and bioactive molecules. MDA and 4-HNE oxidize proteins, forming MDA lysine or 4-HNE cysteine protein adducts that are the major modifications observed in RPE lipofuscin (Schutt et al., 2003). OxLDL is found to be accumulated in AMD lesions (Kamei et al., 2007) and higher in patients' blood with AMD (Javadzadeh et al., 2010). Oxidation of the cholesterol within the LDL particle generates a series of cholesterol oxides, of which 7-ketocholesterol is very toxic to RPE cells (Moreira et al., 2009). Exposure of RPE cells to oxLDL inhibits POS phagocytosis, an important RPE cell function essential for outer segment renewal and survival of photoreceptors, by altering phagosome maturation (Hoppe et al., 2004b) and mis-sorting the principal lysosomal protease cathepsin D (Hoppe et al., 2004a). Moreover, oxLDL induces transcriptional alterations in genes related to lipid metabolism, oxidative stress, inflammation and apoptosis in RPE cells (Yamada et al., 2008; Yu et al., 2009). OxLDL causes RPE cell death, at least in part, through formation of 7-ketocholesterol (Rodriguez et al., 2004). Additionally, oxLDL is ligand for scavenger receptors expressed on macrophages that are recruited to the subretinal sites where oxLDL accumulates, further stressing RPE cells via amplifying inflammatory responses

(Kamei et al., 2007). Collectively, these observations suggest a causal role of oxLDL accumulation in AMD pathogenesis although the precise mechanisms are not well defined

2.3.4 Bis-retinoid pyridinium A2E

A2E, a byproduct of the visual cycle, is formed through the condensation of two molecules of all-trans-retinal with one molecule of phosphatidylethanolamine in the POS upon photoisomerization of 11-*cis* retinal (Mata et al., 2000). A2E accumulates as lipofuscin in RPE cells with ageing since it is resistant to enzymatic degradation. After light, in particular blue light irradiation, A2E is oxidized, initially by addition of light-excited singlet oxygen, and oxidized A2E can then generate free radicals such as superoxide anion and hydroxyl radical, or discompose to reactive dicarbonyls like methylglyoxal, triggering free radical chain reaction (Wu et al., 2010). Light exposure causes death of A2E-loaded RPE cells in other hand A2E-free RPE cells are not (Schutt et al., 2000). Moreover, photooxidation products of A2E have been shown to activate complement system in RPE cells (Zhou et al., 2006), suggesting that sterile inflammation is involved in A2E cytotoxicity. However, a causal role of A2E accumulation in AMD development remains to be confirmed.

3. DAMP receptors

How does the innate immune system distinguish between dead and live cells? The crucial event upon necrotic cell death is the release of intracellular DAMPs and generation of extracellular DAMPs which can be sensed by the receptors on innate immune cells. This section discusses the recent progress in the recognition of DAMPs by pattern recognition receptors and DAMP receptors that are not typically associated with microbial recognition (Figure 1).

3.1 Pattern recognition receptors

Pattern recognition receptors (PRRs) recognize conserved structural moieties called PAMPs found in microorganisms and in turn induce cytokine production, which is important in inflammatory and antimicrobial responses. Up to date, five classes of PRRs have been identified. They are the Toll-like receptors (TLRs), the C-type lectin receptors (CLRs), the nucleotide-binding oligomerization domain (NOD)-like receptors (NLRs), the retinoic acid-inducible gene (RIG)-I-like receptors (RLRs) and absence in melanoma 2 (AIM2). The membrane-bound TLRs and CLRs surveillance the extracellular milieu, whereas RLRs, NLRs and AIM2-like receptors have emerged as pivotal sensors of infection and stress in intracellular compartments (Meylan et al., 2006). Among them, TLRs, CLRs, NLRs and AIM2 participate in DAMP-dependent inflammatory responses.

3.1.1 Toll-like receptors (TLRs)

TLRs have been reported to be activated by intracellular DAMPs including HSPs, S100 proteins, uric acid and HMGB1, as well as extracellular DAMPs such as hyaluronan, heparan sulphate and proteoglycans (Kono & Rock, 2008). RPE cells make up the first line of defense against pathogens by expressing almost all TLR iso-forms except TLR-8 (Kumar et al., 2004). Activation of TLR3 and TLR9 leads to the production of inflammatory mediators including cytokines and adhesion molecules in cultured RPE cells (Ebihara et al., 2007). TLR3 detects mRNA (Kariko et al., 2004) and dsRNA (Dogusan et al., 2008) released from necrotic cells while TLR9 senses endogenous DNA (Zhang et al., 2010), triggering sterile inflammatory response and subsequent toxicity. TLR3 is shown to mediate retinal degeneration caused by impaired clearance of toxic all-trans retinal in mice since TLR3 deficiency confers retina protection (Shiose et al., 2011). Choroidal neovascular membranes from AMD patients expressed higher levels of TLR3 in RPE cells (Maloney et al., 2010) and TLR3 activation by siRNA inhibits CNV as siRNA inhibition is abolished in TLR3-deficient mice (Kleinman et al., 2008). Moreover, dsRNA causes RPE cell death that is mediated by TLR3 and genetic variant in the TLR3 412Phe confers protection against geographic atrophy (Yang et al., 2008). These observations reveal a role of TLR3 in AMD development.

3.1.2 C-type lectin receptors (CLRs)

CLRs including DEC205, Mincle, CLEC9A and DC-SIGN are a family of surface receptors known to recognize carbohydrate moieties on viruses, bacteria and fungi (Cambi & Figdor, 2009). Stimulation of CLRs leads to activation of signaling pathways that elevate cytokine production. Although their ligands are poorly defined, Mincle (also known as CLEC4E) and CLEC9A can sense necrotic cell death (Cambi & Figdor, 2009). Mincle recognizes SAP130 from necrotic cells and triggers intracellular signaling via the associated FcRγ adaptor, leading to the production of inflammatory cytokines (Yamasaki et al., 2008). CLEC9A, a Syk-coupled CLR, can recognize necrotic cells and present dead cell-associated antigens to $CD8^+$ T cells (Sancho et al., 2009). Similar to Mincle, the capability of CLEC9A to recognize necrotic cells makes it a potential receptor that is important for sterile inflammatory responses even though its ligands are unidentified.

3.1.3 NOD-like receptors (NLRs)

NLRs, consisting of the three subfamilies with 14 NALPs, 6 NODs and 2 IPAF/NAIP, are cytosolic PRRs that sense microbial invasion, eliciting an inflammatory response to alert the system to the presence of danger, mainly by assembling inflammasomes that activate caspase-1 for processing immature IL-1β to mature IL-1β (Martinon et al., 2009). NLRs contain a central nucleotide-binding oligomerization domain (NACHT), an N-terminal effector domain (pyrin domain, caspase-recruitment domain or BIR domain) and C-terminal leucine-rich repeats (LRRs). Among the NLRs identified so far, the NOD-, LRR-, and pyrin domain-containing 3 (NLRP3, also termed as NALP3) has been shown to be capable of detecting endogenous danger signals (*See* discussion in NLRP3 inflammasome).

3.1.4 Absence in melanoma 2 (AIM2)

AIM2 is a cytosolic protein containing a C-terminal HIN200 and an N-terminal PYD domain, which is identified to recognize dsDNA derived from virus and bacterial, triggering anti-virus responses (Burckstummer et al., 2009). AIM2 can also be activated by the transfection of synthetic dsDNA (Fernandes-Alnemri et al., 2009), highlighting that the innate response to DNA is regulated by the localization of DNA in concert with the innate receptors rather than the source of DNA. Under physiological conditions, self-DNA is localized in nuclei and mitochondria. However, injured or dying cells can release mitochondrial and genomic DNA into the cytosol where AIM2 resides. Released genomic and mitochondrial DNA have been demonstrated to cause inflammatory responses (Kawashima et al., 2011; Zhang et al., 2010). Whether there is a pathogenic role for AIM2 in sterile inflammation-related diseases remains unclear.

3.2 Non-PRR DAMP receptors

DAMPs can also be recognized by non-PRRs, named as DAMP receptors here. Receptor for AGEs, purinergic $P2X_7$ receptor and scavenger receptor CD36 are currently three relatively appreciated DAMP receptors.

3.2.1 Receptor for AGEs (RAGE)

RAGE is a transmembrane receptor that belongs to the immunoglobulin super-family of cell surface molecules that are constitutively expressed at very low levels in numerous cells, including Muller cells, photoreceptor cells, RPE cells, and vascular endothelial cells (Barile & Schmidt, 2007; Howes et al., 2004). It recognizes AGEs, HMGB1, amyloid-β (Bucciarelli et al., 2002) and the S100 family members (Hofmann et al., 1999). Activation of RAGE by its ligands results in the upregulation of several inflammatory signaling pathways, including NF-κB, phosphoinositide 3-kinase and MAPK signalling pathways, thereby producing inflammatory cytokines (Hofmann et al., 1999). Cellular expression of RAGE increases upon ligand binding, thus amplifying cellular activation. The levels of RAGE *in vivo* are correlated with drusen formation and early development of AMD (Howes et al., 2004). Transgenic expression of RAGE augmented blood-retinal barrier breakdown and leukostasis, accompanied by increased expression of VEGF and ICAM-1 in the retina in a murine diabetic model (Kaji et al., 2007), which were significantly inhibited by systemic administration of a soluble form of RAGE.

3.2.2 Purinergic $P2X_7$ receptor ($P2X_7R$)

The $P2X_7R$ belongs to the P2X receptor subfamily of P2 receptors (receptors for extracellular nucleotides) and is an ATP-gated cation channel that is widely expressed in cells of the immune system (Di Virgilio, 2007). Activation of $P2X_7R$ causes rapid efflux of K^+ with accompanied influx of Ca^{2+} and Na^+. ATP is the preferred agonist for P2X receptor subfamily, however, higher concentration of extracellular ATP is required for $P2X_7R$ activation than that required for the other P2X receptors (Surprenant et al., 1996). The known DAMPs that activate $P2X_7R$ are ATP and uric acid (Riteau et al., 2010). Knockout of $P2X_7R$, or blockade of with antagonist inhibits ATP-dependent lung inflammation (Riteau et al., 2010) or hyperalgesia (Teixeira et al., 2010). Activation of $P2X_7R$ by ATP and synthetic ligand leads to RPE cell death *in vitro*, which is inhibited by $P2X_7R$ antagonist (Yang et al., 2010). Whether ATP- $P2X_7R$ is involved in RPE atrophy *in vivo* is unknown.

3.2.3 Scavenger receptor CD36

CD36 is a cell surface scavenger receptor expressed on RPE cells, which recognizes oxidized POS and facilitates their uptake by RPE cells (Sun et al., 2006). RPE cells can internalize LDL and oxLDL in large quantities *in vitro* and *in vivo* (Gordiyenko et al., 2004). Treatment with oxLDL induces transcriptional alterations in genes related to lipid metabolism, oxidative stress, inflammation and apoptosis in RPE cells (Yamada et al., 2008). Failure in oxLDL clearance further recruits macrophages via cell surface scavenger receptors to the sites where oxLDL accumulates, amplifying inflammatory responses via producing inflammatory cytokines (Kamei et al., 2007). Therefore, efficient recycle of shed POS and clearance of oxLDL are essential for eye health since CD36 deficiency in mice resulted in age-associated accumulation of oxLDL and sub-retinal Bruch's membrane thickening

(Picard et al., 2010) as well as photoreceptor degeneration and choroidal involution (Houssier et al., 2008). Genetic analysis has identified that two common variants, rs3211883 and rs3173798 which do not reside in the coding sequence of *CD36* gene, are associated with neovascular AMD in a Japanese population (Kondo et al., 2009).

4. Mechanisms of sterile inflammation

In response to necrotic cell death, the innate and adaptive immune systems respond with inflammation to contain and remove the offending agents. The mechanisms by which DAMPs trigger inflammatory responses are still not fully understood, however, the outcome of sterile inflammation to structurally diverse DAMPs is quite similar. Discussed here are activation of the NF-κB/AP-1 signaling and the NLRP3/AIM2 inflammasomes for generating inflammatory mediators.

4.1 Generation of inflammatory mediators by activating cell surface DAMP receptors

Production of biologically active inflammatory mediators including cytokines and adhesion molecules during sterile injury-associated cell death is an important mechanism to alert the immune system of tissue damage and to initiate the healing response. Although the mechanistic details of these DAMP receptor signaling are not fully revealed yet, accumulating evidence shows that these DAMP receptors activate transcriptional factor NF-κB and AP-1, driving expression of inflammatory mediators required for initiating and promoting sterile inflammation (Figure 2).

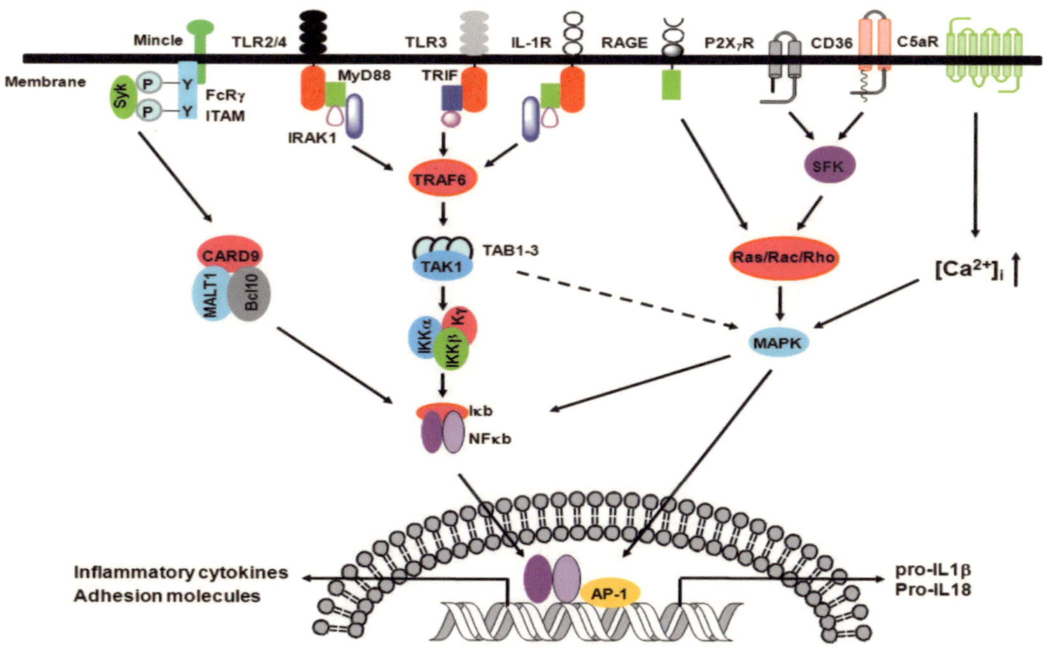

Fig. 2. Overview of cell surface DAMP receptor signaling pathways.

The presentation of DAMP molecules to host cells triggers the sequential activation of signaling cascades that activate transcriptional factors NF-κB and AP-1, leading to production of inflammatory mediators. AP-1, activator protein-1. Bcl10, B cell lymphoma 10. CARD9, caspase recruitment domain-containing protein-9. ITAM, immunoreceptor tyrosine-based activation motif. MyD88, myeloid differentiation primary-response gene 88. IKK, inhibitor of kappa B kinase. IRAK, IL-1 receptor-associated kinase. MAPK, mitogen-activated kinase. NF-κB, nuclear factor kappa B. SFK, src-family kinases. Syk, spleen tyrosine kinase. TAK1, transforming growth factor β–activated kinase 1. TRAF6, TNF receptor-associated factor 6. TRIF, TIR-domain-containing adapter-inducing interferon-β.

The signals relayed from activated TLR2, TLR3, TLR4 and IL-1R convene at TNF receptor-associated factor 6 (TRAF6) that further activates NF-κB through TAK1-IKK or activates AP-1 through TAK1-MAPK (Sloane et al., 2010). On the other hand, CLRs Mincle and CLEC9A couple with FcRγ adaptor and activate transcriptional factor NF-κB through Syk kinase-caspase recruitment domain-containing protein-9 (CARD9) pathway (Drummond et al., 2011). Activated $P2X_7R$ (Skaper et al., 2010) and CD36 (Stuart et al., 2007) first promote activation of src-family kinases that trigger NF-κB- and AP-1-dependent transcription via small G-protein-MAPK pathways. Although the mechanistic details of RAGE signaling and the importance of its various ligands in disease pathology continue to be areas of investigation, activated RAGE by its various ligands also leads to activation of transcription factors NF-κB and AP-1 by ras-MAPK signaling (Glenn & Stitt, 2009). Activated NF-κB and AP-1 finally drive expression of inflammatory mediators, promoting sterile inflammation. Among the inflammatory cytokines synthesized, IL-1β and IL-18 are produced and stored in cytosol as inactive precursors that are then converted into biological active forms by the activated NLRP3 and AIM2 inflammasomes through caspase 1-dependent proteolytic maturation, which will be discussed below.

4.2 Production of active IL-1β by NLRP3 inflammasome

IL-1β is a potent pro-inflammatory cytokine that is important in sterile inflammation by induction of inflammatory mediators (Gabay et al., 2010). IL-1β and IL-18 are synthesized and stored in the cytosol as inactive precursors. The processing and secretion of active IL-1β and IL-18 by inflammatory cells depend largely on the inflammasomes, of which the hallmark is the activation of caspase 1 responsible for processing immature IL-1β and IL-18 into their biologically active forms (Martinon et al., 2009). Among several inflammasomes described up to date, NLRP3 (also named as NALP3) inflammasome has been demonstrated to sense DAMP molecules in sterile inflammatory responses. Understanding how NLRP3 senses diverse sterile stimuli is important for understanding the pathogenesis of possibly many sterile inflammatory disorders and for identifying potential therapeutic targets. NLRP3 inflammasome consists of NLRP3, adaptor protein ASC (apoptosis-associated speck-like protein containing a CARD) and caspase-1 (Martinon et al., 2009). NLRP3 detects the intracellular ligands by its C-terminal LRR domain, triggering oligomerization by NACHT domain interaction in an ATP-dependent manner followed by caspase-1 recruitment and activation by autocleavage. NLRP3 does not sense structurally diverse stimuli individually, but rather senses a common downstream event mainly through three pathways: ROS generation, lysosome rupture and lowering intracellular potassium (Figure 3).

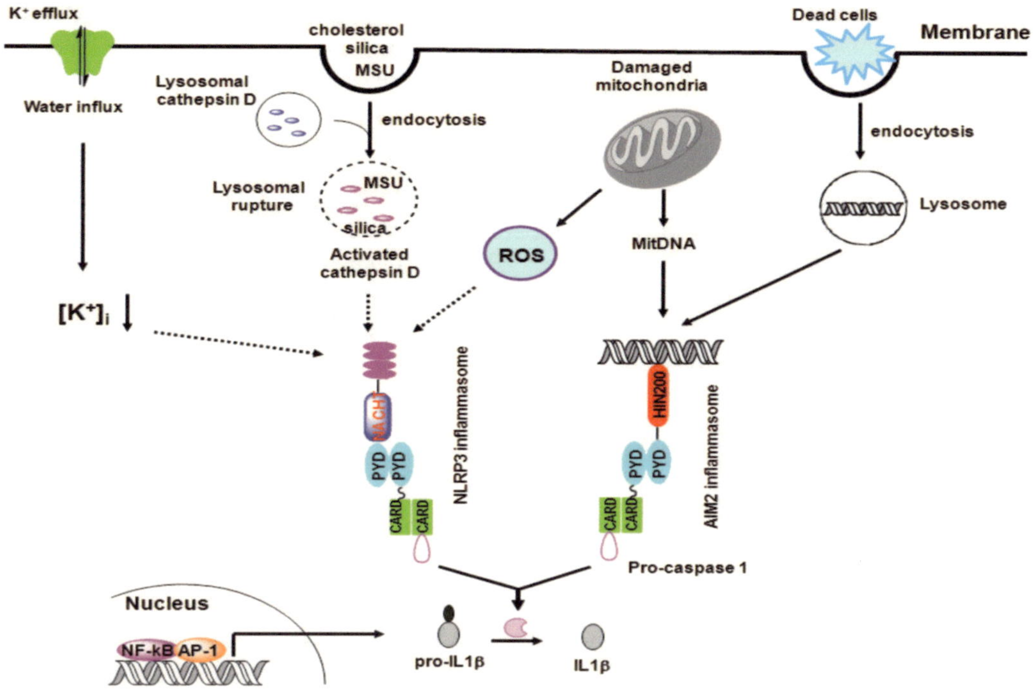

Fig. 3. Intracellular DAMP receptors that sense upcoming danger.

The nucleotide-binding oligomerization domain (NOD)-like receptor NLRP3 (NOD-, LRR- and pyrin domain-containing 3) and the PYHIN (pyrin and HIN200 domain-containing) family protein AIM2 (absent in melanoma 2) are two PRRs that survilliance intracelluar DAMPs. NLRP3 can be activated by lowering intracellular potassium concentration, lysosomal damage-dependent activation of cathepsin B or generation of reactive oxygen species (ROS) during cellular stress or necrosis. On the other hand, intracellular DNA from damaged mitochondria or genomic DNA fragments activates AIM2 via binding to its HIN200 domain. Activated NLRP3 and AIM2 provide binding sites for the adaptor ASC (apoptosis-related speck-like protein) via homotypic pyrin domain (PYD) interactions. Clustered ASC then recruits pro-caspase-1 through caspase recruitment domain (CARD)-CARD interactions for assembling NLRP3 or AIM2 inflammasome. The NLRP3 and AIM2 inflammasomes activate caspase-1 which subsequently processes pro-cytokines interleukin-1β (IL-1β) and IL-18 into their active forms. AP-1, activator protein-1. NF-κB, nuclear factor kappa B.

4.2.1 ROS generation

The detrimental effect of ROS during sterile inflammation depends on the balance between ROS producers and ROS detoxification by antioxidants. ROS are the common integrator across silica, MSU (Dostert et al., 2008) and ATP (Cruz et al., 2007) that activate the NLRP3 inflammasome. ROS removal by *N*-acetyl-L-cysteine, DPI-inhibition of NADPH oxidase and $p22^{phox}$ knockdown resulted in impairment of caspase 1 activation and IL-1β production by these stimuli (Cruz et al., 2007; Dostert et al., 2008). The causal role of ROS in NLRP3 activation is further confirmed by Zhou *et al.* (Zhou et al., 2011) and Nakahira *et al.* (Nakahira et al., 2011), identifying that mitochondrial ROS derived from complex I and III are responsible for NLRP3 activation. Although it is undefined how NLRP3 senses ROS, redox imbalance may be one of the unifying mechanisms by which NLRP3 senses its various activators.

4.2.2 Lowering intracellular potassium

Potassium efflux has been suggested to be an essential upstream signal of NLRP3 activation. Blocking potassium efflux in cultured media abrogates NLRP3 activation by asbestos, MSU and ATP (Dostert et al., 2008). Extracellular ATP is known to open an ATP-gated cation channel that causes potassium efflux via binding to purinergic receptor $P2X_7R$. Antibiotics such as neomycin and gramicidin stimulate NLRP3 inflammasome-dependent secretion of IL-1β, depending on potassium efflux but independent of $P2X_7R$ (Allam et al., 2011). Passive water influx due to sodium overload, which only dilutes cytoplasmic potassium ions, is able to activate NLRP3 inflammasome (Schorn et al., 2011). Thus, NLRP3 senses intracellular K^+ depletion, regardless whether it is due to the activation of specific ion channels or a non-selective increase in ion permeability as a result of cell injury.

4.2.3 Lysosomal rupture

Sterile crystalline and particulate activators of the NLRP3 inflammasome such as urate and cholesterol crystals cause lysosomal destabilization and cathepsin B release, which can be detected by NLRP3. Activation of NLRP3 inflammasome by amyloid-β (Halle et al., 2008) and silica and MSU crystals (Hornung et al., 2008) requires their internalization through endocytosis and lysosomal cathepsin B activation as inhibition of endocytosis or cathepsin B impairs NLRP3-dependent IL-1β production. The same is true to cholesterol crystals that activate NLRP3 inflammasome in a cathepsin B-dependent manner (Rajamaki et al., 2010). Lysosomal damage can occur during cellular injury and necrosis, therefore, lysosomal destabilization may be one of the converging points of divergent danger signals sensed by NRLP3. However, whether there is a common mechanism by which numerous heterogeneous stimuli converge on NLRP3 downstream of ROS generation, potassium efflux and lysosomal rupture, remains to be determined.

4.3 Production of active IL-1β by AIM2 inflammasome

In addition to the NLRP3 inflammasome, the AIM2 inflammasome is the second one indentified so far to be involved in sterile inflammation. In contrast to NLRP3, AIM2 has a highly restricted spectrum of activating stimuli, currently known being involved in sensing cytosolic dsDNA regardless of the DNA source. The HIN200 domain in its C terminus interacts directly with dsDNA and triggers recruitment and activation of caspase-1 in an ASC-dependent manner via its N-terminal pyrin domain, thereby processing IL-1β and IL-18 into their active forms (Hornung et al., 2009). Mitochondrial DNA (Zhang et al., 2010) and genomic DNA fragments (Kawashima et al., 2011) released from cellular injury can trigger inflammatory responses through activation of the AIM2 inflammasome in addition to TLR9.

5. Therapeutic potentials of anti-DAMP for AMD

Cell injury by chronic sterile inflammation leads to progressive loss of cell function and thus contributes to the development of AMD. Protecting retinal cells by neutralizing DAMPs and inhibiting DAMP-initiated inflammatory signaling could potentially delay the onset or progression of this disease. A number of promising anti-DAMP agents are currently under development for AMD therapy, some of them are still in preclinical testing (Table 1).

5.1 Complement alternative pathway inhibitors

As strong association of complement alternative pathway activation with higher AMD risk has been documented, suppressing complement cascade in the retina would be expected to delay or reverse the onset of AMD. Inhibition of complement alternative pathway can be achieved via targeting factor B and factor D which participate in the amplification of the complement alternative pathway, or inhibiting targets downstream the point of conversion for all three complement pathways. TA-106 and TNX-234, anti-Factor B and anti-Factor D antibodies, are in preclinical testing and Phase I/II trial for AMD by Alexion and Genentech, respectively. JPE-1375 is a small molecule peptidomimetic antagonist targeting the C5a receptor (Ricklin & Lambris, 2007) that is in preclinical evaluation for AMD. ARC-1905, a 39-mer oligonucleotide anti-C5 aptamer is in Phase 1 for AMD by Ophthotech. POT-4 is a cyclic peptide capable of binding to human C3, resulting in broad and potent complement activation inhibition (Ricklin & Lambris, 2007). POT-4 is the first complement inhibitor that has entered into a Phase I clinical trial for AMD by Potentia and is now under development by Alcon (Table 1).

Compound	Indications	Company	State of development	Estimated completion day	Mechanism of activation
TA-106	AMD & asthma	Alexion	Pre-clinical testing	Unknown	Anti-factor B antibody
TNX-234	Geographic atrophy	Genentech	Phase I/II	Unknown ongoing	Anti-factor D antibody
JPE-1375	Geographic atrophy	Jerini	Pre-clinical testing	Under development	C5aR antagonist
ARC-1905	AMD	Ophthotech	Phase I	Mar. 2011 ongoing	Anti-C5 aptamer
POT-4	AMD	Alcon	Phase 1	Feb. 2010 completed	C3 inhibitor
Canakinumab	Wet AMD	Novartis	Phase 1	Dec. 2007 completed	Anti-IL1β antibody
Anakinra	Corneal neovascularization	Massachusetts Eye Infirmary	Phase I/II	Under development	IL-1 receptor antagonist
PF-04494700	Alzheimer's dementia	Pfizer	Phase II	Dec. 2010 completed	RAGE inhibitor

Table 1. Developing anti-DAMP therapies for age-related macular degeneration

5.2 IL-1 pathway inhibitor

Given the crucial role for IL-1α and IL-1β in sterile inflammatory responses, blocking IL-1 receptor is expected to benefit patients with sterile inflammatory disorders. Some promising results have been obtained with the application of a recombinant IL-1 receptor antagonist, anakinra. Anakinra is in clinic for the treatment of rheumatoid arthritis (Mertens & Singh, 2009). Phase I/II clinical trials are ongoing for the topical treatment of corneal neovascularization by Massachusetts Eye and Ear Infirmary. Intravitreal delivery of anakinra significantly inhibits experimental CNV in animal model (Olson et al., 2009). A benefit for patients with AMD is expecting with use of anakinra though no clinical trial is initiated. Neutralizing ligands for IL-1 receptor on the other hand would achieve similar outcomes. IL-1β antibody, canakinumab, has been approved for treating cryopyin-associated periodic syndromes. Canakinumab is under Phase I evaluation for choroidal neovascurilization by Norvartis.

5.3 Anti-RAGE

The levels of RAGE, which detects AGEs, S100 proteins, HMGB1 and amyloid-β, are very lower but dramatically increases on the Bruch's membrane around drusen and are associated with early development of AMD. Inhibiting RAGE receptor will block multi-ligand-triggered inflammatory response, thereby delaying or preventing the onset and progression of the disease. Pfizer is conducting a Phase II trial of RAGE inhibitor, PF-04494700, for treating Alzheimer's dementia, which share similar risk factors with AMD.

5.4 Anti-TLR-3

Activation of TLR3 by heterologous RNA from necrotic cells or *Alu* RNA causes RPE cell death and retinal degeneration. TLR3 knockout and TLR3 412Phe provents retinal degeneration in animals and confers protection against geographic atrophy in patients, respectively. TLR3 monoclonal antibody 23C8 is currently in Phase I trial for treatment of inflammation by Innate. No trial has been reported for AMD yet.

6. Conclusion

Cells or tissues incite sterile inflammatory responses to clear and repair the damage by sensing DAMPs derived from necrotic cells. Persistent inflammation causes cell dysfunction and subsequent retinal degeneration. Much progress has been made in identifying sterile inflammatory triggers and understanding the molecule mechanisms, which offers opportunities to design novel targets for delaying and preventing onset of retinal diseases including AMD. However, many questions remain to be answered. As cells contain many DAMPs, which DAMPs are the most important and whether their relative importance depends on cell types or pathophysiological conditions? How do different DAMPs initiate a common sterile inflammatory response and their downstream signaling pathways? Also unknown is the significance of DAMP-receptor interactions in sterile inflammation and disease pathogenesis since some DAMPs bind to several receptors and vice versa. Once the molecular mechanisms by which necrosis triggers sterile inflammation are elucidated and the relative importance of DAMPs is determined, one can manipulate the immune response to treat and manage sterile inflammation-associated diseases.

7. References

Alam MU, Harken JA, Knorn AM, Elford AR, Wigmore K, Ohashi PS & Millar DG (2009) Transgenic expression of Hsc70 in pancreatic islets enhances autoimmune diabetes in response to beta cell damage. J Immunol 183:5728-5737.

Allam R, Darisipudi MN, Rupanagudi KV, Lichtnekert J, Tschopp J & Anders HJ (2011) Cutting edge: Cyclic polypeptide and aminoglycoside antibiotics trigger IL-1beta secretion by activating the NLRP3 inflammasome. J Immunol 186:2714-2718.

Ambati J, Anand A, Fernandez S, Sakurai E, Lynn BC, Kuziel WA, Rollins BJ & Ambati BK (2003) An animal model of age-related macular degeneration in senescent Ccl-2- or Ccr-2-deficient mice. Nat Med 9:1390-1397.

Andersson U, Wang H, Palmblad K, Aveberger AC, Bloom O, Erlandsson-Harris H, Janson A, Kokkola R, Zhang M, Yang H & Tracey KJ (2000) High mobility group 1 protein (HMG-1) stimulates proinflammatory cytokine synthesis in human monocytes. J Exp Med 192:565-570.

Arimura N, Ki-i Y, Hashiguchi T, Kawahara K, Biswas KK, Nakamura M, Sonoda Y, Yamakiri K, Okubo A, Sakamoto T & Maruyama I (2009) Intraocular expression and release of high-mobility group box 1 protein in retinal detachment. Lab Invest 89:278-289.

Asea A, Kraeft SK, Kurt-Jones EA, Stevenson MA, Chen LB, Finberg RW, Koo GC & Calderwood SK (2000) HSP70 stimulates cytokine production through a CD14-dependant pathway, demonstrating its dual role as a chaperone and cytokine. Nat Med 6:435-442.

Babelova A, Moreth K, Tsalastra-Greul W, Zeng-Brouwers J, Eickelberg O, Young MF, Bruckner P, Pfeilschifter J, Schaefer RM, Grone HJ & Schaefer L (2009) Biglycan, a danger signal that activates the NLRP3 inflammasome via toll-like and P2X receptors. J Biol Chem 284:24035-24048.

Barile GR & Schmidt AM (2007) RAGE and its ligands in retinal disease. Curr Mol Med 7:758-765.

Bian ZM, Elner VM, Yoshida A, Kunkel SL & Elner SG (2001) Signaling pathways for glycated human serum albumin-induced IL-8 and MCP-1 secretion in human RPE cells. Invest Ophthalmol Vis Sci 42:1660-1668.

Binder RJ, Kelly JB, 3rd, Vatner RE & Srivastava PK (2007) Specific immunogenicity of heat shock protein gp96 derives from chaperoned antigenic peptides and not from contaminating proteins. J Immunol 179:7254-7261.

Brentano F, Schorr O, Gay RE, Gay S & Kyburz D (2005) RNA released from necrotic synovial fluid cells activates rheumatoid arthritis synovial fibroblasts via Toll-like receptor 3. Arthritis Rheum 52:2656-2665.

Bucciarelli LG, Wendt T, Rong L, Lalla E, Hofmann MA, Goova MT, Taguchi A, Yan SF, Yan SD, Stern DM & Schmidt AM (2002) RAGE is a multiligand receptor of the immunoglobulin superfamily: implications for homeostasis and chronic disease. Cell Mol Life Sci 59:1117-1128.

Burckstummer T, Baumann C, Bluml S, Dixit E, Durnberger G, Jahn H, Planyavsky M, Bilban M, Colinge J, Bennett KL & Superti-Furga G (2009) An orthogonal proteomic-genomic screen identifies AIM2 as a cytoplasmic DNA sensor for the inflammasome. Nat Immunol 10:266-272.

Camara AK, Bienengraeber M & Stowe DF (2011) Mitochondrial approaches to protect against cardiac ischemia and reperfusion injury. Front Physiol 2:13.

Cambi A & Figdor C (2009) Necrosis: C-type lectins sense cell death. Curr Biol 19:R375-378.

Chen CJ, Kono H, Golenbock D, Reed G, Akira S & Rock KL (2007) Identification of a key pathway required for the sterile inflammatory response triggered by dying cells. Nat Med 13:851-856.

Cohen I, Rider P, Carmi Y, Braiman A, Dotan S, White MR, Voronov E, Martin MU, Dinarello CA & Apte RN (2010) Differential release of chromatin-bound IL-1alpha discriminates between necrotic and apoptotic cell death by the ability to induce sterile inflammation. Proc Natl Acad Sci U S A 107:2574-2579.

Cruz CM, Rinna A, Forman HJ, Ventura AL, Persechini PM & Ojcius DM (2007) ATP activates a reactive oxygen species-dependent oxidative stress response and secretion of proinflammatory cytokines in macrophages. J Biol Chem 282:2871-2879.

Decanini A, Nordgaard CL, Feng X, Ferrington DA & Olsen TW (2007) Changes in select redox proteins of the retinal pigment epithelium in age-related macular degeneration. Am J Ophthalmol 143:607-615.

Di Virgilio F (2007) Liaisons dangereuses: P2X(7) and the inflammasome. Trends Pharmacol Sci 28:465-472.

Dogusan Z, Garcia M, Flamez D, Alexopoulou L, Goldman M, Gysemans C, Mathieu C, Libert C, Eizirik DL & Rasschaert J (2008) Double-stranded RNA induces pancreatic beta-cell apoptosis by activation of the toll-like receptor 3 and interferon regulatory factor 3 pathways. Diabetes 57:1236-1245.

Dostert C, Petrilli V, Van Bruggen R, Steele C, Mossman BT & Tschopp J (2008) Innate immune activation through Nalp3 inflammasome sensing of asbestos and silica. Science 320:674-677.

Drummond RA, Saijo S, Iwakura Y & Brown GD (2011) The role of Syk/CARD9 coupled C-type lectins in antifungal immunity. Eur J Immunol 41:276-281.

Ebihara N, Chen L, Tokura T, Ushio H, Iwatsu M & Murakami A (2007) Distinct functions between toll-like receptors 3 and 9 in retinal pigment epithelial cells. Ophthalmic Res 39:155-163.

Ebrahem Q, Renganathan K, Sears J, Vasanji A, Gu X, Lu L, Salomon RG, Crabb JW & Anand-Apte B (2006) Carboxyethylpyrrole oxidative protein modifications stimulate neovascularization: Implications for age-related macular degeneration. Proc Natl Acad Sci U S A 103:13480-13484.

Eigenbrod T, Park JH, Harder J, Iwakura Y & Nunez G (2008) Cutting edge: critical role for mesothelial cells in necrosis-induced inflammation through the recognition of IL-1 alpha released from dying cells. J Immunol 181:8194-8198.

Evans J & Wormald R (1996) Is the incidence of registrable age-related macular degeneration increasing? Br J Ophthalmol 80:9-14.

Fernandes-Alnemri T, Yu JW, Datta P, Wu J & Alnemri ES (2009) AIM2 activates the inflammasome and cell death in response to cytoplasmic DNA. Nature 458:509-513.

Fukuoka Y, Strainic M & Medof ME (2003) Differential cytokine expression of human retinal pigment epithelial cells in response to stimulation by C5a. Clin Exp Immunol 131:248-253.

Gabay C, Lamacchia C & Palmer G (2010) IL-1 pathways in inflammation and human diseases. Nat Rev Rheumatol 6:232-241.

Garg AD, Nowis D, Golab J & Agostinis P (2010) Photodynamic therapy: illuminating the road from cell death towards anti-tumour immunity. Apoptosis 15:1050-1071.

Georgopoulos C & Welch WJ (1993) Role of the major heat shock proteins as molecular chaperones. Annu Rev Cell Biol 9:601-634.

Glenn JV & Stitt AW (2009) The role of advanced glycation end products in retinal ageing and disease. Biochim Biophys Acta 1790:1109-1116.

Gordiyenko N, Campos M, Lee JW, Fariss RN, Sztein J & Rodriguez IR (2004) RPE cells internalize low-density lipoprotein (LDL) and oxidized LDL (oxLDL) in large quantities in vitro and in vivo. Invest Ophthalmol Vis Sci 45:2822-2829.

Gu X, Meer SG, Miyagi M, Rayborn ME, Hollyfield JG, Crabb JW & Salomon RG (2003) Carboxyethylpyrrole protein adducts and autoantibodies, biomarkers for age-related macular degeneration. J Biol Chem 278:42027-42035.

Hageman GS, Luthert PJ, Victor Chong NH, Johnson LV, Anderson DH & Mullins RF (2001) An integrated hypothesis that considers drusen as biomarkers of immune-mediated processes at the RPE-Bruch's membrane interface in aging and age-related macular degeneration. Prog Retin Eye Res 20:705-732.

Halle A, Hornung V, Petzold GC, Stewart CR, Monks BG, Reinheckel T, Fitzgerald KA, Latz E, Moore KJ & Golenbock DT (2008) The NALP3 inflammasome is involved in the innate immune response to amyloid-beta. Nat Immunol 9:857-865.

Heizmann CW, Fritz G & Schafer BW (2002) S100 proteins: structure, functions and pathology. Front Biosci 7:d1356-1368.

Hofmann MA, Drury S, Fu C, Qu W, Taguchi A, Lu Y, Avila C, Kambham N, Bierhaus A, Nawroth P, Neurath MF, Slattery T, Beach D, McClary J, Nagashima M, Morser J, Stern D & Schmidt AM (1999) RAGE mediates a novel proinflammatory axis: a central cell surface receptor for S100/calgranulin polypeptides. Cell 97:889-901.

Hollyfield JG, Bonilha VL, Rayborn ME, Yang X, Shadrach KG, Lu L, Ufret RL, Salomon RG & Perez VL (2008) Oxidative damage-induced inflammation initiates age-related macular degeneration. Nat Med 14:194-198.

Hoppe G, O'Neil J, Hoff HF & Sears J (2004a) Products of lipid peroxidation induce missorting of the principal lysosomal protease in retinal pigment epithelium. Biochim Biophys Acta 1689:33-41.

Hoppe G, O'Neil J, Hoff HF & Sears J (2004b) Accumulation of oxidized lipid-protein complexes alters phagosome maturation in retinal pigment epithelium. Cell Mol Life Sci 61:1664-1674.

Hornung V, Bauernfeind F, Halle A, Samstad EO, Kono H, Rock KL, Fitzgerald KA & Latz E (2008) Silica crystals and aluminum salts activate the NALP3 inflammasome through phagosomal destabilization. Nat Immunol 9:847-856.

Hornung V, Ablasser A, Charrel-Dennis M, Bauernfeind F, Horvath G, Caffrey DR, Latz E & Fitzgerald KA (2009) AIM2 recognizes cytosolic dsDNA and forms a caspase-1-activating inflammasome with ASC. Nature 458:514-518.

Houssier M, Raoul W, Lavalette S, Keller N, Guillonneau X, Baragatti B, Jonet L, Jeanny JC, Behar-Cohen F, Coceani F, Scherman D, Lachapelle P, Ong H, Chemtob S & Sennlaub F (2008) CD36 deficiency leads to choroidal involution via COX2 down-regulation in rodents. PLoS Med 5:e39.

Howes KA, Liu Y, Dunaief JL, Milam A, Frederick JM, Marks A & Baehr W (2004) Receptor for advanced glycation end products and age-related macular degeneration. Invest Ophthalmol Vis Sci 45:3713-3720.

Idzko M, Hammad H, van Nimwegen M, Kool M, Willart MA, Muskens F, Hoogsteden HC, Luttmann W, Ferrari D, Di Virgilio F, Virchow JC, Jr. & Lambrecht BN (2007) Extracellular ATP triggers and maintains asthmatic airway inflammation by activating dendritic cells. Nat Med 13:913-919.

Javadzadeh A, Ghorbanihaghjo A, Bahreini E, Rashtchizadeh N, Argani H & Alizadeh S (2010) Plasma oxidized LDL and thiol-containing molecules in patients with exudative age-related macular degeneration. Mol Vis 16:2578-2584.

Kaji Y, Usui T, Ishida S, Yamashiro K, Moore TC, Moore J, Yamamoto Y, Yamamoto H & Adamis AP (2007) Inhibition of diabetic leukostasis and blood-retinal barrier breakdown with a soluble form of a receptor for advanced glycation end products. Invest Ophthalmol Vis Sci 48:858-865.

Kamei M, Yoneda K, Kume N, Suzuki M, Itabe H, Matsuda K, Shimaoka T, Minami M, Yonehara S, Kita T & Kinoshita S (2007) Scavenger receptors for oxidized lipoprotein in age-related macular degeneration. Invest Ophthalmol Vis Sci 48:1801-1807.

Kaneko H, Dridi S, Tarallo V, Gelfand BD, Fowler BJ, Cho WG, Kleinman ME, Ponicsan SL, Hauswirth WW, Chiodo VA, Kariko K, Yoo JW, Lee DK, Hadziahmetovic M, Song Y, Misra S, Chaudhuri G, Buaas FW, Braun RE, Hinton DR, Zhang Q, Grossniklaus HE, Provis JM, Madigan MC, Milam AH, Justice NL, Albuquerque RJ, Blandford AD, Bogdanovich S, Hirano Y, Witta J, Fuchs E, Littman DR, Ambati BK, Rudin CM, Chong MM, Provost P, Kugel JF, Goodrich JA, Dunaief JL, Baffi JZ & Ambati J (2011) DICER1 deficit induces Alu RNA toxicity in age-related macular degeneration. Nature 471:325-330.

Kariko K, Ni H, Capodici J, Lamphier M & Weissman D (2004) mRNA is an endogenous ligand for Toll-like receptor 3. J Biol Chem 279:12542-12550.

Kawashima A, Tanigawa K, Akama T, Wu H, Sue M, Yoshihara A, Ishido Y, Kobiyama K, Takeshita F, Ishii KJ, Hirano H, Kimura H, Sakai T, Ishii N & Suzuki K (2011) Fragments of genomic DNA released by injured cells activate innate immunity and suppress endocrine function in the thyroid. Endocrinology 152:1702-1712.

Klein R, Klein BE, Jensen SC & Meuer SM (1997) The five-year incidence and progression of age-related maculopathy: the Beaver Dam Eye Study. Ophthalmology 104:7-21.

Kleinman ME, Yamada K, Takeda A, Chandrasekaran V, Nozaki M, Baffi JZ, Albuquerque RJ, Yamasaki S, Itaya M, Pan Y, Appukuttan B, Gibbs D, Yang Z, Kariko K, Ambati BK, Wilgus TA, DiPietro LA, Sakurai E, Zhang K, Smith JR, Taylor EW & Ambati J (2008) Sequence- and target-independent angiogenesis suppression by siRNA via TLR3. Nature 452:591-597.

Kondo N, Honda S, Kuno S & Negi A (2009) Positive association of common variants in CD36 with neovascular age-related macular degeneration. Aging (Albany NY) 1:266-274.

Kono H & Rock KL (2008) How dying cells alert the immune system to danger. Nat Rev Immunol 8:279-289.

Kono H, Chen CJ, Ontiveros F & Rock KL (2010a) Uric acid promotes an acute inflammatory response to sterile cell death in mice. J Clin Invest 120:1939-1949.

Kono H, Karmarkar D, Iwakura Y & Rock KL (2010b) Identification of the cellular sensor that stimulates the inflammatory response to sterile cell death. J Immunol 184:4470-4478.

Kumar MV, Nagineni CN, Chin MS, Hooks JJ & Detrick B (2004) Innate immunity in the retina: Toll-like receptor (TLR) signaling in human retinal pigment epithelial cells. J Neuroimmunol 153:7-15.

Ma W, Lee SE, Guo J, Qu W, Hudson BI, Schmidt AM & Barile GR (2007) RAGE ligand upregulation of VEGF secretion in ARPE-19 cells. Invest Ophthalmol Vis Sci 48:1355-1361.

Maloney SC, Antecka E, Orellana ME, Fernandes BF, Odashiro AN, Eghtedari M & Burnier MN, Jr. (2010) Choroidal neovascular membranes express toll-like receptor 3. Ophthalmic Res 44:237-241.

Martinon F, Mayor A & Tschopp J (2009) The inflammasomes: guardians of the body. Annu Rev Immunol 27:229-265.

Mata NL, Weng J & Travis GH (2000) Biosynthesis of a major lipofuscin fluorophore in mice and humans with ABCR-mediated retinal and macular degeneration. Proc Natl Acad Sci U S A 97:7154-7159.

Matzinger P (1994) Tolerance, danger, and the extended family. Annu Rev Immunol 12:991-1045.

Mertens M & Singh JA (2009) Anakinra for rheumatoid arthritis: a systematic review. J Rheumatol 36:1118-1125.

Meylan E, Tschopp J & Karin M (2006) Intracellular pattern recognition receptors in the host response. Nature 442:39-44.

Mochimaru H, Takahashi E, Tsukamoto N, Miyazaki J, Yaguchi T, Koto T, Kurihara T, Noda K, Ozawa Y, Ishimoto T, Kawakami Y, Tanihara H, Saya H, Ishida S & Tsubota K (2009) Involvement of hyaluronan and its receptor CD44 with choroidal neovascularization. Invest Ophthalmol Vis Sci 50:4410-4415.

Montezuma SR, Sobrin L & Seddon JM (2007) Review of genetics in age related macular degeneration. Semin Ophthalmol 22:229-240.

Moreira EF, Larrayoz IM, Lee JW & Rodriguez IR (2009) 7-Ketocholesterol is present in lipid deposits in the primate retina: potential implication in the induction of VEGF and CNV formation. Invest Ophthalmol Vis Sci 50:523-532.

Nakahira K, Haspel JA, Rathinam VA, Lee SJ, Dolinay T, Lam HC, Englert JA, Rabinovitch M, Cernadas M, Kim HP, Fitzgerald KA, Ryter SW & Choi AM (2011) Autophagy proteins regulate innate immune responses by inhibiting the release of mitochondrial DNA mediated by the NALP3 inflammasome. Nat Immunol 12:222-230.

Nozaki M, Raisler BJ, Sakurai E, Sarma JV, Barnum SR, Lambris JD, Chen Y, Zhang K, Ambati BK, Baffi JZ & Ambati J (2006) Drusen complement components C3a and C5a promote choroidal neovascularization. Proc Natl Acad Sci U S A 103:2328-2333.

Olson JL, Courtney RJ, Rouhani B, Mandava N & Dinarello CA (2009) Intravitreal anakinra inhibits choroidal neovascular membrane growth in a rat model. Ocul Immunol Inflamm 17:195-200.

Picard E, Houssier M, Bujold K, Sapieha P, Lubell W, Dorfman A, Racine J, Hardy P, Febbraio M, Lachapelle P, Ong H, Sennlaub F & Chemtob S (2010) CD36 plays an important role in the clearance of oxLDL and associated age-dependent sub-retinal deposits. Aging (Albany NY) 2:981-989.

Qin S & Rodrigues GA (2010a) Differential roles of AMPKalpha1 and AMPKalpha2 in regulating 4-HNE-induced RPE cell death and permeability. Exp Eye Res 91:818-824.

Qin S & Rodrigues GA (2010b) Role of reactive oxygen species in the oathogenesis of age-related macular degeneration. In: Handbook of Free Radicals: Formation, Types and Effects (Kozyrev D &Slutsky V, eds), pp 167-196. New York: Nova Science Publishers, Inc.

Radu RA, Hu J, Yuan Q, Welch DL, Makshanoff J, Lloyd M, McMullen S, Travis GH & Bok D (2011) Complement system dysregulation and inflammation in the retinal pigment epithelium of a mouse model for stargardt macular degeneration. J Biol Chem.

Rajamaki K, Lappalainen J, Oorni K, Valimaki E, Matikainen S, Kovanen PT & Eklund KK (2010) Cholesterol crystals activate the NLRP3 inflammasome in human macrophages: a novel link between cholesterol metabolism and inflammation. PLoS One 5:e11765.

Relvas LJ, Bouffioux C, Marcet B, Communi D, Makhoul M, Horckmans M, Blero D, Bruyns C, Caspers L, Boeynaems JM & Willermain F (2009) Extracellular nucleotides and interleukin-8 production by ARPE cells: potential role of danger signals in blood-retinal barrier activation. Invest Ophthalmol Vis Sci 50:1241-1246.

Ricklin D & Lambris JD (2007) Complement-targeted therapeutics. Nat Biotechnol 25:1265-1275.

Riteau N, Gasse P, Fauconnier L, Gombault A, Couegnat M, Fick L, Kanellopoulos J, Quesniaux VF, Marchand-Adam S, Crestani B, Ryffel B & Couillin I (2010) Extracellular ATP is a danger signal activating P2X7 receptor in lung inflammation and fibrosis. Am J Respir Crit Care Med 182:774-783.

Rodrigues EB (2007) Inflammation in dry age-related macular degeneration. Ophthalmologica 221:143-152.

Rodriguez IR, Alam S & Lee JW (2004) Cytotoxicity of oxidized low-density lipoprotein in cultured RPE cells is dependent on the formation of 7-ketocholesterol. Invest Ophthalmol Vis Sci 45:2830-2837.

Ryckman C, Vandal K, Rouleau P, Talbot M & Tessier PA (2003) Proinflammatory activities of S100: proteins S100A8, S100A9, and S100A8/A9 induce neutrophil chemotaxis and adhesion. J Immunol 170:3233-3242.

Sancho D, Joffre OP, Keller AM, Rogers NC, Martinez D, Hernanz-Falcon P, Rosewell I & Reis e Sousa C (2009) Identification of a dendritic cell receptor that couples sensing of necrosis to immunity. Nature 458:899-903.

Scaffidi P, Misteli T & Bianchi ME (2002) Release of chromatin protein HMGB1 by necrotic cells triggers inflammation. Nature 418:191-195.

Schaefer L, Babelova A, Kiss E, Hausser HJ, Baliova M, Krzyzankova M, Marsche G, Young MF, Mihalik D, Gotte M, Malle E, Schaefer RM & Grone HJ (2005) The matrix component biglycan is proinflammatory and signals through Toll-like receptors 4 and 2 in macrophages. J Clin Invest 115:2223-2233.

Schleicher ED, Wagner E & Nerlich AG (1997) Increased accumulation of the glycoxidation product N(epsilon)-(carboxymethyl)lysine in human tissues in diabetes and aging. J Clin Invest 99:457-468.

Schorn C, Frey B, Lauber K, Janko C, Strysio M, Keppeler H, Gaipl US, Voll RE, Springer E, Munoz LE, Schett G & Herrmann M (2011) Sodium overload and water influx activate the NALP3 inflammasome. J Biol Chem 286:35-41.

Schutt F, Bergmann M, Holz FG & Kopitz J (2003) Proteins modified by malondialdehyde, 4-hydroxynonenal, or advanced glycation end products in lipofuscin of human retinal pigment epithelium. Invest Ophthalmol Vis Sci 44:3663-3668.

Schutt F, Davies S, Kopitz J, Holz FG & Boulton ME (2000) Photodamage to human RPE cells by A2-E, a retinoid component of lipofuscin. Invest Ophthalmol Vis Sci 41:2303-2308.

Shiose S, Chen Y, Okano K, Roy S, Kohno H, Tang J, Pearlman E, Maeda T, Palczewski K & Maeda A (2011) Toll-like receptor 3 is required for development of retinopathy caused by impaired all-trans-retinal clearance in mice. J Biol Chem.

Skaper SD, Debetto P & Giusti P (2010) The P2X7 purinergic receptor: from physiology to neurological disorders. FASEB J 24:337-345.

Sloane JA, Blitz D, Margolin Z & Vartanian T (2010) A clear and present danger: endogenous ligands of Toll-like receptors. Neuromolecular Med 12:149-163.

Stuart LM, Bell SA, Stewart CR, Silver JM, Richard J, Goss JL, Tseng AA, Zhang A, El Khoury JB & Moore KJ (2007) CD36 signals to the actin cytoskeleton and regulates microglial migration via a p130Cas complex. J Biol Chem 282:27392-27401.

Sun M, Finnemann SC, Febbraio M, Shan L, Annangudi SP, Podrez EA, Hoppe G, Darrow R, Organisciak DT, Salomon RG, Silverstein RL & Hazen SL (2006) Light-induced oxidation of photoreceptor outer segment phospholipids generates ligands for CD36-mediated phagocytosis by retinal pigment epithelium: a potential mechanism for modulating outer segment phagocytosis under oxidant stress conditions. J Biol Chem 281:4222-4230.

Surprenant A, Rassendren F, Kawashima E, North RA & Buell G (1996) The cytolytic P2Z receptor for extracellular ATP identified as a P2X receptor (P2X7). Science 272:735-738.

Taylor KR, Trowbridge JM, Rudisill JA, Termeer CC, Simon JC & Gallo RL (2004) Hyaluronan fragments stimulate endothelial recognition of injury through TLR4. J Biol Chem 279:17079-17084.

Teixeira JM, Oliveira MC, Parada CA & Tambeli CH (2010) Peripheral mechanisms underlying the essential role of P2X7 receptors in the development of inflammatory hyperalgesia. Eur J Pharmacol 644:55-60.

Termeer C, Benedix F, Sleeman J, Fieber C, Voith U, Ahrens T, Miyake K, Freudenberg M, Galanos C & Simon JC (2002) Oligosaccharides of Hyaluronan activate dendritic cells via toll-like receptor 4. J Exp Med 195:99-111.

Tian J, Ishibashi K, Reiser K, Grebe R, Biswal S, Gehlbach P & Handa JT (2005) Advanced glycation endproduct-induced aging of the retinal pigment epithelium and choroid: a comprehensive transcriptional response. Proc Natl Acad Sci U S A 102:11846-11851.

Wang H, Bloom O, Zhang M, Vishnubhakat JM, Ombrellino M, Che J, Frazier A, Yang H, Ivanova S, Borovikova L, Manogue KR, Faist E, Abraham E, Andersson J, Andersson U, Molina PE, Abumrad NN, Sama A & Tracey KJ (1999) HMG-1 as a late mediator of endotoxin lethality in mice. Science 285:248-251.

Wu Y, Yanase E, Feng X, Siegel MM & Sparrow JR (2010) Structural characterization of bisretinoid A2E photocleavage products and implications for age-related macular degeneration. Proc Natl Acad Sci U S A 107:7275-7280.

Yamada Y, Ishibashi K, Bhutto IA, Tian J, Lutty GA & Handa JT (2006) The expression of advanced glycation endproduct receptors in rpe cells associated with basal deposits in human maculas. Exp Eye Res 82:840-848.

Yamada Y, Tian J, Yang Y, Cutler RG, Wu T, Telljohann RS, Mattson MP & Handa JT (2008) Oxidized low density lipoproteins induce a pathologic response by retinal pigmented epithelial cells. J Neurochem 105:1187-1197.

Yamasaki S, Ishikawa E, Sakuma M, Hara H, Ogata K & Saito T (2008) Mincle is an ITAM-coupled activating receptor that senses damaged cells. Nat Immunol 9:1179-1188.

Yang D, Elner SG, Clark AJ, Hughes BA, Petty HR & Elner VM (2010) Activation of P2X Receptors Induces Apoptosis in Human Retinal Pigment Epithelium. Invest Ophthalmol Vis Sci 52:1522-1530.

Yang Z, Stratton C, Francis PJ, Kleinman ME, Tan PL, Gibbs D, Tong Z, Chen H, Constantine R, Yang X, Chen Y, Zeng J, Davey L, Ma X, Hau VS, Wang C, Harmon J, Buehler J, Pearson E, Patel S, Kaminoh Y, Watkins S, Luo L, Zabriskie NA, Bernstein PS, Cho W, Schwager A, Hinton DR, Klein ML, Hamon SC, Simmons E, Yu B, Campochiaro B, Sunness JS, Campochiaro P, Jorde L, Parmigiani G, Zack DJ, Katsanis N, Ambati J & Zhang K (2008) Toll-like Receptor 3 and Geographic Atrophy in Age-Related Macular Degeneration. N Engl J Med.

Yu AL, Lorenz RL, Haritoglou C, Kampik A & Welge-Lussen U (2009) Biological effects of native and oxidized low-density lipoproteins in cultured human retinal pigment epithelial cells. Exp Eye Res 88:495-503.

Zhang Q, Raoof M, Chen Y, Sumi Y, Sursal T, Junger W, Brohi K, Itagaki K & Hauser CJ (2010) Circulating mitochondrial DAMPs cause inflammatory responses to injury. Nature 464:104-107.

Zhou J, Jang YP, Kim SR & Sparrow JR (2006) Complement activation by photooxidation products of A2E, a lipofuscin constituent of the retinal pigment epithelium. Proc Natl Acad Sci U S A 103:16182-16187.

Zhou R, Yazdi AS, Menu P & Tschopp J (2011) A role for mitochondria in NLRP3 inflammasome activation. Nature 469:221-225.

3

Bruch's Membrane: The Critical Boundary in Macular Degeneration

Robert F. Mullins and Elliott H. Sohn
The University of Iowa Institute for Vision Research
The Department of Ophthalmology and Visual Sciences
The University of Iowa Carver College of Medicine
Iowa City, Iowa
USA

1. Introduction

In the early second century A.D., the Roman Empire had reached its zenith. The *pax romana* extended to all the lands touching the Mediterranean, counterclockwise from Northern Africa to Palestine, through Asia Minor, Gaul and Hispania, all the way to modern Wales and England. This last province of Britannia was visited by the emperor Hadrian, where he put on a show of force in response to a recent uprising. Most famously, during this visit Hadrian ordered the construction of a set of earthworks that now bears his name, stretching nearly eighty miles from Carlisle to Newcastle. Studded with fortifications, and manned with highly trained foreign legionnaires, this imposing structure stretched the width of the island and its ruins are impressive still today (Figure 1). While there is disagreement about the principal purpose of Hadrian's Wall—whether primarily as a symbolic marker of the northern extent of the Empire, a defensive fortification, or as a means of regulating commerce—the Historia Augusta states that the wall was constructed *qui barbaros Romanosque divideret;* to separate the Romans from the Barbarians(Magie, 1921).

Whatever the principal motivation for its construction, Hadrian's wall did stand at the frontier between the Roman controlled territory and the Scots, Picts and other uncontrollable northern tribes of reputed violence. To the mind of the most Romanized Britons, who never met one of their northern neighbors, the wall must have represented the safe barrier between civilization and chaos.

Like the boundary between the civilized and barbarian world, a similar barrier stands at the threshold between the neural retina and the blood. The photoreceptor cells of the human retina face a dilemma. These cells are extremely energetic, consuming large quantities of oxygen. Elegant physiological studies by Linsenmeier and colleagues have shown that the oxygen tension from the RPE to the outer nuclear layer plunges over a distance of about 50μm, and that consumption at the level of the inner segment is dramatic(Birol, et al., 2007). Thus, the outer retina has a requirement for a large vascular supply. This requirement is met by the choriocapillaris, a unique vascular bed beneath the RPE. The endothelial cells (EC) of the choriocapillaris, like other EC, appear to use very little of the oxygen they deliver, instead likely relying largely on glycolytic metabolism. The choroid receives the vast majority of the uveal blood supply (in some studies choroidal blood flow was estimated at more than 20x higher than in neural retina(Alm and Bill, 1973)). The proximity of the photoreceptor cells to the choroid is also required to remove wastes from the retina. Each RPE cell turns over many thousands of rod outer segment discs each day(Young, 1971) and this waste material from the RPE must be removed by the vasculature.

However, the juxtaposition of the choroid and retina poses a dilemma: while on one hand the photoreceptor cells have a major vascular requirement, on the other hand the microenvironment of the subretinal space is exquisitely regulated and the presence of subretinal fluid not inherent to this space (i.e., rhegmatogenous retinal detachment) results in rapid and severe vision loss. Having a dense vascular supply adjacent to a tissue that can not tolerate alterations in its interstitial space appears to be a recipe for disaster.

This dilemma is solved through the presence of soluble factors, such as PEDF(Dawson, et al., 1999; Ohno-Matsui, et al., 2001) and insoluble (structural) factors that keep the vasculature in check. In this chapter we will first briefly review the disease age-related macular degeneration (AMD) and then discuss the (normally) insoluble factors that guard the retina against vascular intrusion, namely Bruch's membrane (BrM), that play a role in preserving central vision.

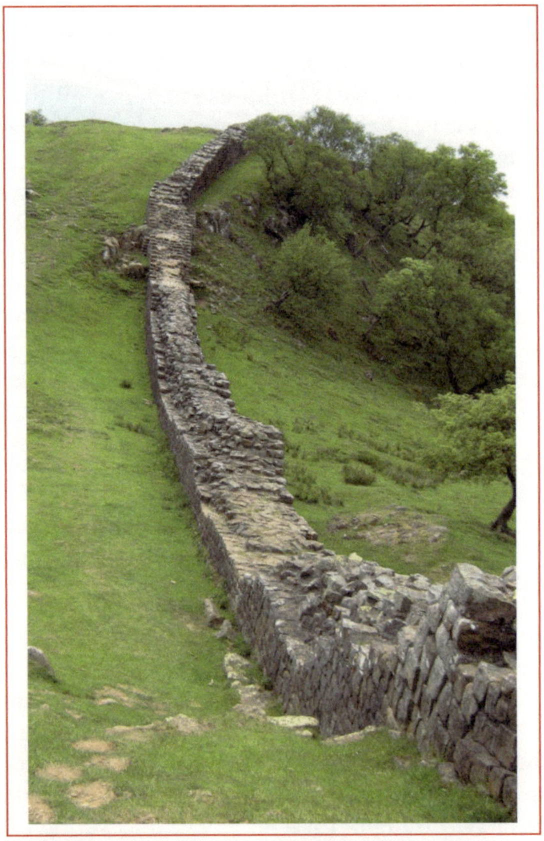

Fig. 1. Section of Hadrian's wall near Carlisle, Cumbria, UK. While sections of stone have been plundered over the hundreds of years of its existence, the wall continues to have an imposing presence. Photo courtesy of Jenna M. Mullins.

2. Clinical relevance of Bruch's membrane dysfunction: Age-related macular degeneration

The most common ocular condition of elderly humans with BrM dysfunction is age-related macular degeneration (AMD). This disease affects the center of the vision by damaging the macula, the critical portion of the retina responsible for fine visual acuity and daily activities such as reading, driving and recognizing faces. It is the most common cause of blindness in the elderly population in the western world(Klein, et al., 1992; Mitchell, et al., 1995; Vingerling, et al., 1995). Genetic variants conferring risk for developing AMD include mutations in complement factor H (*CFH*), complement component 2 (*C2*), *C3, CFB*, and the age-related maculopathy susceptibility 2/HtrA serine peptidase 1 (*ARMS2/HTRA1*)(Bergeron-Sawitzke, et al., 2009; Edwards, et al., 2005; Fritsche, et al., 2008; Hageman, et al., 2005; Haines, et al., 2005; Kanda, et al., 2007; Klein, et al., 2005; Maller, et al., 2007; Rivera, et al., 2005; Yates, et al., 2007); also reviewed in this volume (Dubielecka and Hoh). As AMD is a complex disease, genetic variation accounts for only a portion of risk; environmental influences also play an important role. The most consistently demonstrated factor conferring environmental risk is smoking (Chakravarthy, et al., 2007; de Jong, 2006).

Drusen, focal circular deposits typically located in the macula, are the most commonly identified clinical feature of early AMD. They vary in size and distribution but are usually symmetric between the two eyes. These deposits, along with pigment alterations in the RPE (Figure 2A), increase the risk for development of more advanced stages of AMD associated with visual loss: geographic atrophy (GA) and choroidal neovascularization (CNV) (Figure 2B). Geographic atrophy is the default end-stage of vision loss due to AMD when CNV does not develop. It is recommended that patients with high-risk features (i.e. several medium to large drusen, RPE changes, and or CNV in the fellow eye) take age-related eye disease study (AREDS)-formula vitamins to decrease the chance of CNV.(2001)

Geographic atrophy (GA) refers to a well-circumscribed area of RPE and photoreceptor cell loss in the macula associated with loss of retinal function that correlates clinically to dark spots (scotomas) in the vision. When involving the fovea, visual acuity declines depending on the size of the area affected. Visual loss from GA is indolent, but once present rates of GA progression occur up to 1.52 mm^2/yr to 3.02 mm^2/yr(Holz, et al., 2007; Lindblad, et al., 2009; Sunness, et al., 2007). There is currently no effective treatment for GA but several clinical trials are underway.(Meleth, et al., 2011)

In contrast to GA, CNV is associated with more acute vision change that often presents to the ophthalmologist with metamorphopsia, scotoma, and/or decreased vision. Clinical signs include subretinal hemorrhage, lipid exudate, fluid, and a grey-green lesion (Figure 2B). Classically, dye leakage on fluorescein angiography confirms the growth of the new vessels that occur in the subRPE or subretinal space (Figure 2C). Optical coherence tomography (OCT) characterizes the presence of subretinal fluid, intraretinal edema, RPE detachment, or subRPE/retinal tissue from CNV (Figure 2D,E). Intravitreal injections of anti-VEGF agents are first-line therapy for most CNVs presenting to the retina specialist and almost always stabilize, if not improve, visual acuity.(Brown, et al., 2006; Martin, et al., 2011; Rosenfeld, et al., 2006; Tufail, et al., 2010) Because of its reliability and reproducibility, OCT is used to monitor the CNV and often guides the clinician in the decision-making process for long-term treatment.(Fung, et al., 2007)

The pathologic correlates of BrM changes in AMD is discussed further below. The next sections review the anatomy and early-onset consequences of changes to BrM.

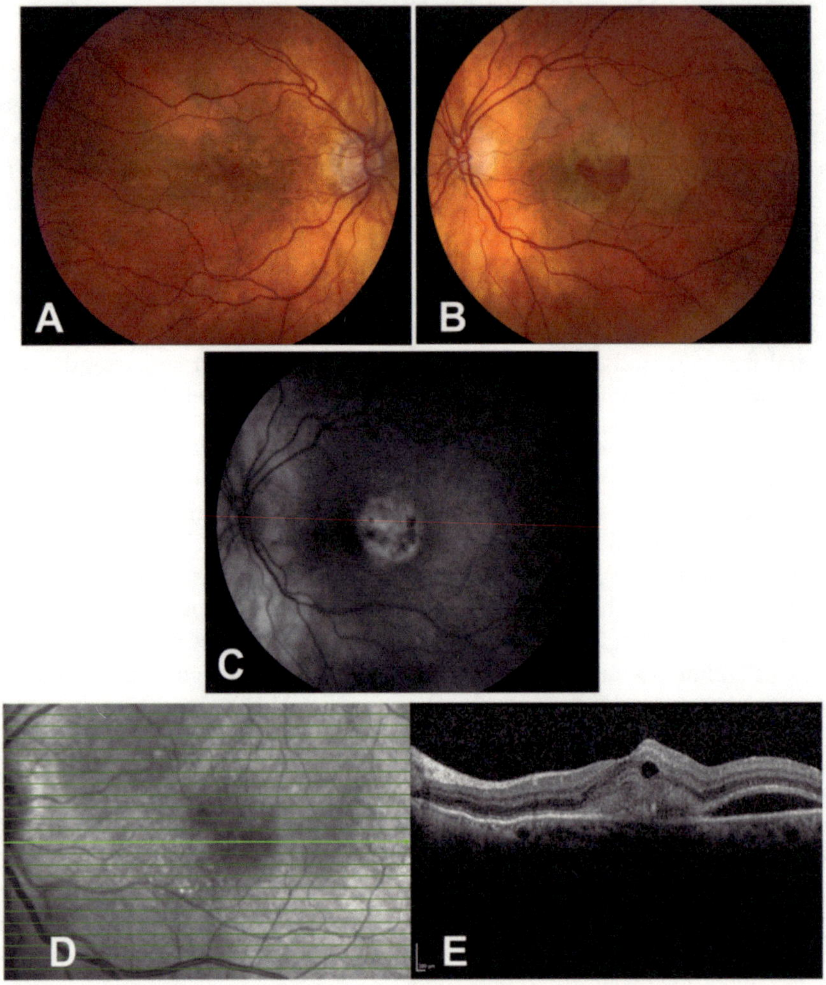

Fig. 2. 87 year-old female presented with a one week history of metamorphopsia in the left eye and visual acuity of 20/80. (A) Fundus photo of the right eye demonstrating non-neovascular AMD. There are two medium sized drusen temporal to the fovea with few small drusen in the superotemporal arcade. RPE changes are most prominent just superior and nasal to the fovea. Visual acuity in this eye was 20/25. (B) The macula of the left eye has a deep gray-green lesion with subretinal hemorrhage consistent with neovascular AMD. (C) Fluorescein angiogram confirms leakage of the CNV centered in the temporal macula but involving the fovea. (D) Infrared image signifying the horizontal scan position of the spectral-domain OCT image of the left eye (E) through the fovea shows subfoveal material, intraretinal edema with a cyst along the temporal edge of the fovea and temporal subretinal fluid.

3. Bruch's membrane: Anatomy

The name "membrane" referring to a refractive band on histological sections has a long history in ophthalmology, and includes the membranes of Descemet and Bowman, as well as the descriptive internal and external limiting membranes. Since the invention of the transmission electron microscope, the term membrane became applied to much smaller structures (plasma membrane, nuclear membrane and basement membrane).

BrM itself is a multilayered, extracellular matrix compartment that includes two basement membranes (more appropriately called basal laminae) at its inner and outer aspects (Figure 3). In addition to the basal laminae of the RPE and choriocapillaris, BrM possesses a central layer of elastin surrounded by two layers of collagen. In normal physiology, BrM appears to function as a robust barrier against neovascularization.

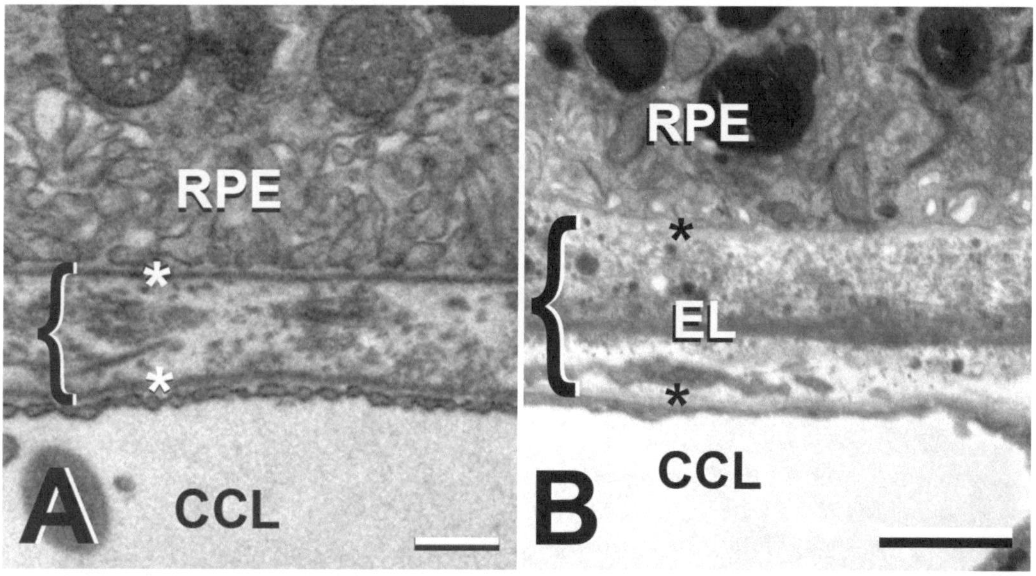

Fig. 3. Ultrastructure of murine (A) and human (B) Bruch's membrane. The basal laminae of the RPE (top) and choriocapillaris (bottom) are indicted by asterisks. Scale bar = 500nm (A) and 2μm (B). Labels indicate Bruch's membrane (bracket), the basal laminae (asterisks), the elastic lamina (EL), and RPE cell and the choriocapillaris lumen (CCL). Scale bar = 2μm. Left panel

Apart from its structural support function, BrM is also highly permeable to fluid and small molecules like oxygen and glucose. This quality likely derives from its sieve like structure appreciated by *en face* electron microscopy(Hogan, et al., 1971). Tracer studies in animals show that BrM (as well as the fenestrated choriocapillaris(Pino and Essner, 1981)) restrict the passage of even modestly sized proteins, while *in vitro* studies of excised human BrM can allow passage of molecules 200kDa or larger(Moore and Clover, 2001), recently discussed(Hussain, et al., 2010). Studies of hydraulic conductivity have invariably shown that the permeability of BrM decreases with increasing age (see below). RPE derived vascular endothelial growth factor also passes through BrM where it influences the structure and function of the choriocapillaris(Saint-Geniez, et al., 2009).

Thus, in normal physiology, there is ready transport of water, nutrients, metabolites, retinoids, and other molecules necessary to maintain retinal health and function in both directions.

4. Classes of Bruch's membrane molecules and their expression

BrM is bounded by two basal laminae (belonging to the RPE and choriocapillaris respectively), which contain the normal array of basal lamina constituents (collagen type IV, laminin, heparan sulfate proteoglycan, and entactin/nidogen)(Kunze, et al., 2010). The specific collagen IV isoforms present within human(Chen, et al., 2003) and mouse(Bai, et al., 2009) eyes differ between the RPE and choriocapillary basal laminae.

Between the two basal laminae, two layers of fibrillar collagens, consisting of types I and III collagen, surround a central core of elastin.(Das, et al., 1990; Nakaizumi, 1964; Nakaizumi, et al., 1964b). The elastic layer, when viewed en face, shows a crisscrossing pattern of web-like fibers with spaces to permit diffusion and allow deformability. This layer has received attention due to its alterations in pathology and biological activity of its degradation products (see below). Elastic fibers in other tissues bind transforming growth factor beta(Karonen, et al., 1997) and endostatin(Miosge, et al., 1999), and a similar association of anti-angiogenic proteins with BrM elastin may therefore "repel" vascular growth into the subretinal space when the elastic layer is intact and when the stimulus for neovascularization is not overwhelming. It is easy to envision that loss of elastin, by whatever mechanism, could lead to removal of a structural and biochemical barrier against choroidal neovascularization. Elastin may also protect against complement mediated injury through its association with the complement regulator decay accelerating factor/CD55(Werth, et al., 1988).

In addition, numerous other ECM molecules have been noted in BrM including the anti-angiogenic glycoprotein thrombospondin(Uno, et al., 2006) and sulfated proteoglycans(Call and Hollyfield, 1990; Clark, et al., 2011; Hewitt, et al., 1989). These molecules likely play important roles in hydration of the matrix, contribute to its barrier function(Prunte and Kain, 1995), the sequestration of growth factors, and may interact with the complement system (see below).

5. Genetic variations affect Bruch's membrane and cause early-onset macular dystrophies

The crucial role of ECM proteins in the macula is underscored by the fact that Bruch's membrane in this region is especially susceptible to mutations in genes with structural or regulatory roles in ECM metabolism. We briefly review a few of these familial macular diseases (i.e. macular dystrophies) with ECM abnormalities below.

Mutations in fibulins: Autosomal dominant radial drusen (also known as Malattia Leventinese, Doyne honeycomb retinal dystrophy, and dominant drusen) is a rare condition caused by a mutation (Arg345Trp) in the *EFEMP1* gene(Stone, et al., 1999). This gene encodes the ECM protein fibulin-3. Patients with this mutation typically have histologically unusual drusen like deposits that radiate from the macula, and may be complicated by neovascularization and/or atrophy(Michaelides, et al., 2006). The fibulin-3 protein is localized to some BrM deposits, as well as photoreceptor outer segments and retinal ganglion cells(Marmorstein, et al., 2002). Mice harboring one or more copies of the mutant *Efemp1* allele develop subRPE deposits resembling basal laminar deposit in human eyes(Fu, et al., 2007; Marmorstein, et al., 2007). In addition to the gene that encodes fibulin-3, mutations in the fibulin-5 gene, that also alter the secretion of the mutant protein(Lotery, et al., 2006), are associated with sporadic cases of AMD(Stone, et al., 2004). This protein regulates elastin assembly(Nakamura, et al., 2002; Yanagisawa, et al., 2002) and is localized to aging BrM and basal deposits in AMD eyes(Mullins, et al., 2007). Notably, fibulin-3 is a binding partner of tissue-inhibitor of metalloproteinase-3 (discussed more fully below)(Klenotic, et al., 2004), serving as a mechanistic link for neovascular membranes through TIMP-3 dysregulation in both conditions. Both fibulin-3 and fibulin-5 are widely expressed, and the reason for macular specific disease—and the pattern of drusen seen with EFEMP1 mutation—remains to be determined. Interestingly, the normal fibulin-5 protein inhibits angiogenesis, and its perturbation could remove a block to pathologic neovascularization(Albig and Schiemann, 2004).

Mutations in TIMP3: Another macular dystrophy, Sorsby fundus dystrophy, is caused by any of several mutations in the tissue inhibitor of metalloproteinases-3 gene, *TIMP3*(Weber, et al., 1994). Like fibulin-3, the TIMP3 protein is localized to BrM and is a major component of drusen(Fariss, et al., 1997). TIMP3 is capable of inhibiting VEGF-mediated angiogenesis by blocking the binding of VEGF to VEGF receptor-2 thereby inhibiting downstream signaling.(Qi, et al., 2003) Histopathology of eyes with Sorby fundus dystrophy shows dramatically thick, confluent deposits with a fragmented elastin layer of BrM (Capon et al., 1989; Chong et al., 2000). Bilateral subretinal neovascular membranes are frequently observed in patients with TIMP3 mutations by the fourth to fifth decades of life(Sivaprasad, et al., 2008; Sorsby and Mason, 1949). The most obvious explanation for grossly abnormal ECM deposits, as well as BrM breaks that permit neovasculrization, is that the TIMP-matrix metalloproteinase balance is disrupted, as TIMP3 substrates are metalloproteinases(Apte, et al., 1995). Interestingly, however, at least for one common TIMP3 mutation (Ser156Cys), the inhibition of MMP activity is not impaired compared to wild type TIMP3(Fogarasi, et al., 2008). Mouse models of SFD with dominant mutations have been generated and these animals show increased deposition of material at the level of BrM(Weber, et al., 2002).

Like the fibulins, TIMP3 is widely expressed(Apte, et al., 1994) and the reason for ocular specific disease is not clear, although it may relate to the unique relationship between the retina and choroidal vasculature. It is also notable that, in contrast to dominant mutations, mice that lack TIMP3 develop abnormal choroidal vasculature, and show loss of intercapillary pillars with large, sinusoidal vessels, indicating that TIMP3 normally functions in the development of the choroidal vasculature(Janssen, et al., 2008). Finally, it is notable that in a very large genome wide association study, an AMD susceptibility locus has been mapped to a region of chromosome 22 near the *TIMP3* gene(Chen, et al., 2011); the functional impact of the variants at this locus are yet to be explored.

Mutations in ABCC6: Whereas EFEMP1 and TIMP3 mutations have not as yet been associated with any pathology outside of the eye, mutations in *ABCC6* cause the systemic elastin disease, pseudoxanthoma elasticum (Bergen, et al., 2000; Le Saux, et al., 2000; Struk, et al., 2000).This disease affects elastic fibers in the skin and vasculature, in addition to BrM. The histopathologic phenotype shows breaks in BrM and elastin calcification and fragmentation(Hagedoorn, 1939). The process of elastin calcification probably makes the brittle BrM susceptible to the fissures referred to clinically as angioid streaks, through which choroidal blood vessels invade the retina.

Thus, genetic conditions that affect the biochemistry of BrM can lead to a phenotype similar to end stage AMD.

6. Bruch's membrane aging changes

BrM undergoes age-related alterations that include anatomical, functional and molecular changes. We briefly review these below.

Ultrastructural changes: Anatomical changes in aging human BrM have been documented extensively and will not be covered to any significant degree here (see for example.(Feeney-Burns and Ellersieck, 1985; Hogan and Alvarado, 1967; Hogan, et al., 1971) These changes include the accumulation of membranous debris on both sides of the elastic lamina(Feeney-Burns and Ellersieck, 1985), accumulation of focal drusen between the RPE basal lamina and inner collagenous layer of BrM(Sarks, et al., 1999), and accumulation of more confluent deposits. These deposits may occupy the same space as drusen and exhibit the appearance of membranous debris (termed basal linear deposits) or may develop between the RPE cell and its basal lamina and have an amorphous or banded structure with a periodicity consistent with that of type VI collagen (referred to as basal laminar deposits)(Curcio and Millican, 1999; Knupp, et al., 2002; Nakaizumi, et al., 1964a; Sarks, et al., 2007). Changes in the elastic lamina are in their own section below.

Functional changes: In addition to the structural alterations that occur in BrM during aging, the function of BrM as a conduit for the passage of material between the RPE and choriocapillaris becomes substantially reduced. Functional changes in aging have been measured primarily through the use of Ussing chambers in which flow of tracer molecules can be assessed. A significant decrease in hydraulic conductivity—a measure of the permeability of tissue—has been described in the aging BrM(Hussain, et al., 2002; Moore, et al., 1995; Starita, et al., 1996). Hydraulic conductivity drops exponentially with advancing age, with greater than 50% reduction occurring every 20 years of age(Starita, et al., 1996). Sequential ablation of different layers of BrM suggests that the major site of resistance that differs between young and old eyes is the inner collagenous layer(Starita, et al., 1997) which also accumulates substantial debris in the aging macula(Newsome, et al., 1987b).

One probable function of elastin in BrM and the choroid is to structurally support this crucial tissue through the approximately 100,000 cycles of the choroidal pulse each day. Notably, in addition to loss of transport facility across BrM with age, a decline in the elasticity (approximately 1% per year after age 21) has also been reported(Ugarte, et al., 2006).

7. Molecular changes in Bruch's membrane also occur during aging

Lipids: An increased lipid content has been demonstrated using a variety of histochemical(Pauleikhoff, et al., 1990) and biochemical(Sheraidah, et al., 1993) approaches. Lipid content of BrM varies regionally between macular and extramacular samples(Gulcan, et al., 1993; Holz, et al., 1994).

Photoreceptor cells are extremely enriched for some classes of lipids, including the omega-3 fatty acid docosahexaenoic acid (DHA). This molecule can be metabolized to the neuroprotective molecule NPD1(Bazan, 2005) or oxidized to form a reactive, proinflammatory, angiogenic mediator carboxyethylpyrrole (CEP)(Hollyfield, et al., 2008). At least in the case of CEP, which is deposited in BrM in AMD(Gu, et al., 2003), photoreceptor outer segments are the most likely source. The photoreceptor origin of BrM lipids has been advanced for other classes as well(Pauleikhoff, et al., 1994). Some classes of lipids, including esterified and unesterified cholesterol(Haimovici, et al., 2001; Rudolf and Curcio, 2009), are assembled into distinct lipoprotein complexes and secreted by the RPE(Li, et al., 2005; Malek, et al., 2003; Wang, et al., 2011; Wang, et al., 2009). The provenance of all classes of lipids that accumulate in aging BrM is not entirely resolved, however, as recently reviewed(Ebrahimi and Handa, 2011).

Membrane attack complex of complement: In addition to lipidic changes, activation of the complement system has received considerable attention, particularly in view of the compelling genetic evidence that polymorphisms in the complement inhibitor complement factor H (*CFH*) (in addition to other genes whose products regulate the complement system) (Bergeron-Sawitzke, et al., 2009; Edwards, et al., 2005; Fritsche, et al., 2008; Hageman, et al., 2005; Haines, et al., 2005; Kanda, et al., 2007; Klein, et al., 2005; Maller, et al., 2007; Rivera, et al., 2005; Yates, et al., 2007) is strongly associated with AMD (discussed above). Studies on the membrane attack complex of complement show that the majority of labeling is found in BrM and particularly around the choriocapillaris(Gerl, et al., 2002; Hageman, et al., 2005; Mullins, et al., 2011b; Seth, et al., 2008; Skeie, et al., 2010). In one study, this labeling was found to be statistically higher in aged ($\geq$69) as compared to young ($\leq$56) donors, indicating an increased complement load during aging(Seth, et al., 2008). The aberrant activation of the complement system may result in endothelial cell loss in the choriocapillaris(Mullins, et al., 2011b), increased VEGF synthesis by the RPE(Nozaki, et al., 2006), upregulated ICAM-1 RNA and protein by the choriocapillaris(Skeie, et al., 2010), and abnormal T cell activation(Liu, et al., 2011). The pathology that follows these challenges by the RPE and choroid are likely to worsen with aging. While there is generally not strong histological evidence that the membrane attack complex complement places a significant challenge to the RPE, it is noteworthy that expression of CD46 decreases in the pathogenesis of geographic atrophy(Vogt, et al., 2011). Since CD46 is a negative regulator of complement activity, playing a similar function at the cell surface that CFH plays in the extracellular space, even small or histochemically undetectable levels of complement could injure the RPE in this weakened state.

In addition to age, genotype of *CFH* appears to regulate the amount of membrane attack complex in the BrM/choriocapillaris. In a small study of genotyped eyes, we found that donors homozygous for the high risk allele (H at codon 402) had on average over 50% more membrane attack complex than age matched donors who were homozygous for the low risk allele(Mullins, et al., 2011a). Thus both genotype and age contribute to the deposition of potentially cytolytic membrane attack complexes in the aging choroid.

Extracellular matrix: ECM structural molecules also show age- and AMD-related changes. We will briefly review these changes, with special emphasis on elastin. Studies in mice show increased deposition of basal lamina proteins in BrM with age(Kunze, et al., 2010). While drusen themselves contain few classic extracellular matrix molecules(Hageman, et al., 1999;

Newsome, et al., 1987a) aging BrM may show increased type IV collagen that contributes to its thickening(Marshall, et al., 1994). Basal lamina constituents are also present in granular basal laminar deposit material(van der Schaft, et al., 1994). In eyes with early AMD, the abundance of thrombospondin has been shown to be decreased(Uno, et al., 2006)—in view of the role of this protein in suppressing angiogenesis, its reduction may create a permissive environment for neovascularization. The altered homeostasis of ECM observed in aging and AMD may be in part due to the age-dependent reduction in matrix metalloproteinase activity(Guo, et al., 1999) and in the available pool of MMPs(Kumar, et al., 2010) that has been observed in human eyes. Proteomic studies of combined BrM/choroid layers from human donor eyes further reveal increases in some matrix proteins (e.g., MMP3, collagen I) and decreases in other proteins (e.g., nidogen-2, fibulin-1) during the progression of AMD(Yuan, et al., 2010).

Other age-related changes include the accumulation of iron and advanced glycation endproducts in BrM. While outside the scope of this article, the reader is referred to several excellent articles and reviews(Glenn, et al., 2009; Handa, et al., 1999; He, et al., 2007; Wong, et al., 2007), including in the current volume (Kaji et al.).

Elastin metabolism in AMD: Elastin is a hydrophobic glycoprotein of approximately 72kDa. It has an unusual primary sequence in which about one third of its amino acid composition is comprised of glycine. Unlike fibrillar collagens, which also contain glycines at every third amino acid, elastin does not form into triple helices. Instead, elastin monomers (tropoelastin molecules) are assembled into cross-linked networks by enzymatic modification of lysine residues by lysyl oxidases (Figure 4). The resulting network of hydrophobic elastin polymers is responsible for the elastic recoil of arteries, and indeed participates in maintenance of diastolic blood pressure(Faury, 2001). Elastin is found in multiple tissues including skin, large blood vessels, and BrM of the eye.

Several studies suggest that abnormal elastin physiology is involved in the pathogenesis of AMD, and especially neovascular AMD. One of the first indications of widespread elastin changes came from studies linking dermatologic changes with neovascular AMD. Whereas elastotic degeneration of sun-exposed skin is a typical finding, Blumenkranz and colleagues reported histopathologic evidence of elastotic degeneration of sun-protected skin in patients with CNV(Blumenkranz, et al., 1986). Second, Spraul and Grossniklaus, in performing morphometric studies on a series of human donor eyes with neovascular AMD, noted that calcification and fragmentation of the elastic lamina was a frequent finding(Spraul and Grossniklaus, 1997; Spraul, et al., 1999) suggesting elastin breakdown within BrM as a cause or consequence of AMD pathology. Third, Chong et al. made similar findings at the ultrastructural scale, in which we observed a relative paucity of macular elastin and noted that eyes with neovascular AMD tended to have a thinner and more porous elastic lamina of BrM than controls(Chong, et al., 2005) The thinning of the elastic lamina is in contrast to the general "thickening" of BrM during aging (which is actually accumulation of debris rather than expansion of its matrix components)(Feeney-Burns and Ellersieck, 1985). Fourth, genetic variations in genes associated with elastin biology are associated with macular disease, including *ABCC6* and *FBLN5* (discussed above) and polymorphisms in the elastin gene (*ELN*) that have been described in association with polypoidal choroidal vasculopathy(Kondo, et al., 2008). Mice deficient for the elastin crosslinking protein LOXL1 show disrupted BrM elastin and increased severity of experimental neovascularization(Yu, et al., 2008). In addition, significantly elevated serum levels of elastin derived peptides (EDPs) have been found in the serum of CNV patients, with higher levels in CNV than in dry AMD, and higher levels in dry AMD than controls(Sivaprasad, et al., 2005). In this study, the authors noted that a sustained elevated level of EDPs could not be solely due to BrM degradation, and is instead likely to be due to systemic elastin abnormalities, consistent with those described by Blumenkranz et al. Finally, the breakdown products of elastin itself (elastin derived peptides) induce some angiogenic behaviors of choroidal endothelial cells(Skeie and Mullins, 2008)(Figure 4). Thus, the breakdown of elastin in BrM may simultaneously (a) remove a critical structural and chemical barrier to neovascularization and (b) actively induce the growth of pathologic blood vessels into the retina. Taken together, these studies provide strong support for the notion that abnormalities in elastin metabolism, both in ocular and extraocular tissues, are associated with the pathogenesis of neovascular AMD.

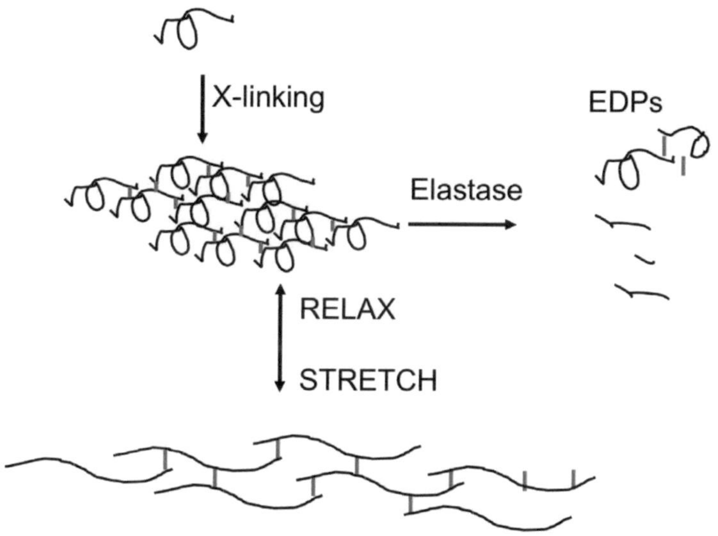

Fig. 4. Elastin monomers are crosslinked by lysyl oxidases into insoluble elastic networks that can repeatedly stretch and relax, essential for tissues like the choroid. Degradation of elastin by matrix metalloproteinases/elastases leads to the loss of integrity of the elastin network and the release of biologically active elastin derived peptides (EDPs) which can promote neovascularization. Adapted from Alberts et al., 2008

8. Consequences of ECM abnormalities

The development of either excessive material in Bruch's membrane or erosion of Bruch's membrane may have serious consequences whether congenital or age-related. Some events, such as membrane attack complex deposition, may lead to choroidal endothelial cell loss(Mullins, et al., 2011b) and place ischemic stress on the oxygen hungry photoreceptor cells. Vascular loss may exacerbate the development of drusen, as the ability of the choroid to remove debris is further compromised; in this context it is notable that drusen form preferentially in eyes and in regions of eyes depleted of capillary lumens(Lengyel, et al., 2004; Mullins, et al., 2011b; Sarks, et al., 1999)(Figure 5).

In addition, the interposition of lipid rich material between the retina and its vascular supply, even with a healthy choriocapillaris, can compromise the normal trafficking between these tissues(Curcio, et al., 2010). The accumulation of lipids in BrM (consistent with the reduced ability to move water through the aging BrM--discussed above) has led some investigators to the attractive hypothesis that normal pumping of fluid through the RPE, combined with a nonpermeable BrM, could cause pigment epithelial detachments(Pauleikhoff, et al., 1990). Moreover, the molecules that accumulate in aging Bruch's membrane—including CEP-modified proteins and advanced glycation endproducts—may themselves be toxic, pro-inflammatory, and pro-angiogenic(Ebrahem, et al., 2006; Glenn, et al., 2009; Ma, et al., 2007).

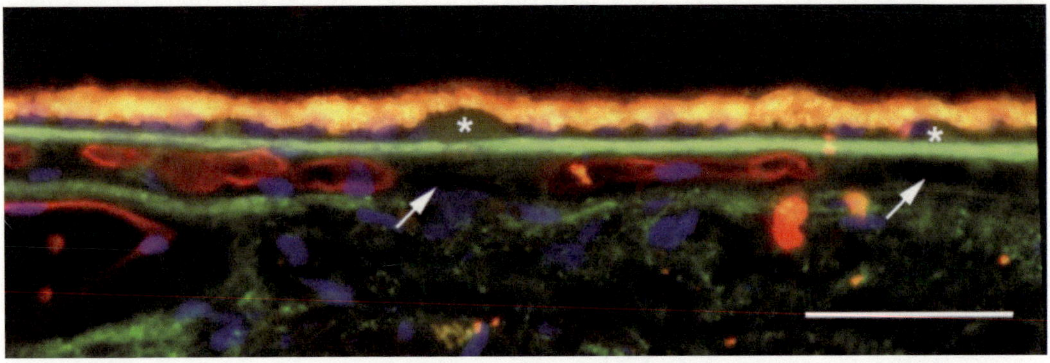

Fig. 5. In human eyes, formation of deposits in the ECM, such as drusen (asterisks) occur preferentially in areas of choroid without capillary lumens, suggesting that the clearance of extracellular debris by the choriocapillaris may be preventative against drusen formation. Arrows, indicate "ghost" capillary vessels. Green immunoreactivity, anti-elastin; red labeling, UEA-I (a vascular marker); orange autofluorescence in the RPE is due to lipofuscin; blue fluorescence is due to a nuclear counterstain. Scale bar = 50μm.

While atrophic changes in AMD may be most easily attributed to excess material deposited in BrM, at some point in the development of neovascular AMD the structure of BrM becomes compromised. That defects in BrM permit angiogenesis into the retina is clear from both genetic diseases in which large cracks appear in the calcified BrM (i.e., pseudoxanthoma elasticum, discussed above) as well as animal models of CNV in which rupture of BrM is sufficient to induce neovascular AMD-like pathology(Ryan, 1980). The molecular changes in early and late AMD that include loss of anti-angiogenic proteins(Bhutto, et al., 2008) and calcification and fragmentation of BrM elastin(Chong, et al., 2005; Spraul and Grossniklaus, 1997) show that breakdown of BrM elastin occurs during the progression of AMD and provides opportunities for neovascular events. These may be especially problematic since, as noted above, fragments of elastin are sufficient to promote the migration of choroidal EC(Skeie and Mullins, 2008).

9. Potential ECM mediated therapeutics

In view of the many roles of the extracellular matrix in macular health and disease, several potential areas exist for ameliorating the pathogenesis of AMD. Current early-phase clinical trials for non-neovascular AMD directed at extracellular matrix dysfunction are limited to the complement system and summarized in recent reviews. (Yehoshua et al., 2011; Meleth et al., 2011). Ameliorating AMD by modulating other changes that occur in the ECM remains to be explored. This discussion is not intended to be inclusive but to highlight a few areas in which a better understanding of ECM pathobiology of AMD may be helpful.

As discussed above, aberrant elastin metabolism and perhaps signaling are associated with AMD, especially neovascular AMD. Systemic elastin abnormalities occur in AMD, and the local changes in BrM likely at once both remove a barrier to neovascualization and promote growth of new blood vessels from the choroid. A better understanding of the molecules involved in this signaling may provide additional targets of neovascular AMD to accompany anti-VEGF drugs in some cases. This is vital in the cases of neovascular AMD that do not fully respond to anti-VEGF therapy or that develop 'tachyphylaxis' to anti-VEGF drugs.(Gasperini, et al., 2011; Schaal, et al., 2008)

In addition to the pro-angiogenic effects of the elastin components of BrM, other components of BrM are often anti-angiogenic. This has been noted for several molecules including thrombospondin, as discussed above, endostatin(Marneros, et al., 2007; Mori, et al., 2001) a fragment of collagen type XVIII, and fragments of collagen IV(Lima, et al., 2006). Enhancing the expression of these anti-angiogenic molecules through gene delivery or systemic administration shows promise as another tool against neovascular AMD, especially since decreased expression of these inhibitors occurs during pathogenesis(Bhutto, et al., 2008). A caution for these studies is that increases in BrM collagen IV have been linked to thickening of BrM and the development of subRPE deposits, as noted above.

Apart from interfering with signaling events in the aging macula, it may also be possible and necessary to reconstruct BrM in some cases. With the promise of stem cell mediated therapies for AMD and other maculopathies, having a substrate on which transplanted cells can attach and perform their normal physiologic functions is a considerable challenge. Replacing defective RPE cells has been proposed as a mechanism to ameliorate both neovascular(Tezel, et al., 2007) and atrophic(Du, et al., 2011) AMD. Elegant experiments at delivering RPE cells from a variety of potential sources(da Cruz, et al., 2007) indicate that modifying BrM to accept transplanted cells(Gullapalli, et al., 2004) and/or delivering cells on degradable scaffolds(Thomson, et al., 2010) will be necessary for successful transplantation. Advances in combining materials science with cell biology will be essential for the next generation of treatments for AMD.

In summary, the relationship between the photoreceptor cells/RPE and the vascular supply is complex, and the intervening layer of extracellular matrix is especially susceptible to genetic and age-related changes that impair its function. A better understanding of this complex boundary will provide novel opportunities for therapy.

10. Abbreviations

RPE, retinal pigment epithelium; EC, endothelial cell; BrM, Bruch's membrane; ECM, extracellular matrix; AMD, age-related macular degeneration; GA, geographic atrophy; CNV, choroidal neovascularization; OCT, optical coherence tomography; VEGF, vascular endothelial growth factor

11. Acknowledgments

The authors wish to thank Ms. Aditi Khanna for technical assistance. Supported by NEI-017451, the Macula Vision Research Foundation, and the Hansjoerg EJW, MD, PhD Professorship in Best Disease Research.

12. References

2001. A randomized, placebo-controlled, clinical trial of high-dose supplementation with vitamins C and E, beta carotene, and zinc for age-related macular degeneration and vision loss. Arch Ophthalmol 119:1417-36.

Alberts B, Johnson A, Lewis J, Raff M, Roberts K, Walter P, 2002. NYGS. 2008. Molecular Biology of the Cell. 4th edition. New York: Garland Science.

Albig AR, Schiemann WP. 2004. Fibulin-5 antagonizes vascular endothelial growth factor (VEGF) signaling and angiogenic sprouting by endothelial cells. DNA Cell Biol 23(6):367-79.

Alm A, Bill A. 1973. Ocular and optic nerve blood flow at normal and increased intraocular pressures in monkeys (Macaca irus): a study with radioactively labelled microspheres including flow determinations in brain and some other tissues. Exp Eye Res 15(1):15-29.

Apte SS, Hayashi K, Seldin MF, Mattei MG, Hayashi M, Olsen BR. 1994. Gene encoding a novel murine tissue inhibitor of metalloproteinases (TIMP), TIMP-3, is expressed in developing mouse epithelia, cartilage, and muscle, and is located on mouse chromosome 10. Developmental Dynamics 200(3):177-97.

Apte SS, Olsen BR, Murphy G. 1995. The gene structure of tissue inhibitor of metalloproteinases (TIMP)-3 and its inhibitory activities define the distinct TIMP gene family. J Biol Chem 270(24):14313-8.

Bai X, Dilworth DJ, Weng YC, Gould DB. 2009. Developmental distribution of collagen IV isoforms and relevance to ocular diseases. Matrix Biol 28(4):194-201.

Bazan NG. 2005. Neuroprotectin D1 (NPD1): a DHA-derived mediator that protects brain and retina against cell injury-induced oxidative stress. Brain Pathol 15(2):159-66.

Bergen AA, Plomp AS, Schuurman EJ, Terry S, Breuning M, Dauwerse H, Swart J, Kool M, van Soest S, Baas F and others. 2000. Mutations in ABCC6 cause pseudoxanthoma elasticum. Nat Genet 25(2):228-31.

Bergeron-Sawitzke J, Gold B, Olsh A, Schlotterbeck S, Lemon K, Visvanathan K, Allikmets R, Dean M. 2009. Multilocus analysis of age-related macular degeneration. Eur J Hum Genet 17(9):1190-9.

Bhutto IA, Uno K, Merges C, Zhang L, McLeod DS, Lutty GA. 2008. Reduction of endogenous angiogenesis inhibitors in Bruch's membrane of the submacular region in eyes with age-related macular degeneration. Arch Ophthalmol 126(5):670-8.

Birol G, Wang S, Budzynski E, Wangsa-Wirawan ND, Linsenmeier RA. 2007. Oxygen distribution and consumption in the macaque retina. Am J Physiol Heart Circ Physiol 293(3):H1696-704.

Blumenkranz M, Russell S, Robey M, Kott-Blumenkranz R, Penneys N. 1986. Risk factors in age-related maculopathy complicated by choroidal neovascularization. Ophthalmology 93:552-558.

Brown DM, Kaiser PK, Michels M, Soubrane G, Heier JS, Kim RY, Sy JP, Schneider S. 2006. Ranibizumab versus verteporfin for neovascular age-related macular degeneration. N Engl J Med 355(14):1432-44.

Call TW, Hollyfield JG. 1990. Sulfated proteoglycans in Bruch's membrane of the human eye: localization and characterization using cupromeronic blue. Exp Eye Res 51(4):451-62.

Chakravarthy U, Augood C, Bentham GC, de Jong PT, Rahu M, Seland J, Soubrane G, Tomazzoli L, Topouzis F, Vingerling JR and others. 2007. Cigarette smoking and age-related macular degeneration in the EUREYE Study. Ophthalmology 114(6):1157-63.

Chen L, Miyamura N, Ninomiya Y, Handa JT. 2003. Distribution of the collagen IV isoforms in human Bruch's membrane. Br J Ophthalmol 87(2):212-5.

Chen W, Stambolian D, Edwards AO, Branham KE, Othman M, Jakobsdottir J, Tosakulwong N, Pericak-Vance MA, Campochiaro PA, Klein ML and others. 2011. Genetic variants near TIMP3 and high-density lipoprotein-associated loci influence susceptibility to age-related macular degeneration. Proc Natl Acad Sci U S A 107(16):7401-6.

Chong N, Keonin J, Luthert P, Frennesson C, Weingeist D, Wolfe R, Mullins R, Hageman G. 2005. Decreased thickness and integrity of the macular elastic layer of Bruch's membrane correspond to distribution of lesions associated with AMD. Am J Pathol 166(1):241-51.

Clark SJ, Keenan TD, Fielder HL, Collinson LJ, Holley RJ, Merry CL, van Kuppevelt TH, Day AJ, Bishop PN. 2011. Mapping the differential distribution of glycosaminoglycans in the adult human retina, choroid, and sclera. Invest Ophthalmol Vis Sci 52(9):6511-21.

Curcio C, Millican C. 1999. Basal linear deposit and large drusen are specific for early age-related maculopathy. Archives of Ophthalmology 117:329-39.

Curcio CA, Johnson M, Huang JD, Rudolf M. 2010. Apolipoprotein B-containing lipoproteins in retinal aging and age-related macular degeneration. J Lipid Res 51(3):451-67.

da Cruz L, Chen FK, Ahmado A, Greenwood J, Coffey P. 2007. RPE transplantation and its role in retinal disease. Prog Retin Eye Res 26(6):598-635.

Das A, Frank RN, Zhang NL, Turczyn TJ. 1990. Ultrastructural localization of extracellular matrix components in human retinal vessels and Bruch's membrane. Arch Ophthalmol 108(3):421-9.

Dawson D, Volpert O, Gillis P, Crawford S, Xu H, Benedict W, Bouck N. 1999. Pigment epithelium-derived factor: a potent inhibitor of angiogenesis. Science 285:245-8.

de Jong PT. 2006. Age-related macular degeneration. N Engl J Med 355(14):1474-85.

Du H, Lim SL, Grob S, Zhang K. 2011. Induced pluripotent stem cell therapies for geographic atrophy of age-related macular degeneration. Semin Ophthalmol 26(3):216-24.

Ebrahem Q, Renganathan K, Sears J, Vasanji A, Gu X, Lu L, Salomon RG, Crabb JW, Anand-Apte B. 2006. Carboxyethylpyrrole oxidative protein modifications stimulate neovascularization: Implications for age-related macular degeneration. Proc Natl Acad Sci U S A 103(36):13480-4.

Ebrahimi KB, Handa JT. 2011. Lipids, lipoproteins, and age-related macular degeneration. J Lipids 2011:802059.

Edwards A, Ritter R, Abel K, Manning A, Panhuysen C, Farrer L. 2005. Complement factor H polymorphism and age-related macular degeneration. Science 308:421-4.

Fariss RN, Apte SS, Olsen BR, Iwata K, Milam AH. 1997. Tissue inhibitor of metalloproteinases-3 is a component of Bruch's membrane of the eye. American Journal of Pathology 150(1):323-8.

Faury G. 2001. Function-structure relationship of elastic arteries in evolution: from microfibrils to elastin and elastic fibres. Pathol Biol (Paris) 49:310-25.

Feeney-Burns L, Ellersieck M. 1985. Age-related changes in the ultrastructure of Bruch's membrane. American Journal of Ophthalmology 100:686-697.

Fogarasi M, Janssen A, Weber BH, Stohr H. 2008. Molecular dissection of TIMP3 mutation S156C associated with Sorsby fundus dystrophy. Matrix Biol 27(5):381-92.

Fritsche LG, Loenhardt T, Janssen A, Fisher SA, Rivera A, Keilhauer CN, Weber BH. 2008. Age-related macular degeneration is associated with an unstable ARMS2 (LOC387715) mRNA. Nat Genet 40(7):892-6.

Fu L, Garland D, Yang Z, Shukla D, Rajendran A, Pearson E, Stone E, Zhang K, Pierce E. 2007. The R345W mutation in EFEMP1 is pathogenic and causes AMD-like deposits in mice. Hum Mol Genet 15:2411-22.

Fung AE, Lalwani GA, Rosenfeld PJ, Dubovy SR, Michels S, Feuer WJ, Puliafito CA, Davis JL, Flynn HW, Jr., Esquiabro M. 2007. An optical coherence tomography-guided, variable dosing regimen with intravitreal ranibizumab (Lucentis) for neovascular age-related macular degeneration. Am J Ophthalmol 143(4):566-83.

Gasperini JL, Fawzi AA, Khondkaryan A, Lam L, Chong LP, Eliott D, Walsh AC, Hwang J, Sadda SR. 2011. Bevacizumab and ranibizumab tachyphylaxis in the treatment of choroidal neovascularisation. Br J Ophthalmol.

Gerl V, Bohl J, Pitz S, Stoffelns B, Pfeiffer N, Bhakdi S. 2002. Extensive deposits of complement C3d and C5b-9 in the choriocapillaris of eyes of patients with diabetic retinopathy. Invest Ophthalmol Vis Sci 43:1104-1108.

Glenn JV, Mahaffy H, Wu K, Smith G, Nagai R, Simpson DA, Boulton ME, Stitt AW. 2009. Advanced glycation end product (AGE) accumulation on Bruch's membrane: links to age-related RPE dysfunction. Invest Ophthalmol Vis Sci 50(1):441-51.

Gu X, Meer SG, Miyagi M, Rayborn ME, Hollyfield JG, Crabb JW, Salomon RG. 2003. Carboxyethylpyrrole protein adducts and autoantibodies, biomarkers for age-related macular degeneration. J Biol Chem 278(43):42027-35.

Gulcan HG, Alvarez RA, Maude MB, Anderson RE. 1993. Lipids of human retina, retinal pigment epithelium, and Bruch's membrane/choroid: comparison of macular and peripheral regions. Invest Ophthalmol Vis Sci 34(11):3187-93.

Gullapalli VK, Sugino IK, Van Patten Y, Shah S, Zarbin MA. 2004. Retinal pigment epithelium resurfacing of aged submacular human Bruch's membrane. Trans Am Ophthalmol Soc 102:123-37; discussion 137-8.

Guo L, Hussain A, Limb G, Marshall J. 1999. Age-dependent variation in metalloproteinase activity of isolated human Bruch's membrane and choroid. Invest Ophthalmol Vis Sci 40:2676-82.

Hagedoorn A. 1939. Report of a case of the syndrome of Gronblad and Strandberg (angioid streaks and pseudoxanthoma elasticum). Arch Ophthalmol 21:746-74.

Hageman G, Anderson D, Johnson L, Hancox L, Taiber A, Hardisty L, Hageman J, Stockman H, Borchardt J, Gehrs K and others. 2005. A common haplotype in the complement regulatory gene factor H (HF1/CFH) predisposes individuals to age-related macular degeneration. Proc Natl Acad Sci U S A 102:7227-32.

Hageman G, Mullins R, Russell S, Johnson L, Anderson D. 1999. Vitronectin is a constituent of ocular drusen and the vitronectin gene is expressed in human retinal pigmented epithelial cells. FASEB Journal 13(3):477-84.

Haimovici R, Gantz DL, Rumelt S, Freddo TF, Small DM. 2001. The lipid composition of drusen, Bruch's membrane, and sclera by hot stage polarizing light microscopy. Invest Ophthalmol Vis Sci 42(7):1592-9.

Haines J, Hauser M, Schmidt S, Scott W, Olson L, Gallins P, Spencer K, Kwan S, Noureddine M, Gilbert J and others. 2005. Complement factor H variant increases the risk of age-related macular degeneration. Science 308:419-21.

Handa JT, Verzijl N, Matsunaga H, Aotaki-Keen A, Lutty GA, te Koppele JM, Miyata T, Hjelmeland LM. 1999. Increase in the advanced glycation end product pentosidine in Bruch's membrane with age. Invest Ophthalmol Vis Sci 40(3):775-9.

He X, Hahn P, Iacovelli J, Wong R, King C, Bhisitkul R, Massaro-Giordano M, Dunaief JL. 2007. Iron homeostasis and toxicity in retinal degeneration. Prog Retin Eye Res 26(6):649-73.

Hewitt A, Nakazawa K, Newsome D. 1989. Analysis of newly synthesized Bruch's membrane proteoglycans. Investigative Ophthalmology & Visual Science 30(3):478-86.

Hogan M, Alvarado J. 1967. Studies on the human macula. Aging changes in Bruch's membrane. Archives of Ophthalmology 77:410-420.

Hogan M, Alvarado J, Weddell J. 1971. Histology of the Human Eye. Philadelphia.: Saunders Company.

Hollyfield JG, Bonilha VL, Rayborn ME, Yang X, Shadrach KG, Lu L, Ufret RL, Salomon RG, Perez VL. 2008. Oxidative damage-induced inflammation initiates age-related macular degeneration. Nat Med 14(2):194-8.

Holz F, Sheraiadah G, Pauleikhoff D, Marshall J, Bird A. 1994. Analysis of lipid deposits extracted from human macular and peripheral Bruch's membrane. Archives of Ophthalmology 112:402-406.

Holz FG, Bindewald-Wittich A, Fleckenstein M, Dreyhaupt J, Scholl HP, Schmitz-Valckenberg S. 2007. Progression of geographic atrophy and impact of fundus autofluorescence patterns in age-related macular degeneration. Am J Ophthalmol 143(3):463-72.

Hussain A, Rowe L, Marshall J. 2002. Age-related alterations in the diffusional transport of amino acids across the human Bruch's-choroid complex. Journal of the Optical Society of America 19:166-72.

Hussain AA, Starita C, Hodgetts A, Marshall J. 2010. Macromolecular diffusion characteristics of ageing human Bruch's membrane: implications for age-related macular degeneration (AMD). Exp Eye Res 90(6):703-10.

Janssen A, Hoellenriegel J, Fogarasi M, Schrewe H, Seeliger M, Tamm E, Ohlmann A, May CA, Weber BH, Stohr H. 2008. Abnormal vessel formation in the choroid of mice lacking tissue inhibitor of metalloprotease-3. Invest Ophthalmol Vis Sci 49(7):2812-22.

Kanda A, Chen W, Othman M, Branham KE, Brooks M, Khanna R, He S, Lyons R, Abecasis GR, Swaroop A. 2007. A variant of mitochondrial protein LOC387715/ARMS2, not HTRA1, is strongly associated with age-related macular degeneration. Proc Natl Acad Sci U S A 104(41):16227-32.

Karonen T, Jeskanen L, Keski-Oja J. 1997. Transforming growth factor beta 1 and its latent form binding protein-1 associate with elastic fibres in human dermis: accumulation in actinic damage and absence in anetoderma. Br J Dermatol 137:51-8.

Klein R, Klein B, Linton K. 1992. Prevalence of age-related maculopathy. The Beaver Dam Eye Study. Ophthalmology 99:933-43.

Klein R, Zeiss C, Chew E, Tsai J, Sackler R, Haynes C, Henning A, Sangiovanni J, Mane S, Mayne S and others. 2005. Complement factor H polymorphism in age-related macular degeneration. Science 308:385-9.

Klenotic PA, Munier FL, Marmorstein LY, Anand-Apte B. 2004. Tissue inhibitor of metalloproteinases-3 (TIMP-3) is a binding partner of epithelial growth factor-containing fibulin-like extracellular matrix protein 1 (EFEMP1). Implications for macular degenerations. J Biol Chem 279(29):30469-73.

Knupp C, Amin S, Munro P, Luthert P, Squire J. 2002. Collagen VI assemblies in age-related macular degeneration. J Struct Biol 139:181-9.

Kondo N, Honda S, Ishibashi K, Tsukahara Y, Negi A. 2008. Elastin gene polymorphisms in neovascular age-related macular degeneration and polypoidal choroidal vasculopathy. Invest Ophthalmol Vis Sci 49(3):1101-5.

Kumar A, El-Osta A, Hussain AA, Marshall J. 2010. Increased sequestration of matrix metalloproteinases in ageing human Bruch's membrane: implications for ECM turnover. Invest Ophthalmol Vis Sci 51(5):2664-70.

Kunze A, Abari E, Semkova I, Paulsson M, Hartmann U. 2010. Deposition of nidogens and other basement membrane proteins in the young and aging mouse retina. Ophthalmic Res 43(2):108-12.

Le Saux O, Urban Z, Tschuch C, Csiszar K, Bacchelli B, Quaglino D, Pasquali-Ronchetti I, Pope FM, Richards A, Terry S and others. 2000. Mutations in a gene encoding an ABC transporter cause pseudoxanthoma elasticum. Nat Genet 25(2):223-7.

Lengyel I, Tufail A, Hosaini HA, Luthert P, Bird AC, Jeffery G. 2004. Association of drusen deposition with choroidal intercapillary pillars in the aging human eye. Invest Ophthalmol Vis Sci 45(9):2886-92.

Li CM, Chung BH, Presley JB, Malek G, Zhang X, Dashti N, Li L, Chen J, Bradley K, Kruth HS and others. 2005. Lipoprotein-like particles and cholesteryl esters in human Bruch's membrane: initial characterization. Invest Ophthalmol Vis Sci 46(7):2576-86.

Lima ESR, Kachi S, Akiyama H, Shen J, Aslam S, Yuan Gong Y, Khu NH, Hatara MC, Boutaud A, Peterson R and others. 2006. Recombinant non-collagenous domain of alpha2(IV) collagen causes involution of choroidal neovascularization by inducing apoptosis. J Cell Physiol 208(1):161-6.

Lindblad AS, Lloyd PC, Clemons TE, Gensler GR, Ferris FL, 3rd, Klein ML, Armstrong JR. 2009. Change in area of geographic atrophy in the Age-Related Eye Disease Study: AREDS report number 26. Arch Ophthalmol 127(9):1168-74.

Liu B, Wei L, Meyerle C, Tuo J, Sen HN, Li Z, Chakrabarty S, Agron E, Chan CC, Klein ML and others. 2011. Complement component C5a Promotes Expression of IL-22 and IL-17 from Human T cells and its Implication in Age-related Macular Degeneration. J Transl Med 9:111.

Lotery AJ, Baas D, Ridley C, Jones RP, Klaver CC, Stone E, Nakamura T, Luff A, Griffiths H, Wang T and others. 2006. Reduced secretion of fibulin 5 in age-related macular degeneration and cutis laxa. Hum Mutat 27(6):568-74.

Ma W, Lee S, Guo J, Qu W, Hudson B, Schmidt A, Barile G. 2007. RAGE ligand upregulation of VEGF secretion in ARPE-19 cells. Invest Ophthalmol Vis Sci 48:1355-61.

Magie D. 1921. Historia Augusta. Loeb Classical Library.

Malek G, Li CM, Guidry C, Medeiros NE, Curcio CA. 2003. Apolipoprotein B in cholesterol-containing drusen and basal deposits of human eyes with age-related maculopathy. Am J Pathol 162(2):413-25.

Maller JB, Fagerness JA, Reynolds RC, Neale BM, Daly MJ, Seddon JM. 2007. Variation in complement factor 3 is associated with risk of age-related macular degeneration. Nat Genet 39(10):1200-1.

Marmorstein L, Munier F, Arsenijevic Y, Schorderet D, McLaughlin P, Chung D, Traboulsi E, Marmorstein A. 2002. Aberrant accumulation of EFEMP1 underlies drusen formation in Malattia Leventinese and age-related macular degeneration. Proc Natl Acad Sci U S A 99:13067-13072.

Marmorstein LY, McLaughlin PJ, Peachey NS, Sasaki T, Marmorstein AD. 2007. Formation and progression of sub-retinal pigment epithelium deposits in Efemp1 mutation knock-in mice: a model for the early pathogenic course of macular degeneration. Hum Mol Genet 16(20):2423-32.

Marneros AG, She H, Zambarakji H, Hashizume H, Connolly EJ, Kim I, Gragoudas ES, Miller JW, Olsen BR. 2007. Endogenous endostatin inhibits choroidal neovascularization. FASEB J 21(14):3809-18.

Marshall GE, Konstas AG, Reid GG, Edwards JG, Lee WR. 1994. Collagens in the aged human macula. Graefes Arch Clin Exp Ophthalmol 232(3):133-40.

Martin DF, Maguire MG, Ying GS, Grunwald JE, Fine SL, Jaffe GJ. 2011. Ranibizumab and bevacizumab for neovascular age-related macular degeneration. N Engl J Med 364(20):1897-908.

Meleth AD, Wong WT, Chew EY. 2011. Treatment for atrophic macular degeneration. Curr Opin Ophthalmol 22(3):190-3.

Michaelides M, Jenkins SA, Brantley MA, Jr., Andrews RM, Waseem N, Luong V, Gregory-Evans K, Bhattacharya SS, Fitzke FW, Webster AR. 2006. Maculopathy due to the R345W substitution in fibulin-3: distinct clinical features, disease variability, and extent of retinal dysfunction. Invest Ophthalmol Vis Sci 47(7):3085-97.

Miosge N, Sasaki T, Timpl R. 1999. Angiogenesis inhibitor endostatin is a distinct component of elastic fibers in vessel walls. The FASEB Journal 13:1743-50.

Mitchell P, Smith W, Attebo K, Wang J. 1995. Prevalence of age-related maculopathy in Australia. The Blue Mountains Eye Study. Ophthalmology 102:1450-60.

Moore D, Clover G. 2001. The effect of age on the macromolecuar permeability of human Bruch's membrane. Invest Ophthalmol Vis Sci 42:2970-5.

Moore D, Hussain A, Marshall J. 1995. Age-related variation in the hydraulic conductivity of Bruch's membrane. Invest Ophthalmol Vis Sci 36:1290-1297.

Mori K, Ando A, Gehlbach P, Nesbitt D, Takahashi K, Goldsteen D, Penn M, Chen CT, Melia M, Phipps S and others. 2001. Inhibition of choroidal neovascularization by intravenous injection of adenoviral vectors expressing secretable endostatin. Am J Pathol 159(1):313-20.

Mullins RF, Dewald AD, Streb LM, Wang K, Kuehn MH, Stone EM. 2011a. Elevated membrane attack complex in human choroid with high risk complement factor H genotypes. Exp Eye Res.

Mullins RF, Johnson MN, Faidley EA, Skeie JM, Huang J. 2011b. Choriocapillaris vascular dropout related to density of drusen in human eyes with early age-related macular degeneration. Invest Ophthalmol Vis Sci 52(3):1606-12.

Mullins RF, Olvera MA, Clark AF, Stone EM. 2007. Fibulin-5 distribution in human eyes: relevance to age-related macular degeneration. Exp Eye Res 84(2):378-80.

Nakaizumi Y. 1964. The Ultrastructure of Bruch's Membrane. I. Human, Monkey, Rabbit, Guinea Pig, and Rat Eyes. Arch Ophthalmol 72:380-7.

Nakaizumi Y, Hogan M, Feeney L. 1964a. The ultrastructure of Bruch's membrane. III. The macular region of the human eye. Archives of Ophthalmology 72:395-.

Nakaizumi Y, Hogan MJ, Feeney L. 1964b. The Ultrastructure of Bruch's Membrane. 3. The Macular Area of the Human Eye. Arch Ophthalmol 72:395-400.

Nakamura T, Lozano P, Ikeda Y, Iwanaga Y, Hinek A, Minamisawa S, Cheng C, Kobuke K, Dalton N, Takada Y and others. 2002. Fibulin-5/DANCE is essential for elastogenesis in vivo. Nature 415:171-5.

Newsome D, Hewitt A, Huh W, Robey P, Hassell J. 1987a. Detection of specific extracellular matrix molecules in drusen, Bruch's membrane, and ciliary body. American Journal of Ophthalmology 104:373-381.

Newsome D, Huh W, Green W. 1987b. Bruch's membrane age-related changes vary by region. Current Eye Research 6:1211-1221.

Nozaki M, Raisler BJ, Sakurai E, Sarma JV, Barnum SR, Lambris JD, Chen Y, Zhang K, Ambati BK, Baffi JZ and others. 2006. Drusen complement components C3a and C5a promote choroidal neovascularization. Proc Natl Acad Sci U S A.

Ohno-Matsui K, Morita I, Tombran-Tink J, Mrazek D, Onodera M, Uetama T, Hayano M, Murota SI, Mochizuki M. 2001. Novel mechanism for age-related macular

degeneration: an equilibrium shift between the angiogenesis factors VEGF and PEDF. J Cell Physiol 189(3):323-33.
Pauleikhoff D, Harper C, Marshall J, Bird A. 1990. Aging changes in Bruch's membrane. A histochemical and morphologic study. Ophthalmology 97:171-178.
Pauleikhoff D, Sheraidah G, Marshall J, Bird A, Wessing A. 1994. Biochemical and histochemical analysis of age related lipid deposits in Bruch's membrane. Ophthalmologe 91(6):730-4.
Pino RM, Essner E. 1981. Permeability of rat choriocapillaris to hemeproteins. Restriction of tracers by a fenestrated endothelium. J Histochem Cytochem 29(2):281-90.
Prunte C, Kain HL. 1995. Enzymatic digestion increases permeability of the outer blood-retinal barrier for high-molecular-weight substances. Graefes Arch Clin Exp Ophthalmol 233(2):101-11.
Qi JH, Ebrahem Q, Moore N, Murphy G, Claesson-Welsh L, Bond M, Baker A, Anand-Apte B. 2003. A novel function for tissue inhibitor of metalloproteinases-3 (TIMP3): inhibition of angiogenesis by blockage of VEGF binding to VEGF receptor-2. Nat Med 9(4):407-15.
Rivera A, Fisher SA, Fritsche LG, Keilhauer CN, Lichtner P, Meitinger T, Weber BH. 2005. Hypothetical LOC387715 is a second major susceptibility gene for age-related macular degeneration, contributing independently of complement factor H to disease risk. Hum Mol Genet 14(21):3227-36.
Rosenfeld PJ, Heier JS, Hantsbarger G, Shams N. 2006. Tolerability and efficacy of multiple escalating doses of ranibizumab (Lucentis) for neovascular age-related macular degeneration. Ophthalmology 113(4):623 e1.
Rudolf M, Curcio CA. 2009. Esterified cholesterol is highly localized to Bruch's membrane, as revealed by lipid histochemistry in wholemounts of human choroid. J Histochem Cytochem 57(8):731-9.
Ryan S. 1980. Subretinal neovascularization after argon laser photocoagulation. Albrecht Von Graefes Arch Klin Exp Ophthalmol 215(1):29-42.
Saint-Geniez M, Kurihara T, Sekiyama E, Maldonado AE, D'Amore PA. 2009. An essential role for RPE-derived soluble VEGF in the maintenance of the choriocapillaris. Proc Natl Acad Sci U S A 106(44):18751-6.
Sarks S, Arnold J, Killingsworth M, Sarks J. 1999. Early drusen formation in the normal and aging eye and their relation to age-related maculopathy: a clinicopathological study. British Journal of Ophthalmology 83:358-68.
Sarks S, Cherepanoff S, Killingsworth M, Sarks J. 2007. Relationship of Basal laminar deposit and membranous debris to the clinical presentation of early age-related macular degeneration. Invest Ophthalmol Vis Sci 48:968-77.
Schaal S, Kaplan HJ, Tezel TH. 2008. Is there tachyphylaxis to intravitreal anti-vascular endothelial growth factor pharmacotherapy in age-related macular degeneration? Ophthalmology 115(12):2199-205.
Seth A, Cui J, To E, Kwee M, Matsubara J. 2008. Complement-associated deposits in the human retina. Invest Ophthalmol Vis Sci 49(2):743-50.

Sheraidah G, Steinmetz R, Maguire J, Pauleikhoff D, Marshall J, Bird A. 1993. Correlation between lipids extracted from Bruch's membrane and age. Ophthalmology 100:47-51.

Sivaprasad S, Chong N, Bailey T. 2005. Serum elastin-derived peptides in age-related macular degeneration. Invest Ophthalmol Vis Sci 46:3046-51.

Sivaprasad S, Webster AR, Egan CA, Bird AC, Tufail A. 2008. Clinical course and treatment outcomes of Sorsby fundus dystrophy. Am J Ophthalmol 146(2):228-234.

Skeie JM, Fingert J, Russell S, Stone EM, Mullins RF. 2010. Complement Component C5a Activates ICAM-1 Expression on Human Choroidal Endothelial Cells. Invest Ophthalmol Vis Sci 51:5336-42.

Skeie JM, Mullins RF. 2008. Elastin-mediated choroidal endothelial cell migration: possible role in age-related macular degeneration. Invest Ophthalmol Vis Sci 49:5574-80.

Sorsby A, Mason ME. 1949. A fundus dystrophy with unusual features. Br J Ophthalmol 33(2):67-97.

Spraul C, Grossniklaus H. 1997. Characteristics of drusen and Bruch's membrane in postmortem eyes with age-related macular degeneration. Archives of Ophthalmology 115:267-73.

Spraul C, Lang G, Grossniklaus H, Lang G. 1999. Histologic and morphometric analysis of the choroid, Bruch's membrane, and retinal pigment epithelium in postmortem eyes with age-related macular degeneration and histologic examination of surgically excised choroidal neovascular membranes. Survey of Ophthalmology 44(1):S10-32.

Starita C, Hussain A, Pagliarini S, Marshall J. 1996. Hydrodynamics of ageing Bruch's membrane: implications for macular disease. Experimental Eye Research 62:565-572.

Starita C, Hussain AA, Patmore A, Marshall J. 1997. Localization of the site of major resistance to fluid transport in Bruch's membrane. Invest Ophthalmol Vis Sci 38(3):762-7.

Stone E, Braun T, Russell S, Kuehn M, Lotery A, Moore P, Eastman C, Casavant T, Sheffield V. 2004. Missense variations in the fibulin 5 gene and age-related macular degeneration. N Engl J Med 351:346-53.

Stone E, Lotery A, Munier F, Heon E, Piguet B, Guymer R, Vandenburgh K, Cousin P, Nishimura D, Swiderski R and others. 1999. A single EFEMP1 mutation associated with both Malattia Leventinese and Doyne honeycomb retinal dystrophy. Nature Genetics 22:199-202.

Struk B, Cai L, Zach S, Ji W, Chung J, Lumsden A, Stumm M, Huber M, Schaen L, Kim CA and others. 2000. Mutations of the gene encoding the transmembrane transporter protein ABC-C6 cause pseudoxanthoma elasticum. J Mol Med 78(5):282-6.

Sunness JS, Margalit E, Srikumaran D, Applegate CA, Tian Y, Perry D, Hawkins BS, Bressler NM. 2007. The long-term natural history of geographic atrophy from age-related macular degeneration: enlargement of atrophy and implications for interventional clinical trials. Ophthalmology 114(2):271-7.

Tezel TH, Del Priore LV, Berger AS, Kaplan HJ. 2007. Adult retinal pigment epithelial transplantation in exudative age-related macular degeneration. Am J Ophthalmol 143(4):584-95.

Thomson HA, Treharne AJ, Walker P, Grossel MC, Lotery AJ. 2010. Optimisation of polymer scaffolds for retinal pigment epithelium (RPE) cell transplantation. Br J Ophthalmol 95(4):563-8.

Tufail A, Patel PJ, Egan C, Hykin P, da Cruz L, Gregor Z, Dowler J, Majid MA, Bailey C, Mohamed Q and others. 2010. Bevacizumab for neovascular age related macular degeneration (ABC Trial): multicentre randomised double masked study. BMJ 340:c2459.

Ugarte M, Hussain AA, Marshall J. 2006. An experimental study of the elastic properties of the human Bruch's membrane-choroid complex: relevance to ageing. Br J Ophthalmol 90(5):621-6.

Uno K, Bhutto IA, McLeod DS, Merges C, Lutty GA. 2006. Impaired expression of thrombospondin-1 in eyes with age related macular degeneration. Br J Ophthalmol 90(1):48-54.

van der Schaft T, Mooy C, de Bruijn W, Bosman F, de Jong P. 1994. Immunohistochemical light and electron microscopy of basal laminar deposit. Graefe's Archives for Clinical and Experimental Ophthalmology 232:40-46.

Vingerling J, Dielemans I, Hofman A, Grobbee D, Hijmering M, Kramer C, de Jong P. 1995. The prevalence of age-related maculopathy in the Rotterdam Study. Ophthalmology 102:205-10.

Vogt SD, Curcio CA, Wang L, Li CM, McGwin G, Jr., Medeiros NE, Philp NJ, Kimble JA, Read RW. 2011. Retinal pigment epithelial expression of complement regulator CD46 is altered early in the course of geographic atrophy. Exp Eye Res.

Wang L, Clark ME, Crossman DK, Kojima K, Messinger JD, Mobley JA, Curcio CA. 2011. Abundant lipid and protein components of drusen. PLoS ONE 5(4):e10329.

Wang L, Li CM, Rudolf M, Belyaeva OV, Chung BH, Messinger JD, Kedishvili NY, Curcio CA. 2009. Lipoprotein particles of intraocular origin in human Bruch membrane: an unusual lipid profile. Invest Ophthalmol Vis Sci 50(2):870-7.

Weber B, Lin B, White K, Kohler K, Soboleva G, Herterich S, Seeliger M, Jaissle G, Grimm C, Reme C and others. 2002. A mouse model for Sorsby fundus dystrophy. Invest Ophthalmol Vis Sci 43:2732-40.

Weber B, Vogt G, Pruett R, Stohr H, Felbor U. 1994. Mutations in the tissue inhibitor of metalloproteinases-3 (TIMP3) in patients with Sorsby's fundus dystrophy. Nature Genetics 8(4):352-6.

Werth V, Ivanov I, Nussenzweig V. 1988. Decay-accelerating factor in human skin is associated with elastic fibers. J Invest Dermatol 91:511-6.

Wong RW, Richa DC, Hahn P, Green WR, Dunaief JL. 2007. Iron toxicity as a potential factor in AMD. Retina 27(8):997-1003.

Yanagisawa H, Davis EC, Starcher BC, Ouchi T, Yanagisawa M, Richardson JA, Olson EN. 2002. Fibulin-5 is an elastin-binding protein essential for elastic fibre development in vivo. Nature 415(6868):168-71.

Yates JR, Sepp T, Matharu BK, Khan JC, Thurlby DA, Shahid H, Clayton DG, Hayward C, Morgan J, Wright AF and others. 2007. Complement C3 variant and the risk of age-related macular degeneration. N Engl J Med 357(6):553-61.

Yehoshua Z, Rosenfeld P, TA. A. 2011. Current Clinical Trials in Dry AMD and the Definition of Appropriate Clinical Outcome Measures. Semin Ophthalmol. 26:167-80.

Young RW. 1971. The renewal of rod and cone outer segments in the rhesus monkey. J Cell Biol 49(2):303-18.

Yu H, Liu X, Kiss S, Connolly E, Gragoudas E, Michaud N, Bulgakov O, Adamian M, DeAngelis M, Miller J and others. 2008. Increased Choroidal Neovascularization Following Laser Induction in Mice Lacking Lysyl oxidase-like 1. Invest Ophthalmol Vis Sci 49:2599-605.

Yuan X, Gu X, Crabb JS, Yue X, Shadrach K, Hollyfield JG, Crabb JW. 2010. Quantitative proteomics: comparison of the macular Bruch membrane/choroid complex from age-related macular degeneration and normal eyes. Mol Cell Proteomics 9(6):1031-46.

4

Non-Enzymatic Post-Translational Modifications in the Development of Age-Related Macular Degeneration

Yuichi Kaji[1], Tetsuro Oshika[1] and Noriko Fujii[2]
[1]*Department of Pathophysiology of Vision and Ophthalmology, University of Tsukuba Graduate School of Comprehensive and Human Scicences, Tsukuba, Ibaraki,*
[2]*Research Reactor Institute, Kyoto University, Kumatori, Sennan, Osaka, Japan*

1. Introduction

Age-related macular degeneration (AMD) is a leading cause of blindness among Caucasians in various countries.1-3 In addition, cases of AMD are increasing among non-Caucasians, and AMD has become one of the major causes of blindness worldwide. To address this problem, several etiological, pathological, and basic science studies are being conducted. Etiological studies have revealed that the risk factors of AMD include smoking,4 increasing age, and the presence of cardiovascular disorders.5 However, the molecular mechanisms linking these risk factors to AMD are still unclear.

Pathoclinical studies have revealed macular drusen, which are small lumps of abnormally accumulated proteins beneath the retinal pigment of epithelial cells, to be a sign of AMD (Figure 1).6 Proteomics analysis of drusen has revealed that it is composed of various proteins, including clusterin, albumin, TIMP3, vitronectin, complement components, and crystallin. However, the pathological role of drusen in the development of AMD is still unclear.

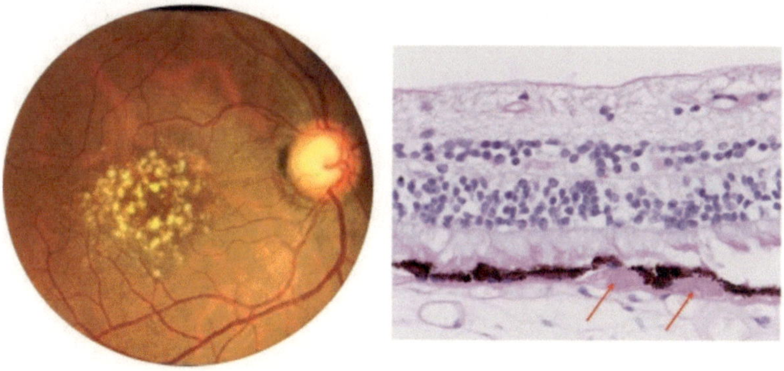

Fig. 1. **Drusen as an early sign of age-related macular degeneration**
Drusen are seen as yellow to white materials especially in the macular area (Left). Histologically, drusen are recognized as extracellular deposits that form between the retinal pigmented epithelium (RPE) and Bruch's membrane (arrows in the right Fig.).

AMD and other aging-related changes in the body have certain common characteristics, including the aggregation of abnormal proteins, seen in the lens and brain of patients with cataract and Alzheimer's disease, respectively. Post-translational modifications of proteins are also aging-related changes commonly seen in the target organ. For example, advanced glycation of proteins and racemization of amino acids with resultant D-amino acid formation in proteins are well-documented changes related to aging. Post-translational modification of proteins occurs because of aging, and it contributes to the aging changes of organs.

In order to elucidate the molecular mechanism of AMD, we evaluated the role of post-translational modifications of proteins in the development of AMD, particularly the formation of advanced glycation end products (AGEs) and D-amino acids in the development of drusen.

2. Post-translational modifications in age-related disorders

Post-translational modification of proteins is a molecular characteristic of the aging process. This is of 2 types as follows: enzymatic post-translational modification, which includes phosphorylation and glycosylation and is essential for protein function; and non-enzymatic post-translational modification that includes advanced glycation, racemization (and the resultant D-amino acid formation), and truncation, which impairs protein function, contributing to the aging process at the molecular level in various organs (Figure 2).

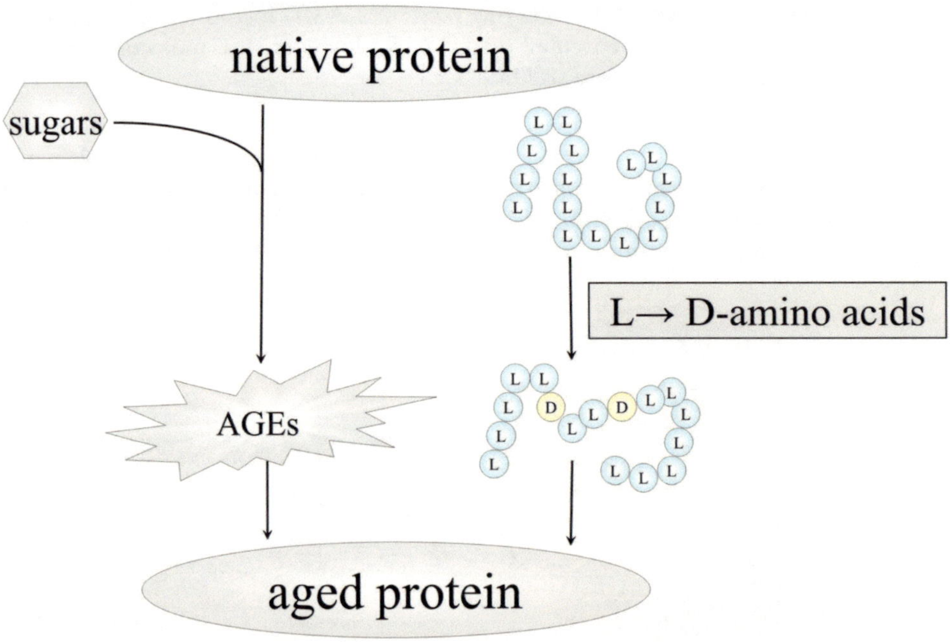

Fig. 2. **Aging of proteins at the molecular level**
Non-enzymatic post-translational modifications of proteins, including formation of AGEs and D-amino acids, are recognized as an aging process of proteins at the molecular level.

2.1 Advanced glycation end products

Advanced glycation end products (AGEs) are the final reaction products of proteins and reducing sugars. The reaction of reducing sugars (glucose and fructose) with Lys and Arg residues in proteins leads to the formation of Schiff base and Amadori products, which slowly undergo oxidation, dehydration, and condensation to form AGEs (Figure 3). The final products vary depending on the proteins, sugars, and the reactions involved. However, common structures called AGE motifs are seen in the products, irrespective of the proteins and sugars involved. Recently, a number of AGE motifs, including N^{ε}-(carboxy) methyl-L-lysine, imidazoline, pyrraline, and pentosidine, have been revealed.

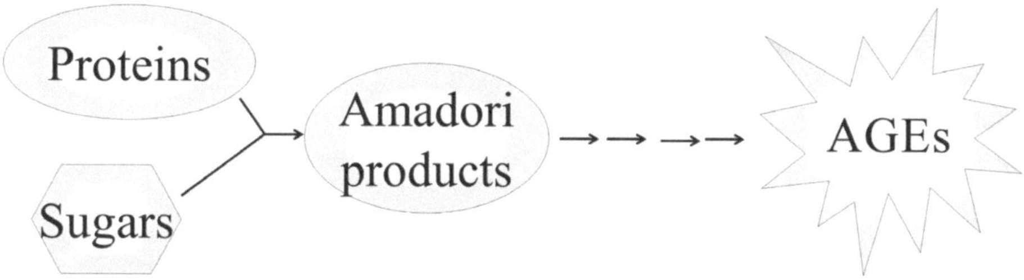

Fig. 3. **Multistep reactions of AGE formation**
Proteins and reducing sugars react with each other to form Amadori products. After multistep reactions, including oxidation, dehydration, and condensation, AGEs are generated.

Our body is like an incubator containing sugars and proteins, in which AGEs are naturally formed, particularly in the tissues with a low turnover rate such as bone, teeth, dura mater, and lens. AGEs tend to accumulate with age, and they are known to do so in the target organ of age-related disorders such as Alzheimer's disease and atherosclerosis. Thus, accumulation of AGEs in tissues is thought to be a biomarker of the aging process.

Formation of AGEs increases in diabetes partly because the concentration of reducing sugars increases in the blood. An accumulation of AGEs is seen in the thickened basement membrane and sclerotic lesions of the glomerulus in diabetic nephropathy. Furthermore, AGEs in the vitreous body and cornea are involved in the development of diabetic retinopathy and keratopathy, respectively.11-14

AGEs, along with being the accessory products of the aging process and diabetes, also possibly contribute to the aging process and diabetic complications. AGEs are known to alter the structure of proteins by intra- and inter-molecular crosslinking, consequently disrupting their function. For example, naïve laminin has a figure of the cross, but AGE-modified laminin is deformed, and thus, loses its adhesion property to epithelial cells.

2.2 D-amino acids

Proteins of all living organism on earth are composed of 20 types of amino acids. Among them, 19 amino acids other than glycine have chiral carbon atoms in the molecule.

Depending on the configuration of the side chains around the chiral carbon atoms, amino acids are either l- or d-amino acids. If amino acids were synthesized chemically, the quantity of l- and d-amino acids would be equal. However, proteins in all living organisms are composed exclusively of l-amino acids.

L-amino acids are converted to D-amino acids with a half-life of several thousand years, thus creating an equal amount of L- and D-amino acids over a particular period. This amount of D-amino acids is used for the age determination of fossils. Thus, D-amino acids are regarded as the products of post-mortal change and are irrelevant to living organisms. However, biologically uncommon D-amino acids that are enantiomers of L-amino acids have been found in the lenses16-19, teeth20, bones, brains21, skin22, aortas23, erythrocytes24, lungs25, and ligaments of elderly donors.26 The presence of D-amino acids in aged tissues of the living body is considered to be a result of racemization of L-amino acids in proteins in metabolically inert tissues during one's lifetime (Figure 4).

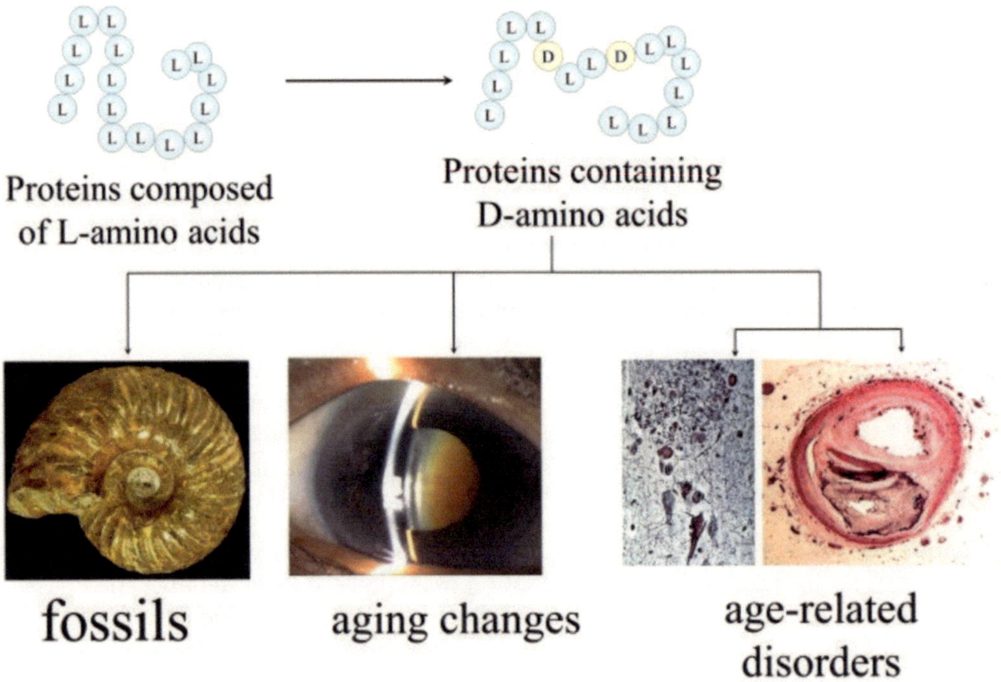

Fig. 4. **Significance of D-amino acids in proteins**
D-amino acids in proteins are seen in fossils as well as in the target organs of aging changes and age related disorders such as cataract, Alzheimer's disease, and atherosclerosis.

2.3 Co-localization of advanced glycation end products and D-amino acids in age-related macular degeneration

To reveal the role of AGEs and D-amino acids in the development of AMD, we analyzed the immunohistochemical localization of AGE and D-amino acid-containing proteins in human ocular samples of various ages.

Eye samples: Nine eyes from 9 donors of 18 to 88 years of age were obtained at the time of necropsy and used as samples for this study. Among them, 4 eyes from donors older than 68 years had drusen.

Antibodies: N^{ε}-(carboxy) methyl-L-lysine (CML) is the major component of AGEs in the body. A monoclonal antibody to CML was purchased (Transgenic Co. Ltd, Kumamoto, Japan).

The preparation and characterization of the primary antibody of D-β-Asp containing proteins was as described previously.27 The polyclonal antibody to the synthetic peptide called peptide 3R(Gly-Leu-D-β-Asp-Ala-Thy-Gly-Leu-D-β-Asp-Ala-Thy-Gly-Leu-D-β-Asp-Ala-Thy) corresponding to 3 repeats of positions 149–153 of the human α-A-crystallin was prepared and purified.

Immunohistochemistry: Immunohistochemical localization of CML and D-β-Asp containing proteins was investigated using the antibodies mentioned above. After fixation with 10% formalin solution, 4-μm-thick sections of the paraffin-embedded ocular samples were prepared. After deparaffinization, the sections were treated with 2 mg/mL of monoclonal antibody to CML or 1:500 diluted polyclonal antibody to D-β-Asp-containing proteins. After washing with phosphate-buffered saline, the sections were treated with secondary antibodies labeled with a polymer of horse radish peroxidase (Hitofine, Max-PO kit, Nichirei Co. Ltd, Tokyo, Japan). The final products were visualized using diaminobenzidine solution dissolved in phosphate-buffered saline.

No immunoreactivity to CML was seen in the retinas, choroids, or scleras of 5 eyes of donors younger than 18 years of age. In contrast, moderate immunoreactivity was seen in the retinal nerve fiber layers, and strong immunoreactivity was seen in the drusen and the thickened Bruch's membrane of the 5 eyes of donors older than 68 years (Figure 5).

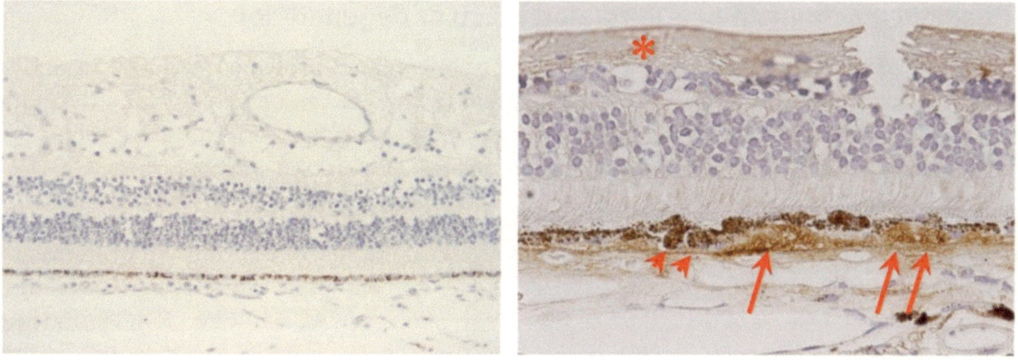

Fig. 5. **Immunohistochemical localization of AGE in human retina and choroid**
No immunoreactivity to CML, a major component of AGEs, is noted in young donor eyes. In contrast, immunoreactivity to CML is seen in the retinal nerve fiber layer (*), drusen (arrows), and thickened Bruch's membrane (arrowheads).

Similarly, no immunoreactivity to the D-β-Asp containing proteins was seen in the retinas, choroids, or scleras of donors younger than 18 years. In contrast, strong immunoreactivity was seen in the drusen seen in donors older than 68 years. In addition, moderate immunoreactivity to D-β-Asp containing proteins was seen in the sclera, the internal limiting membrane of retinal vessels, and Bruch membranes (Figure 6).

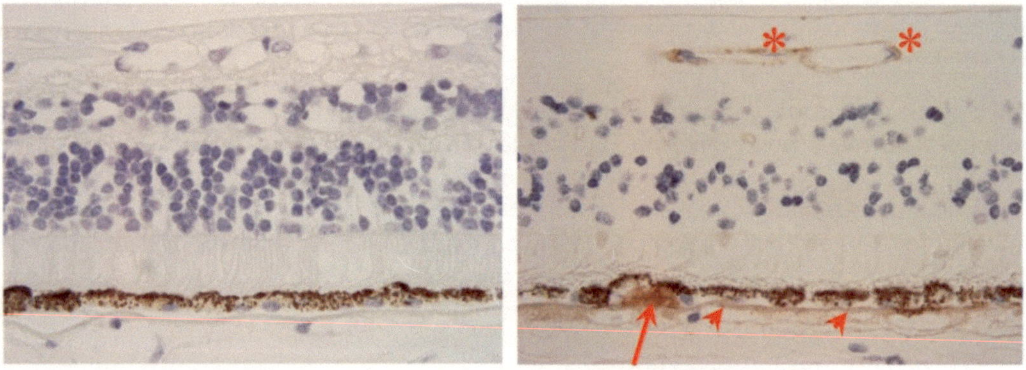

Fig. 6. **Immunohistochemical localization of D-amino acid-containing proteins in human retina and choroid**
No immunoreactivity to D-β-Asp-containing proteins, one of the major components of D-amino acids, is noted in young donor eyes. In contrast, the immunoreactivity to D-β-Asp-containing proteins is seen in the vessel walls (*), drusen (arrows), and thickened Bruch's membrane (arrowheads).

3. Possible mechanism of age-related macular degeneration

Drusen, an early sign of AMD, are small lumps of aggregated proteins rich in AGEs and D-amino acid containing proteins, which, in addition to being accessory products of the aging process, also possibly accelerate the aging process, suggesting that AGEs and D-amino acids in drusen play a central role in the development of AMD via various mechanisms.

One possible mechanism involves the interaction of AGEs and AGE receptors, which increases inflammation and accelerates neovascularization. AGE-modified proteins are recognized by the receptor for AGE (RAGE),30 galectin-3,31 macrophage scavenger receptors, and CD36.32 Particularly, the interaction of AGEs with RAGE induces inflammatory cytokines such as TNF-α and VEGF.33 RAGEs are expressed on the surface of retinal pigment epithelial cells. Furthermore, the interaction of AGE and RAGE increases the expression of RAGE, which serves as a positive feedback for the reaction. Thus, the constant interaction of AGEs in drusen with RAGE on retinal pigment epithelial cells would increase the expression of VEGF and induce neovascularization, resulting in AMD (Figure 7).

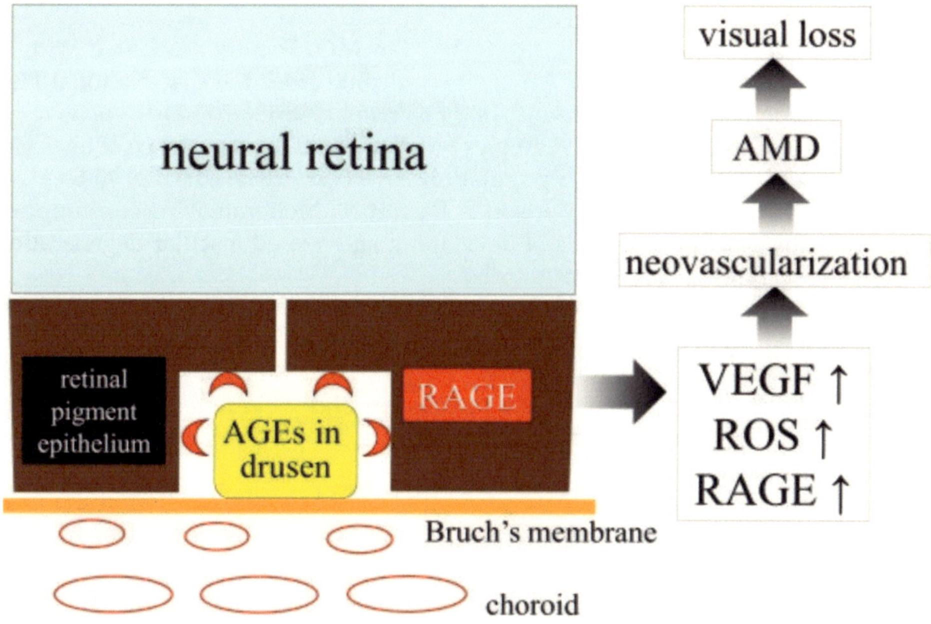

Fig. 7. **Possible mechanism of AMD in relation to AGEs in drusen**
The constant interaction of RAGE with AGEs in retinal pigment epithelial cells and drusen leads to the expression of VEGF, reactive oxygen species, and the increased expression of RAGE. This process then leads to neovascularization of the retina, which is a typical clinicopathological finding of AMD.

Another possible mechanism involves autoantibodies to AGE-modified proteins that have been detected in the elderly or in patients with rheumatic arthritis, which may induce inflammatory changes. Thus, autoimmune reactions may occur in tissues containing AGEs. In fact, proteomic analysis of drusen in human and animal models of AMD has revealed the deposition of IgG and complement factors. In addition, Becerra *et al.* have reported that the pathogenesis of AMD involves inflammatory changes.37 Based on these findings, intravitreal injection of corticosteroids to reduce the inflammation is clinically used to treat AMD.38 At present, the pathological role of D-amino acid containing proteins in the development of AMD is unknown. However, AGEs and D-amino acids need to be targeted for the prevention and treatment of AMD. For example, pyridoxamine inhibits the formation of AGEs in the body, and it has been used in clinical trials for the treatment of diabetic nephropathy. In addition, D-aspartyl endopeptidase has been shown to digest some D-amino acid containing proteins,41 suggesting that an increased expression of the intrinsic D-aspartyl endopeptidase would decrease the amount of D-amino acids-containing proteins in the target organ of the aging process. We suggest that the accumulating data on AGEs and D-amino acids will pave the way for new therapies for AMD in the near future.

4. Acknowledgement

This work was supported by Grants for Scientific Research 21592216 (2009-2011) from the Ministry of Education, Culture, Sports, Science, and Technology of Japan.

5. References

[1] Goldberg J, Flowerdew G, Smith E, Brody JA, Tso MO. Factors associated with age-related macular degeneration. An analysis of data from the first National Health and Nutrition Examination Survey. *Am J Epidemiol* 1988;128:700-710.

[2] Klein R, Chou CF, Klein BE, Zhang X, Meuer SM, Saaddine JB. Prevalence of age-related macular degeneration in the US population. *Arch Ophthalmol* 2011;129:75-80.

[3] Obisesan TO, Hirsch R, Kosoko O, Carlson L, Parrott M. Moderate wine consumption is associated with decreased odds of developing age-related macular degeneration in NHANES-1. *J Am Geriatr Soc* 1998;46:1-7.

[4] Seddon JM, Willett WC, Speizer FE, Hankinson SE. A prospective study of cigarette smoking and age-related macular degeneration in women. *JAMA* 1996;276:1141-1146.

[5] Vingerling JR, Dielemans I, Bots ML, Hofman A, Grobbee DE, de Jong PT. Age-related macular degeneration is associated with atherosclerosis. The Rotterdam Study. *Am J Epidemiol* 1995;142:404-409.

[6] Sarks SH, Arnold JJ, Killingsworth MC, Sarks JP. Early drusen formation in the normal and aging eye and their relation to age related maculopathy: a clinicopathological study. *Br J Ophthalmol* 1999;83:358-368.

[7] Crabb JW, Miyagi M, Gu X, et al. Drusen proteome analysis: an approach to the etiology of age-related macular degeneration. *Proc Natl Acad Sci U S A* 2002;99:14682-14687.

[8] Umeda S, Suzuki MT, Okamoto H, et al. Molecular composition of drusen and possible involvement of anti-retinal autoimmunity in two different forms of macular degeneration in cynomolgus monkey (Macaca fascicularis). *FASEB J* 2005;19:1683-1685.

[9] Grillari J, Grillari-Voglauer R, Jansen-Durr P. Post-translational modification of cellular proteins by ubiquitin and ubiquitin-like molecules: role in cellular senescence and aging. *Adv Exp Med Biol* 2010;694:172-196.

[10] Harding JJ, Beswick HT, Ajiboye R, Huby R, Blakytny R, Rixon KC. Non-enzymic post-translational modification of proteins in aging. A review. *Mech Ageing Dev* 1989;50:7-16.

[11] Stitt AW. Advanced glycation: an important pathological event in diabetic and age related ocular disease. *Br J Ophthalmol* 2001;85:746-753.

[12] Stitt AW. The maillard reaction in eye diseases. *Ann N Y Acad Sci* 2005;1043:582-597.

[13] Kaji Y, Usui T, Ishida S, et al. Inhibition of diabetic leukostasis and blood-retinal barrier breakdown with a soluble form of a receptor for advanced glycation end products. *Invest Ophthalmol Vis Sci* 2007;48:858-865.

[14] Kaji Y, Usui T, Oshika T, et al. Advanced glycation end products in diabetic corneas. *Invest Ophthalmol Vis Sci* 2000;41:362-368.

[15] Charonis AS, Reger LA, Dege JE, et al. Laminin alterations after in vitro nonenzymatic glycosylation. *Diabetes* 1990;39:807-814.

[16] Fujii N, Harada K, Momose Y, Ishii N, Akaboshi M. D-amino acid formation induced by a chiral field within a human lens protein during aging. *Biochem Biophys Res Commun* 1999;263:322-326.

[17] Fujii N, Shimo-Oka T, Ogiso M, et al. Localization of biologically uncommon D-beta-aspartate-containing alphaA-crystallin in human eye lens. *Mol Vis* 2000;6:1-5.

[18] Fujii N, Takemoto LJ, Momose Y, Matsumoto S, Hiroki K, Akaboshi M. Formation of four isomers at the asp-151 residue of aged human alphaA-crystallin by natural aging. *Biochem Biophys Res Commun* 1999;265:746-751.
[19] Kaji Y, Oshika T, Takazawa Y, Fukayama M, Takata T, Fujii N. Localization of D-beta-aspartic acid-containing proteins in human eyes. *Invest Ophthalmol Vis Sci* 2007;48:3923-3927.
[20] Masters PM. Stereochemically altered noncollagenous protein from human dentin. *Calcif Tissue Int* 1983;35:43-47.
[21] Shapira R, Chou CH. Differential racemization of aspartate and serine in human myelin basic protein. *Biochem Biophys Res Commun* 1987;146:1342-1349.
[22] Fujii N, Tajima S, Tanaka N, Fujimoto N, Takata T, Shimo-Oka T. The presence of D-beta-aspartic acid-containing peptides in elastic fibers of sun-damaged skin: a potent marker for ultraviolet-induced skin aging. *Biochem Biophys Res Commun* 2002;294:1047-1051.
[23] Powell JT, Vine N, Crossman M. On the accumulation of D-aspartate in elastin and other proteins of the ageing aorta. *Atherosclerosis* 1992;97:201-208.
[24] McFadden PN, Clarke S. Methylation at D-aspartyl residues in erythrocytes: possible step in the repair of aged membrane proteins. *Proc Natl Acad Sci U S A* 1982;79:2460-2464.
[25] Shapiro SD, Endicott SK, Province MA, Pierce JA, Campbell EJ. Marked longevity of human lung parenchymal elastic fibers deduced from prevalence of D-aspartate and nuclear weapons-related radiocarbon. *J Clin Invest* 1991;87:1828-1834.
[26] Ritz-Timme S, Laumeier I, Collins M. Age estimation based on aspartic acid racemization in elastin from the yellow ligaments. *Int J Legal Med* 2003;117:96-101.
[27] Yang D, Fujii N, Takata T, et al. Immunological detection of D-beta-aspartate-containing protein in lens-derived cell lines. *Mol Vis* 2003;9:200-204.
[28] Ishibashi T, Murata T, Hangai M, et al. Advanced glycation end products in age-related macular degeneration. *Arch Ophthalmol* 1998;116:1629-1632.
[29] Kaji Y, Oshika T, Takazawa Y, Fukayama M, Fujii N. Accumulation of D-beta-aspartic acid-containing proteins in age-related ocular diseases. *Chem Biodivers* 2010;7:1364-1370.
[30] Wautier JL, Wautier MP, Schmidt AM, et al. Advanced glycation end products (AGEs) on the surface of diabetic erythrocytes bind to the vessel wall via a specific receptor inducing oxidant stress in the vasculature: a link between surface-associated AGEs and diabetic complications. *Proc Natl Acad Sci U S A* 1994;91:7742-7746.
[31] Vlassara H, Li YM, Imani F, et al. Identification of galectin-3 as a high-affinity binding protein for advanced glycation end products (AGE): a new member of the AGE-receptor complex. *Mol Med* 1995;1:634-646.
[32] Ohgami N, Nagai R, Ikemoto M, et al. Cd36, a member of the class b scavenger receptor family, as a receptor for advanced glycation end products. *J Biol Chem* 2001;276:3195-3202.
[33] Ma W, Lee SE, Guo J, et al. RAGE ligand upregulation of VEGF secretion in ARPE-19 cells. *Invest Ophthalmol Vis Sci* 2007;48:1355-1361.
[34] Zhou J, Cai B, Jang YP, Pachydaki S, Schmidt AM, Sparrow JR. Mechanisms for the induction of HNE- MDA- and AGE-adducts, RAGE and VEGF in retinal pigment epithelial cells. *Exp Eye Res* 2005;80:567-580.

[35] Shibayama R, Araki N, Nagai R, Horiuchi S. Autoantibody against N(epsilon)-(carboxymethyl)lysine: an advanced glycation end product of the Maillard reaction. *Diabetes* 1999;48:1842-1849.

[36] Tai AW, Newkirk MM. An autoantibody targeting glycated IgG is associated with elevated serum immune complexes in rheumatoid arthritis (RA). *Clin Exp Immunol* 2000;120:188-193.

[37] Klein R, Knudtson MD, Klein BE, et al. Inflammation, complement factor h, and age-related macular degeneration: the Multi-ethnic Study of Atherosclerosis. *Ophthalmology* 2008;115:1742-1749.

[38] Becerra EM, Morescalchi F, Gandolfo F, et al. Clinical evidence of intravitreal triamcinolone acetonide in the management of age-related macular degeneration. *Curr Drug Targets* 2011;12:149-172.

[39] Metz TO, Alderson NL, Thorpe SR, Baynes JW. Pyridoxamine, an inhibitor of advanced glycation and lipoxidation reactions: a novel therapy for treatment of diabetic complications. *Arch Biochem Biophys* 2003;419:41-49.

[40] Williams ME, Bolton WK, Khalifah RG, Degenhardt TP, Schotzinger RJ, McGill JB. Effects of pyridoxamine in combined phase 2 studies of patients with type 1 and type 2 diabetes and overt nephropathy. *Am J Nephrol* 2007;27:605-614.

[41] Kinouchi T, Nishio H, Nishiuchi Y, et al. Isolation and characterization of mammalian D-aspartyl endopeptidase. *Amino Acids* 2007;32:79-85.

5

Experimental Treatments for Neovascular Age-Related Macular Degeneration

C. V. Regatieri[1,3], J. L. Dreyfuss[2,4] and H. B. Nader[2]
[1]Departmento de Oftalmologia,
[2]Departmento de Bioquímica,
Escola Paulista de Medicina, Universidade Federal de São Paulo, UNIFESP, São Paulo,
[3]Schepens Eye Research Institute,
Harvard Medical School, Department of Ophthalmology, Boston,
[4]Harvard-MIT Division of Health Sciences and Technology,
Massachusetts Institute of Technology, Cambridge,
[1,2]Brazil
[3,4]USA

1. Introduction

Age related macular degeneration (AMD) is the leading cause of severe visual loss in adults older than 60 years (1, 2). It is estimated that approximately 30% of adults older than 75 years have some sign of AMD and around 10% develop advanced stages of the disease. More than 1.6 million people in the United States currently have one or both eyes affected by an advanced stage of AMD and it is estimated that there are another 7 million individuals "at risk" (1). Due to rapid aging of the population in many developed countries, this number is expected to double by the year of 2020 (1, 3). Although neovascular AMD only accounts for about 10–20% of the overall AMD incidence, this subtype is responsible for 90% of cases of severe vision loss (20/200 or worse) (4, 5).

Neovascular AMD is characterized by the presence of choroidal neovascularization (CNV) and is associated with retinal pigment epithelium detachment (PED), retinal pigment epithelium (RPE) tears, fibrovascular disciform scarring, and vitreous hemorrhage(4).

Choroidal neovascularization is an intricate process controlled by myriad angiogenic agents such as growth factors, cytokines, and extracellular matrix (ECM) components. Several growth factors have been implicated in pathologic vessel formation in ocular diseases, such as age-related macular degeneration, including fibroblast growth factor (FGF), platelet-derived growth factor (PEDF), tumor necrosis factor (TNF-α) and vascular endothelial growth factor (VEGF)(6). Additionally, it is hypothesized that an inflammatory process is behind the pathogenesis of AMD. It was found that extracellular depositions of diffuse basal laminar and linear deposits (BLD) between the cytoplasmic and basement membrane of the RPE are significantly associated with CNV formation (4, 5, 7). Histological studies of these BLDs proved the presence of complement complexes C3, C5b-9, MMP- 2, MMP-9, and vitronectin (8). Further support of this hypothesis came from genetic studies where mutations/polymorphisms were found in genes coding for the alternative complement pathway regulator (Factor H and Factor H related proteins) and complement pathway proteins (complement component C2, factor B, and toll-like receptor 4).

Several focal treatments have been proposed and extensively studied to prevent the severe visual loss in neovascular AMD patients including laser photocoagulation (9), photodynamic therapy (PDT) (10) and the combination of PDT with intraocular injections of triamcinolone acetonide. Despite anatomical success, there is a low chance for visual improvement when these treatments are used. In recent years, research has provided new insights into the pathogenesis of macular disease. Today less destructive treatments directly targeting CNV and its pathogenic cascade have become available (8, 11). Antibodies against VEGF uniquely offer a significant chance of increase in visual acuity to patients affected by neovascular AMD.

Currently, inhibition of VEGF-A is the first choice of therapy for neovascular AMD, which not only stabilizes, but also improves visual acuity. The most effective preparations, bevacizumab (Avastin, Genentech Inc, South San Francisco, California) or ranibizumab (Lucentis, Genentech Inc), are recombinant monoclonal antibodies (Fab) that neutralize all biologically active forms of VEGF (12). Two Phase III clinical trials (MARINA and ANCHOR) studied ranibizumab for the treatment of CNV associated with neovascular AMD (13-15). In both of these studies, ranibizumab was administered every 4 weeks (fixed schedule) for up to two years without monthly imaging. Both trials demonstrated prevention of substantial vision loss (lost < 15 letters) in more than 90% of subjects. Additionally, approximately 30% to 40% of the subjects experienced substantial visual acuity gains (gain > 15 letters). Though these dramatic results have revolutionized the treatment of neovascular AMD, the monthly treatment schedule used in the clinical trials has a number of drawbacks including the high number of injections and the lack of efficiency in some patients who do not respond to anti-VEGF therapy (12).

Therefore it is important to continue the study of the CNV physiopathology in order to find new molecules involved in the angiogenesis. In this way it will be possible to develop new drugs to reduce the treatment frequency and to treat patients that don't respond to anti-VEGF therapy.

2. Animal models of choroidal neovascularization

The development of animal models of CNV has paralleled and contributed to the understanding of the biology of this condition. In addition, these models have also been developed in order to test new treatments.

a. Laser induced models of CNV

The first CNV model was developed in primates (16), and coworkers later developed a rat model of CNV in 1989 (17). Those authors created argon laser photocoagulation spots (647 nm, 100 mm, 50e100 mW, 0.1 s) through a dilated pupil with a coverslip over the cornea. The created spots break the Bruch's membrane, with a central bubble formation with or without intraretinal or choroidal hemorrhage. There was fluorescein angiographic evidence of CNV in 24% of the created lesions. Examination of enucleated eyes by light and electron microscopy showed pathologic evidence of CNV in 60% of the lesions. Frank and coworkers also developed a rat model of CNV in 1989 (18). Also, a diode laser may be used to create the CNV (532 nm, 100 mm 50e100 mW, 0.1 s) and this model has been used to assess aging as it relates to CNV formation.

b. Surgically induced models of CNV

Subretinal and/or choroidal neovascularization has been immunologically and mechanically induced in rat and mouse models, primarily by injection of synthetic peptides, viral vectors containing VEGF, cells and inert synthetic materials (19-21).

c. Transgenic and knockout mouse models of CNV

Although there are several transgenic mouse models AMD (22), only a relatively few of the models spontaneously develop CNV. It has become apparent that overexpression of VEGF by the retina or RPE is not enough to elicit CNV in these models and there is a central role of compromised Bruch's membrane in the development of CNV (22). The advantages of these models are the ability to study various biologic components of CNV by comparing with controls and cross breeding experiments. Disadvantages relate to the length of time for the CNV to develop, the relatively small percentages of eyes that develop CNV and the small size of the CNV.

3. Retina cytotoxicity assays for new drugs

a. "In vitro" assays

Toxicity is a complex event *in vivo*, where there may be direct cellular damage, physiological effects, inflammatory effects and other systemic effects. Currently, it is difficult to monitor systemic and physiological effects *in vitro*, so most assays determine effects at cellular level, or cytotoxicity (23).

New drugs have to go through extensive cytotoxicity testing before they are released for the use (24, 25). Today there is a continuous search for methods to determine the toxicity by using *in vitro* tests, trying to reduce the number of experiments involving animals (26). Important live-cell functions, including apoptosis, cell adhesion, cell migration and cell proliferation, can be monitored with various *in vitro* tests by using colorimetric and fluorescence assays (27, 28). The most frequently used cell lines are: human retinal pigment epithelial cells (ARPE-19), rat neurosensory retinal cells (R28), rat retinal ganglion cells (RGC-5)(29, 30), the immortalized Muller cell line (MIO-M1) (31) and human umbilical vein endothelial cells (HUVEC) and rabbit aorta endothelial cells (6, 32, 33).

Many of these processes lead to changes in intracellular and membrane components that can be followed with appropriately responsiveness by indicators that could be detected by microscopy, flow cytometry or with a microplate reader. Because cytotoxicity could not be easily defined in terms of a single physiological or morphological parameter, it is often desirable to combine several different measures, such as enzymatic activity, membrane permeability or oxidation-reduction potential. The most common assay to determine the cytotoxicity is the viability assay. The viability is principally used to measure the proportion of viable (life and function) cells after a drug exposure. Most tests verify the cell membrane integrity by dye exclusion, as Naphtalene Black and Trypan Blue as well as by dye uptake as fluorescein diacetate and propidium iodide (PI) (34, 35). In the first one viable cells are impermeable to the dye, and the analysis is performed by light microscopy. In the second test viable cells uptake diacetyl fluorescein and hydrolyze (esterase) in fluorescein that fluoresce in green, and the nucleus of the non-viable cells are stained by the PI that fluoresce in red, the analysis could be performed both by fluorescence microscopy and flow cytometry (36).

Cell viability also can also be measured by MTT reduction (37) using a microtitration assay in 96 multiwell plates. The reduction of tetrazolium salt (yellow) is reduced in metabolically active cells to form insoluble purple formazan crystals. Other assays include acidotropic stain using acridine orange that concentrates in acidic organelles in a pH-dependent manner. Under fluorescence microscope it is possible to see the metachromatic green or red fluorescence of acridine orange to assess cell viability (38).

Besides viability the apoptosis research is a powerful tool for drug toxicity screening. Apoptosis is the programmed cell death and is characterized morphologically by compaction of the nuclear chromatin, cell-permeability and production of apoptotic bodies. The characteristic observed in apoptotic cells is the fragmentation of the chromatin, degradation of the nuclear envelope and nuclear blebbing, resulting in the formation of micronuclei. A different assay frequently used is the APO-BrdU TUNEL (Terminal Deoxynucleotide Transferase dUTP Nick End Labeling) where DNA strands of apoptotic cells are labeled with BrdUTP, once incorporated into the DNA, BrdU can be detected by an anti-BrdU antibody conjugated with a enzyme or a fluorescent probe using immunohistochemistry or immunofluorescence (39).

Annexin V is a protein that binds phosphatidylserine located at the cell surface and used to detect apoptotic cells. In apoptotic cells phosphatidylserine is exposed to the outer of the plasma membrane being detected by the annexin V conjugated with a fluorophor. Fluorescent cells could be observed in fluorescence microscope or flow cytometer (33, 40).

b. "In vivo" assays

Retinal toxicity can be evaluated by intravitreal injections of drugs in rats, mice, rabbits and non-human primates. The safety and efficacy of intravitreal drugs can be analyzed in choroidal neovascularization (CNV) in the laser-induced rat model (6, 41). The investigation of toxicity in animal models using the standard tools of light microscopy (LM) and histopathological analysis makes critical benchmarks for the study of development of the angioproliferative disease. In this way is possible to observe the functional and morphological alteration results of drug toxicity *in vivo*.

Microscopic studies using light, electron or confocal microscopy are common methods used for retinal biocompatibility studies. For microscopy analysis, it is essential to know the normal retina morphology of the animal species analyzed. Histological studies, using light or electron microscopies could be descriptive or analytical.

Clinical evaluation is also an important method to evaluate the retinal toxicity of new drugs. The occurrence of a transient or permanent toxic reaction can be documented by the retinal appearance, function or histological findings in experimental eyes (42). Ocular examinations include slitlamp for anterior segment and detailed dilated fundus examinations (42, 43).

Electrophysiological testing is an effective and objective method to assess the status of the visual pathways. The electroretinogram (ERG) is obtained by recording, through a contact lens electrode on the cornea, the electrical potential generated by the retina in response to a brief stimulus (flash or flicker) of light. ERG is one of the most important examinations for retinal biocompatibility in experimental models, since it is a functional and objective test. In animals, behavioral assessment of visual function is a difficult parameter to be evaluated. Currently, the basis of retinal evaluation for pharmacological and toxicological effects of intravitreally-administered drugs in animals consists of ERG associated with histopathology by light and electron microscopy (44, 45). Toxicity testing can be obtained in rodent as well as non-rodent species for extrapolation to humans for determining risk and safety (46).

4. Therapeutic Monoclonal Antibodies

Monoclonal antibodies (mAbs) can be used therapeutically due to the binding to molecular targets with high specificity. In ophthalmology, therapeutic mAbs have been introduced recently to treat inflammatory and angiogenic diseases. The rationale for mAb application in ophthalmology also is based on a recent understanding of the molecular biology of various ocular diseases (12).

a. Monoclonal Antibody anti-tumor necrosis alpha

Recent evidences have shown that the cytokine TNF-α participates actively in the pathogenesis of inflammatory, edematous, neovascular and neurodegenerative ocular, and extra ocular diseases. In addition, the central pathogenic role of TNF in medicine is supported by the clinical efficacy of TNF-α antagonists such as infliximab in randomized controlled trials for various diseases including rheumatoid arthritis (RA) and Crohn's disease (47). Furthermore, although TNF-α is barely detectable in the serum of healthy humans at levels of 10 fg/ml, in patients with systemic inflammatory or neoplastic diseases, the levels increase markedly to 50 pg/ml (48).

Consecutive studies have described the role of infliximab in the treatment of ocular inflammation. Single or multiple infusions of infliximab at concentrations of 3–10 mg/kg within a 2- to 36-month period have been efficacious in preventing ocular attacks, decreasing relapses, diminishing concomitant corticosteroid use, and controlling disease activity in patients with idiopathic uveitis or uveitis associated with juvenile arthritis, ankylosing spondylitis, Behcet's disease, sarcoidosis, or Crohn's disease (12).

Regarding ocular neovascularization, one patient with Behcet's disease with uveitis and retinal neovascularization treated with systemic infliximab had regression of new vessels after 8 months. A series of patients receiving 5 mg/kg of infliximab infusions for inflammatory arthritis had remarkable regression of CNV due to AMD (49, 50). The preventive and therapeutic effects of infliximab and etanercept have been studied in a rat model of laser-induced CNV as reported previously by other reports and by our research group (6, 51). In the study by Olson et al., both anti-TNF agents given prophylactically decreased the size and leakage of CNV lesions in these animal models, although in one study only etanercept induced reduction of CNV (52). We performed intravitreal injection of escalating doses of infliximab from 10 to 320 μg in rats after laser-induced CNV. At lower doses, infliximab promoted significant reduction of neovascular complex. However, at higher doses, it induced no effect compared to the control group. These results suggested that either the pro-angiogenic effect of anti-TNF mAb might occur only at higher doses or that in a lower dose some antiangiogenic indirect effect may be seen. Clinical studies have shown a marked elevation in vitreous levels of TNF-α in patients with PDR (53, 54). Experimental studies in a rat RD (retinal detachment) model showed that anti-TNF agents might reduce leukocyte adhesion, blood–retina barrier breakdown, and endothelial injury. The association between TNF-α and pathologic intraocular neovascularization may be explained by direct transmembrane-TNF stimulation of blood vessel growth, or TNF-α-induced expression of isoform VEGF-C, which may protect retinal endothelial cells from apoptosis (55).

b. Monoclonal Antibody anti-platelet derived growth factor

Vascular endothelial cells release PDGF-B, which in turn induce recruitment, proliferation, and survival of pericytes, glial cells, and RPE cells (56). Newly established pericytes along with retinal cells provide survival signals for endothelial cells, and more importantly, pericytes may promote the scarring process following CNV (57). Mural cell recruitment to the growing endothelial tube is regulated by PDGF-B signaling; interference with this pathway causes disruption of endothelial cell–mural cell interactions and loss of mural cells. Therefore, antagonists of PDGFs with or without VEGF antagonists may reduce scarring and neovascularization. Moreover, inhibition of both VEGF-A and PDGF-B signaling may be more effective than blocking VEGF-A alone in causing vessel regression in multiple models of neovascular growth (58-60). A clinical trial phase 1 is evaluating the safety of a monoclonal antibody anti PDGF injected intravitreously for the treatment of neovascular AMD (E10030- Ophthotech Corporation, clinical trial NCT00569140) (61).

c. Monoclonal Antibody anti-integrin $\alpha5\beta1$

Components of the ECM play an important role in angiogenesis and CNV formation by helping to facilitate endothelial cell migration. Integrins are heterodimeric transmembrane proteins, composed of alpha and beta subunits, which interact with the ECM. Both $\alpha v\beta3$ and $\alpha5\beta1$ integrins have been shown to play a role in angiogenesis and their expression is upregulated in activated vascular endothelial cells (62). Inhibition of $\alpha5\beta1$ integrin may be of particular interest for the treatment of neovascular AMD because of its expression in RPE, macrophages, and fibroblasts in addition to endothelial cells. Wang et al. demonstrated that an integrin $\alpha5\beta1$ inhibitor (ATN-161) was able to inhibit CNV leakage and neovascularization in a laser induced CNV model (63).

d. Monoclonal Antibody anti-basic fibroblast growth factor (b-FGF)

FGFs are a family of heparin-binding growth factors involved in wound healing and embryonic development. The basic-FGF form, also referred to as b-FGF, may be a more potent angiogenic factor than VEGF or PDGF (64). In the eye, FGF is localized within the lacrimal gland, retina, lens, photoreceptors, aqueous humor, vitreous, and corneal epithelium. In both retina and RPE cells, FGF induces changes in cellular proliferation and *in vivo* angiogenesis. Most uveal melanoma cell lines express FGF subtypes including b-FGF to various extents, and increased FGF expression along with other growth factors was reported in an animal model of retinal detachment (65, 66).

An anti-FGF mAb (no registered brand name to date, BioWa, Princeton, NJ, USA) was developed recently for future application on the treatment of various cancers. Although no study has reported if that anti- FGF agent is useful in ocular pharmacology, some potential indications for the application of anti-FGF mAb based on FGF function can be proposed as adjuvant chemotherapy for ocular melanoma, in conjunction with other mAbs such as anti-TNF to treat PVR associated with rhegmatogenous retinal detachment, and to reduce the chance of PCO after cataract surgery (12, 67). More investigation should unravel the usefulness of anti-FGF mAbs in PCO or PVR, because so far the absence of a cause–effect relationship has not been settled. In addition, other mediators may play a more important role than FGF in these entities.

5. Angiostatic compounds

a. Heparin mimetics

Choroidal neovascularization is a complex process controlled by numerous angiogenic agents such as growth factors, cytokines and ECM components, including glycosaminoglycans (GAGs) (68, 69). GAGs can interact with a diverse range of proteins leading to various biological activities, including angiogenesis (69). Among the sulfated GAGs, heparin and heparan sulfate (HS) have been involved in the modulation of the neovascularization that takes place in different physiological and pathological conditions (70-73). This modulation occurs through the interaction of GAGs with angiogenic growth factors, such as VEGF, FGF, TGF-β, IFN-γ and TNF-α. This property of GAGs to bind and modulate angiogenic growth factors provides a strong reason for studying and designing new synthetic GAG analogs, or discovering GAG-like natural compounds, endowed with angiostatic properties. Sulfated oligosaccharides, which are structural mimics of HS or heparin, are potential drug candidates because these compounds may interfere with the role HS plays in the process of angiogenesis. Heparin is known for its anticoagulant activity, but it also has a strong anti-inflammatory effect also (74, 75).

Recently, we have shown that a heparinoid isolated from marine shrimp presenting negligible anticoagulant and hemorrhagic activities was able to reduce over 60% the neovascularization areas in the laser induced CNV after intravitreal injection. Also this compound is capable of reducing acute inflammatory processes in an animal model (76).

Studies using intravitreal injection of PI88 (phosphomannopentaose sulfate) showed that this compound is capable to reduce the neovascularization area in laser induced experimental CNV in 50% (77). Intravitreal injection of heparin also can reduce the size of the CNV, but the hemorrhagic complications are imminent (33, 78).

The pharmacological and biochemical properties of the heparinoids point to these compounds as compelling drug candidates for treating neovascular AMD.

b. Blockage of complement cascade

Immunological factors are involved not only in the pathogenesis of AMD, but also in its treatment of this disease. Genetic polymorphisms in different complement proteins can increase the risk for developing AMD (e.g., lack of factor H in patients with Y402H mutations) (79). There are three pathways of complement activation and all of them activate a final common pathway (C3). Lipofucsin and basal lipid deposits between Bruch's membrane and the retinal pigment epithelium (RPE) cell layer may act as a stimulus for the local activation of the complement system. This may lead to a further growth of the deposits due to the strong chemotactic activity of complement activation products with an influx of inflammatory cells (80). Furthermore these activated RPE cells release angiogenic stimuli leading to choroidal neovascularization (81).

Several agents that modulate different parts of the complement system are in clinical trials. In general, these agents work either by replacing a defective complement component as factor H, that is the central soluble activation inhibitor of the alternative complement pathway, or by blocking the complement pathway C3, the POT-4 (79, 82).

c. Kinase inhibitors

Another approach to inhibit angiogenic growth factors as VEGF is through inhibition of the downstream signaling pathways targeting the tyrosine kinases. Several inhibitors were tested and a case in point is the intravitreally administered Vatalanib, a VEGF receptor inhibitor that binds to the intracellular kinase domain (83). Other kinases inhibitors currently in development include pazopanib, sorafenib, motesanib, TG100801, as well as AG013736 (84-86).

Sorafenib is an orally active multikinase inhibitor that inhibits the serine/threonine kinases activity of the VEGF receptor. The CNV area in sorafenib-treated rats was significantly reduced in a dose-dependent manner (85). Sorafenib is in phase III trials for renal-cell carcinoma patients.

6. Small interference RNA (siRNA)

RNA interference is a technology that allows the silencing of genes in animals using therapeutic double-stranded RNA molecules. siRNA molecules induce gene silencing by binding to complementary target RNA molecules in association with the nucleolytic cytoplasmic protein complex known as the RNA-induced silencing complex (87). Nowadays, siRNA is being designed to reduce the production of angiogenic molecules providing potent therapies for ocular neovascularization in patients with AMD. siRNA can be injected into the vitreous cavity or at the subretinal space to treat choroidal neovascularization. This delivery produces local silencing of a gene with small chance for a systemic effect on the same gene (88, 89).

The targeted genes for CNV treatment are mostly VEGF and VEGF receptors (90-92). The silencing of hypoxia inducible factor-1alpha (HIF-1alpha), that regulates the VEGF expression in hypoxic conditions of ocular angiogenesis is also under investigation to treat CNV (93). siRNA targeting the TGF-β, involved in fibrotic scars, seems to be another great potential to treat AMD (94). Furthermore genes associated to photoreceptors degeneration (apoptosis mediators) *c-Jun*, and *Bax* are being tested for futures therapies (95).

A phase I study to investigate the safety, tolerability, pharmacokinetics of a single intravitreous injection of Sirna-027 (siRNA-mediated VEGF silencing) in 26 patients with choroidal neovascularization was completed, and stabilization or improvement in visual acuity and foveal thickness was observed (90).

7. Gene therapy

Gene-based therapy is defined as the introduction, using a vector, of nucleic acids into cells with the objective of changing gene expression to prevent or reverse a pathological process (96). Pro- and antiangiogenic factors regulate the pathogenesis of the ocular neovascularization. Gene transfer to increase expression of endogenous antiangiogenic proteins has the potential to provide long-term stability in patients with AMD (97). There are two routes of administration of viral vectors: intravitreous injection and subretinal injection. The main vectors used for gene transfer are adenovirus, adeno-associated virus (AAV) and lentivirus (96).

Genes encoding antiangiogenic proteins are genetically inserted in viral vectors. The viral vectors infect animal cells and the overexpression of the antiangiogenic protein can be detected. Pigment epithelium-derived factor (PEDF) is a serine proteinase inhibitor from cultured retinal pigmented epithelial cells, which posses a combination of neurotrophic, antitumoral and antiangiogenic activities. Intravitreous or subretinal injection of adenoviral vector expressing human PEDF suppressed the development of retinal neovascularization (98). In the rat CNV model, the gene transfer of PEDF using ultrasound-mediated microbubbles was able to inhibit effectively the CNV (99).

The secreted extracellular domain of VEGF receptor-1, sFlt-1, a soluble form of the Flt-1 VEGF receptor has been used effectively in recombinant adenovirus (Ad)- and recombinant adeno-associated virus (AAV)-mediated antiangiogenic gene therapy to inhibit angiogenesis in CNV animal models (100, 101). The expression of sFlt-1 was associated with the long-term regression of neovascular vessels in mice and monkey (102).

Endostatin is C-terminal fragment derived from collagen XVIII that inhibits tumor angiogenesis (103). Systemic injection of adenoviral vectors containing a sequence coding for murine endostatin, and the mice injected had the serum levels of endostatin raised up to 10-fold and had nearly complete prevention of CNV (104). Subconjunctival injection of recombinant adeno-associated viral vector expressing human angiostatin reduced alkali burn-induced corneal angiogenesis (105).

Intravitreal adenovirus-mediated gene transfer of 15-Lipoxygenase-1, an oxidizing enzyme producing reactive lipid hydroperoxides, efficiently inhibited VEGF induced neovascularization and pathological changes in rabbit eyes (106).

8. Conclusions

The treatment of AMD up to 2000 was limited to vessel destructive procedures that did not improve the visual acuity. The development and testing of therapeutic agents that prevent or delay the progression of AMD is urgently needed, from the standpoint of patient care and quality of life, as well as cost savings. The development of new therapies targeting the angiogenic components of CNV could have a significant impact on the health and quality of life of AMD patients. Moreover combination therapy will possibly replace monotherapy as the treatment of choice in order to reduce the frequency of treatment and prevent the late-stage complications of neovascular AMD.

9. References

[1] Friedman DS, O'Colmain BJ, Munoz B, Tomany SC, McCarty C, de Jong PT, et al. Prevalence of age-related macular degeneration in the United States. Arch Ophthalmol. 2004 Apr;122(4):564-72.

[2] Klein R, Klein BE, Linton KL. Prevalence of age-related maculopathy. The Beaver Dam Eye Study. Ophthalmology. 1992 Jun;99(6):933-43.

[3] Thylefors B. A global initiative for the elimination of avoidable blindness. Indian J Ophthalmol. 1998 Sep;46(3):129-30.

[4] Bressler NM, Bressler SB, Fine SL. Age-related macular degeneration. Surv Ophthalmol. 1988 May-Jun;32(6):375-413.

[5] Votruba M, Gregor Z. Neovascular age-related macular degeneration: present and future treatment options. Eye (Lond). 2001 Jun;15(Pt 3):424-9.

[6] Regatieri CV, Dreyfuss JL, Melo GB, Lavinsky D, Farah ME, Nader HB. Dual role of intravitreous infliximab in experimental choroidal neovascularization: effect on the expression of sulfated glycosaminoglycans. Invest Ophthalmol Vis Sci. 2009 Nov;50(11):5487-94.

[7] Argon laser photocoagulation for neovascular maculopathy. Five-year results from randomized clinical trials. Macular Photocoagulation Study Group. Arch Ophthalmol. 1991 Aug;109(8):1109-14.

[8] Ferrara N, Gerber HP, LeCouter J. The biology of VEGF and its receptors. Nat Med. 2003 Jun;9(6):669-76.

[9] Bressler NM, Arnold J, Benchaboune M, Blumenkranz MS, Fish GE, Gragoudas ES, et al. Verteporfin therapy of subfoveal choroidal neovascularization in patients with age-related macular degeneration: additional information regarding baseline lesion composition's impact on vision outcomes-TAP report No. 3. Arch Ophthalmol. 2002 Nov;120(11):1443-54.

[10] Chen Y, Vuong LN, Liu J, Ho J, Srinivasan VJ, Gorczynska I, et al. Three-dimensional ultrahigh resolution optical coherence tomography imaging of age-related macular degeneration. Opt Express. 2009 Mar 2;17(5):4046-60.

[11] Brown DM, Kaiser PK, Michels M, Soubrane G, Heier JS, Kim RY, et al. Ranibizumab versus verteporfin for neovascular age-related macular degeneration. N Engl J Med. 2006 Oct 5;355(14):1432-44.

[12] Rodrigues EB, Farah ME, Maia M, Penha FM, Regatieri C, Melo GB, et al. Therapeutic monoclonal antibodies in ophthalmology. Prog Retin Eye Res. 2009 Mar;28(2):117-44.

[13] Boyer DS, Antoszyk AN, Awh CC, Bhisitkul RB, Shapiro H, Acharya NR. Subgroup analysis of the MARINA study of ranibizumab in neovascular age-related macular degeneration. Ophthalmology. 2007 Feb;114(2):246-52.

[14] Kaiser PK, Blodi BA, Shapiro H, Acharya NR. Angiographic and optical coherence tomographic results of the MARINA study of ranibizumab in neovascular age-related macular degeneration. Ophthalmology. 2007 Oct;114(10):1868-75.

[15] Kaiser PK, Brown DM, Zhang K, Hudson HL, Holz FG, Shapiro H, et al. Ranibizumab for predominantly classic neovascular age-related macular degeneration: subgroup analysis of first-year ANCHOR results. Am J Ophthalmol. 2007 Dec;144(6):850-7.

[16] Ryan SJ. The development of an experimental model of subretinal neovascularization in disciform macular degeneration. Trans Am Ophthalmol Soc. 1979;77:707-45.

[17] Dobi ET, Puliafito CA, Destro M. A new model of experimental choroidal neovascularization in the rat. Arch Ophthalmol. 1989 Feb;107(2):264-9.
[18] Frank RN, Das A, Weber ML. A model of subretinal neovascularization in the pigmented rat. Curr Eye Res. 1989 Mar;8(3):239-47.
[19] Schmack I, Berglin L, Nie X, Wen J, Kang SJ, Marcus AI, et al. Modulation of choroidal neovascularization by subretinal injection of retinal pigment epithelium and polystyrene microbeads. Mol Vis. 2009;15:146-61.
[20] Baba T, Bhutto IA, Merges C, Grebe R, Emmert D, McLeod DS, et al. A rat model for choroidal neovascularization using subretinal lipid hydroperoxide injection. Am J Pathol. 2010 Jun;176(6):3085-97.
[21] Grossniklaus HE, Kang SJ, Berglin L. Animal models of choroidal and retinal neovascularization. Prog Retin Eye Res. 2010 Nov;29(6):500-19.
[22] van Eeden PE, Tee LB, Lukehurst S, Lai CM, Rakoczy EP, Beazley LD, et al. Early vascular and neuronal changes in a VEGF transgenic mouse model of retinal neovascularization. Invest Ophthalmol Vis Sci. 2006 Oct;47(10):4638-45.
[23] Freshney RI. Culture of animal cells: A manual of basic technique. Liss AR, editor. 2005;4.
[24] Brasnu E, Brignole-Baudouin F, Riancho L, Guenoun JM, Warnet JM, Baudouin C. In vitro effects of preservative-free tafluprost and preserved latanoprost, travoprost, and bimatoprost in a conjunctival epithelial cell line. Curr Eye Res. 2008 Apr;33(4):303-12.
[25] Baudouin C, Riancho L, Warnet JM, Brignole F. In vitro studies of antiglaucomatous prostaglandin analogues: travoprost with and without benzalkonium chloride and preserved latanoprost. Invest Ophthalmol Vis Sci. 2007 Sep;48(9):4123-8.
[26] Slater K. Cytotoxicity tests for high-throughput drug discovery. Curr Opin Biotechnol. 2001 Feb;12(1):70-4.
[27] Kummar S, Gutierrez M, Doroshow JH, Murgo AJ. Drug development in oncology: classical cytotoxics and molecularly targeted agents. Br J Clin Pharmacol. 2006 Jul;62(1):15-26.
[28] Stalmans P, Van Aken EH, Veckeneer M, Feron EJ, Stalmans I. Toxic effect of indocyanine green on retinal pigment epithelium related to osmotic effects of the solvent. Am J Ophthalmol. 2002 Aug;134(2):282-5.
[29] Jin Y, Uchida S, Yanagi Y, Aihara M, Araie M. Neurotoxic effects of trypan blue on rat retinal ganglion cells. Exp Eye Res. 2005 Oct;81(4):395-400.
[30] Narayanan R, Kenney MC, Kamjoo S, Trinh TH, Seigel GM, Resende GP, et al. Trypan blue: effect on retinal pigment epithelial and neurosensory retinal cells. Invest Ophthalmol Vis Sci. 2005 Jan;46(1):304-9.
[31] Limb GA, Salt TE, Munro PM, Moss SE, Khaw PT. In vitro characterization of a spontaneously immortalized human Muller cell line (MIO-M1). Invest Ophthalmol Vis Sci. 2002 Mar;43(3):864-9.
[32] Bargagna-Mohan P, Ravindranath PP, Mohan R. Small molecule anti-angiogenic probes of the ubiquitin proteasome pathway: potential application to choroidal neovascularization. Invest Ophthalmol Vis Sci. 2006 Sep;47(9):4138-45.
[33] Dreyfuss JL, Regatieri CV, Lima MA, Paredes-Gamero EJ, Brito AS, Chavante SF, et al. A heparin mimetic isolated from a marine shrimp suppresses neovascularization. J Thromb Haemost. 2010 Aug;8(8):1828-37.

[34] Edwards BS, Ivnitski-Steele I, Young SM, Salas VM, Sklar LA. High-throughput cytotoxicity screening by propidium iodide staining. Curr Protoc Cytom. 2007 Jul;Chapter 9:Unit9 24.
[35] Chang YS, Wu CL, Tseng SH, Kuo PY, Tseng SY. In vitro benzyl alcohol cytotoxicity: implications for intravitreal use of triamcinolone acetonide. Exp Eye Res. 2008 Jun;86(6):942-50.
[36] Reynolds CP, Kang MH, Keshelava N, Maurer BJ. Assessing combinations of cytotoxic agents using leukemia cell lines. Curr Drug Targets. 2007 Jun;8(6):765-71.
[37] Mosmann T. Rapid colorimetric assay for cellular growth and survival: application to proliferation and cytotoxicity assays. J Immunol Methods. 1983 Dec 16;65(1-2):55-63.
[38] Nascimento FD, Rizzi CC, Nantes IL, Stefe I, Turk B, Carmona AK, et al. Cathepsin X binds to cell surface heparan sulfate proteoglycans. Arch Biochem Biophys. 2005 Apr 15;436(2):323-32.
[39] Ammons WS, Wang JW, Yang Z, Tidmarsh GF, Hoffman RM. A novel alkylating agent, glufosfamide, enhances the activity of gemcitabine in vitro and in vivo. Neoplasia. 2007 Aug;9(8):625-33.
[40] Queiroz AF, Silva RA, Moura RM, Dreyfuss JL, Paredes-Gamero EJ, Souza AC, et al. Growth inhibitory activity of a novel lectin from Cliona varians against K562 human erythroleukemia cells. Cancer Chemother Pharmacol. 2009 May;63(6):1023-33.
[41] El Bradey M, Cheng L, Bartsch DU, Appelt K, Rodanant N, Bergeron-Lynn G, et al. Preventive versus treatment effect of AG3340, a potent matrix metalloproteinase inhibitor in a rat model of choroidal neovascularization. J Ocul Pharmacol Ther. 2004 Jun;20(3):217-36.
[42] Dierks D, Lei B, Zhang K, Hainsworth DP. Electroretinographic effects of an intravitreal injection of triamcinolone in rabbit retina. Arch Ophthalmol. 2005 Nov;123(11):1563-9.
[43] Husain D, Kim I, Gauthier D, Lane AM, Tsilimbaris MK, Ezra E, et al. Safety and efficacy of intravitreal injection of ranibizumab in combination with verteporfin PDT on experimental choroidal neovascularization in the monkey. Arch Ophthalmol. 2005 Apr;123(4):509-16.
[44] Weymouth AE, Vingrys AJ. Rodent electroretinography: methods for extraction and interpretation of rod and cone responses. Prog Retin Eye Res. 2008 Jan;27(1):1-44.
[45] Rosolen SG, Rigaudiere F, Le Gargasson JF, Brigell MG. Recommendations for a toxicological screening ERG procedure in laboratory animals. Doc Ophthalmol. 2005 Jan;110(1):57-66.
[46] Lu F, Adelman RA. Are intravitreal bevacizumab and ranibizumab effective in a rat model of choroidal neovascularization? Graefes Arch Clin Exp Ophthalmol. 2009 Feb;247(2):171-7.
[47] Scott DL, Kingsley GH. Tumor necrosis factor inhibitors for rheumatoid arthritis. N Engl J Med. 2006 Aug 17;355(7):704-12.
[48] Edrees AF, Misra SN, Abdou NI. Anti-tumor necrosis factor (TNF) therapy in rheumatoid arthritis: correlation of TNF-alpha serum level with clinical response and benefit from changing dose or frequency of infliximab infusions. Clin Exp Rheumatol. 2005 Jul-Aug;23(4):469-74.

[49] Pessler F, Monash B, Rettig P, Forbes B, Kreiger PA, Cron RQ. Sjogren syndrome in a child: favorable response of the arthritis to TNFalpha blockade. Clin Rheumatol. 2006 Sep;25(5):746-8.
[50] Vazquez-Cobian LB, Flynn T, Lehman TJ. Adalimumab therapy for childhood uveitis. J Pediatr. 2006 Oct;149(4):572-5.
[51] Olson JL, Courtney RJ, Mandava N. Intravitreal infliximab and choroidal neovascularization in an animal model. Arch Ophthalmol. 2007 Sep;125(9):1221-4.
[52] Shi X, Semkova I, Muther PS, Dell S, Kociok N, Joussen AM. Inhibition of TNF-alpha reduces laser-induced choroidal neovascularization. Exp Eye Res. 2006 Dec;83(6):1325-34.
[53] Limb GA, Soomro H, Janikoun S, Hollifield RD, Shilling J. Evidence for control of tumour necrosis factor-alpha (TNF-alpha) activity by TNF receptors in patients with proliferative diabetic retinopathy. Clin Exp Immunol. 1999 Mar;115(3):409-14.
[54] Doganay S, Evereklioglu C, Er H, Turkoz Y, Sevinc A, Mehmet N, et al. Comparison of serum NO, TNF-alpha, IL-1beta, sIL-2R, IL-6 and IL-8 levels with grades of retinopathy in patients with diabetes mellitus. Eye (Lond). 2002 Mar;16(2):163-70.
[55] Zhao B, Smith G, Cai J, Ma A, Boulton M. Vascular endothelial growth factor C promotes survival of retinal vascular endothelial cells via vascular endothelial growth factor receptor-2. Br J Ophthalmol. 2007 Apr;91(4):538-45.
[56] Campochiaro PA, Glaser BM. Platelet-derived growth factor is chemotactic for human retinal pigment epithelial cells. Arch Ophthalmol. 1985 Apr;103(4):576-9.
[57] Bergers G, Song S. The role of pericytes in blood-vessel formation and maintenance. Neuro Oncol. 2005 Oct;7(4):452-64.
[58] Campochiaro PA. Targeted pharmacotherapy of retinal diseases with ranibizumab. Drugs Today (Barc). 2007 Aug;43(8):529-37.
[59] Campochiaro PA. Seeing the light: new insights into the molecular pathogenesis of retinal diseases. J Cell Physiol. 2007 Nov;213(2):348-54.
[60] Campochiaro PA. Molecular targets for retinal vascular diseases. J Cell Physiol. 2007 Mar;210(3):575-81.
[61] Ciulla TA, Rosenfeld PJ. Antivascular endothelial growth factor therapy for neovascular age-related macular degeneration. Curr Opin Ophthalmol. 2009 May;20(3):158-65.
[62] Avraamides CJ, Garmy-Susini B, Varner JA. Integrins in angiogenesis and lymphangiogenesis. Nat Rev Cancer. 2008 Aug;8(8):604-17.
[63] Wang W, Wang F, Lu F, Xu S, Hu W, Huang J, et al. The Anti-angiogenic Effects of Integrin {alpha}5{beta}1 Inhibitor (ATN-161) in Vitro and in Vivo. Invest Ophthalmol Vis Sci. 2010 Aug 3.
[64] Cross MJ, Claesson-Welsh L. FGF and VEGF function in angiogenesis: signalling pathways, biological responses and therapeutic inhibition. Trends Pharmacol Sci. 2001 Apr;22(4):201-7.
[65] Nguyen M, Arnheiter H. Signaling and transcriptional regulation in early mammalian eye development: a link between FGF and MITF. Development. 2000 Aug;127(16):3581-91.
[66] Nakazawa T, Matsubara A, Noda K, Hisatomi T, She H, Skondra D, et al. Characterization of cytokine responses to retinal detachment in rats. Mol Vis. 2006;12:867-78.

[67] Chamberlain CG, McAvoy JW. Evidence that fibroblast growth factor promotes lens fibre differentiation. Curr Eye Res. 1987 Sep;6(9):1165-9.
[68] Campochiaro PA. Retinal and choroidal neovascularization. J Cell Physiol. 2000 Sep;184(3):301-10.
[69] Dreyfuss JL, Regatieri CV, Jarrouge TR, Cavalheiro RP, Sampaio LO, Nader HB. Heparan sulfate proteoglycans: structure, protein interactions and cell signaling. An Acad Bras Cienc. 2009 Sep;81(3):409-29.
[70] Mataveli FD, Han SW, Nader HB, Mendes A, Kanishiro R, Tucci P, et al. Long-term effects for acute phase myocardial infarct VEGF165 gene transfer cardiac extracellular matrix remodeling. Growth Factors. 2009 Feb;27(1):22-31.
[71] Tkachenko E, Rhodes JM, Simons M. Syndecans: new kids on the signaling block. Circ Res. 2005 Mar 18;96(5):488-500.
[72] Soler R, Bruschini H, Martins JR, Dreyfuss JL, Camara NO, Alves MT, et al. Urinary glycosaminoglycans as biomarker for urothelial injury: is it possible to discriminate damage from recovery? Urology. 2008 Oct;72(4):937-42.
[73] Dreyfuss JL, Veiga SS, Coulson-Thomas VJ, Santos IA, Toma L, Coletta RD, et al. Differences in the expression of glycosaminoglycans in human fibroblasts derived from gingival overgrowths is related to TGF-beta up-regulation. Growth Factors. 2010 Feb;28(1):24-33.
[74] Dietrich CP. Novel heparin degradation products. Isolation and characterization of novel disaccharides and oligosaccharides produced from heparin by bacterial degradation. Biochem J. 1968 Jul;108(4):647-54.
[75] Young E. The anti-inflammatory effects of heparin and related compounds. Thromb Res. 2008;122(6):743-52.
[76] Brito AS, Arimateia DS, Souza LR, Lima MA, Santos VO, Medeiros VP, et al. Anti-inflammatory properties of a heparin-like glycosaminoglycan with reduced anti-coagulant activity isolated from a marine shrimp. Bioorg Med Chem. 2008 Nov 1;16(21):9588-95.
[77] Tang WQ, He SZ, Liang XM, Hou BK. [The preliminary study of Phosphomannopentaose sulfate (PI-88) on the experimental choroidal neovascularization]. Zhonghua Yan Ke Za Zhi. 2008 Sep;44(9):813-9.
[78] Tomida D, Nishiguchi KM, Kataoka K, Yasuma TR, Iwata E, Uetani R, et al. Suppression of choroidal neovascularization and quantitative and qualitative inhibition of VEGF and CCL2 by heparin. Invest Ophthalmol Vis Sci. 2011 May;52(6):3193-9.
[79] Zarbin MA, Rosenfeld PJ. Pathway-based therapies for age-related macular degeneration: an integrated survey of emerging treatment alternatives. Retina. 2010 Oct;30(9):1350-67.
[80] Rohrer B, Coughlin B, Kunchithapautham K, Long Q, Tomlinson S, Takahashi K, et al. The alternative pathway is required, but not alone sufficient, for retinal pathology in mouse laser-induced choroidal neovascularization. Mol Immunol. Mar;48(6-7):e1-8.
[81] Kijlstra A, La Heij E, Hendrikse F. Immunological factors in the pathogenesis and treatment of age-related macular degeneration. Ocul Immunol Inflamm. 2005 Feb;13(1):3-11.

[82] Ni Z, Hui P. Emerging pharmacologic therapies for wet age-related macular degeneration. Ophthalmologica. 2009;223(6):401-10.
[83] Chappelow AV, Kaiser PK. Neovascular age-related macular degeneration: potential therapies. Drugs. 2008;68(8):1029-36.
[84] Maier P, Unsoeld AS, Junker B, Martin G, Drevs J, Hansen LL, et al. Intravitreal injection of specific receptor tyrosine kinase inhibitor PTK787/ZK222 584 improves ischemia-induced retinopathy in mice. Graefes Arch Clin Exp Ophthalmol. 2005 Jun;243(6):593-600.
[85] Park YH, Roh SY, Lee YC. Effect of sorafenib on experimental choroidal neovascularization in the rat. Clin Experiment Ophthalmol. Oct;38(7):718-26.
[86] Mousa SA, Mousa SS. Current status of vascular endothelial growth factor inhibition in age-related macular degeneration. BioDrugs. Jun;24(3):183-94.
[87] Jost D, Nowojewski A, Levine E. Small RNA biology is systems biology. BMB Rep. Jan;44(1):11-21.
[88] Campochiaro PA. Potential applications for RNAi to probe pathogenesis and develop new treatments for ocular disorders. Gene Ther. 2006 Mar;13(6):559-62.
[89] Tolentino M. Interference RNA technology in the treatment of CNV. Ophthalmol Clin North Am. 2006 Sep;19(3):393-9, vi-vii.
[90] Kaiser PK, Symons RC, Shah SM, Quinlan EJ, Tabandeh H, Do DV, et al. RNAi-based treatment for neovascular age-related macular degeneration by Sirna-027. Am J Ophthalmol. Jul;150(1):33-9 e2.
[91] Campa C, Harding SP. Anti-VEGF compounds in the treatment of neovascular age related macular degeneration. Curr Drug Targets. Feb;12(2):173-81.
[92] Gu L, Chen H, Tuo J, Gao X, Chen L. Inhibition of experimental choroidal neovascularization in mice by anti-VEGFA/VEGFR2 or non-specific siRNA. Exp Eye Res. Sep;91(3):433-9.
[93] Jiang J, Xia XB, Xu HZ, Xiong Y, Song WT, Xiong SQ, et al. Inhibition of retinal neovascularization by gene transfer of small interfering RNA targeting HIF-1alpha and VEGF. J Cell Physiol. 2009 Jan;218(1):66-74.
[94] Nakamura H, Siddiqui SS, Shen X, Malik AB, Pulido JS, Kumar NM, et al. RNA interference targeting transforming growth factor-beta type II receptor suppresses ocular inflammation and fibrosis. Mol Vis. 2004 Oct 4;10:703-11.
[95] Lingor P, Koeberle P, Kugler S, Bahr M. Down-regulation of apoptosis mediators by RNAi inhibits axotomy-induced retinal ganglion cell death in vivo. Brain. 2005 Mar;128(Pt 3):550-8.
[96] Kay MA. State-of-the-art gene-based therapies: the road ahead. Nat Rev Genet. 2011 May;12(5):316-28.
[97] Campochiaro PA. Gene transfer for neovascular age-related macular degeneration. Hum Gene Ther. 2011 May;22(5):523-9.
[98] Mori K, Duh E, Gehlbach P, Ando A, Takahashi K, Pearlman J, et al. Pigment epithelium-derived factor inhibits retinal and choroidal neovascularization. J Cell Physiol. 2001 Aug;188(2):253-63.
[99] Zhou XY, Liao Q, Pu YM, Tang YQ, Gong X, Li J, et al. Ultrasound-mediated microbubble delivery of pigment epithelium-derived factor gene into retina inhibits choroidal neovascularization. Chin Med J (Engl). 2009 Nov 20;122(22):2711-7.

[100] Bainbridge JW, Mistry A, De Alwis M, Paleolog E, Baker A, Thrasher AJ, et al. Inhibition of retinal neovascularisation by gene transfer of soluble VEGF receptor sFlt-1. Gene Ther. 2002 Mar;9(5):320-6.
[101] Lai CM, Brankov M, Zaknich T, Lai YK, Shen WY, Constable IJ, et al. Inhibition of angiogenesis by adenovirus-mediated sFlt-1 expression in a rat model of corneal neovascularization. Hum Gene Ther. 2001 Jul 1;12(10):1299-310.
[102] Lai CM, Shen WY, Brankov M, Lai YK, Barnett NL, Lee SY, et al. Long-term evaluation of AAV-mediated sFlt-1 gene therapy for ocular neovascularization in mice and monkeys. Mol Ther. 2005 Oct;12(4):659-68.
[103] Folkman J. Antiangiogenesis in cancer therapy--endostatin and its mechanisms of action. Exp Cell Res. 2006 Mar 10;312(5):594-607.
[104] Mori K, Ando A, Gehlbach P, Nesbitt D, Takahashi K, Goldsteen D, et al. Inhibition of choroidal neovascularization by intravenous injection of adenoviral vectors expressing secretable endostatin. Am J Pathol. 2001 Jul;159(1):313-20.
[105] Cheng HC, Yeh SI, Tsao YP, Kuo PC. Subconjunctival injection of recombinant AAV-angiostatin ameliorates alkali burn induced corneal angiogenesis. Mol Vis. 2007;13:2344-52.
[106] Viita H, Kinnunen K, Eriksson E, Lahteenvuo J, Babu M, Kalesnykas G, et al. Intravitreal adenoviral 15-lipoxygenase-1 gene transfer prevents vascular endothelial growth factor A-induced neovascularization in rabbit eyes. Hum Gene Ther. 2009 Dec;20(12):1679-86.

6

Basic Research and Clinical Application of Drug Delivery Systems for the Treatment of Age-Related Macular Degeneration

Giuseppe Lo Giudice and Alessandro Galan
San Paolo Ophthalimc Center, San Antonio Hospital
Italy

1. Introduction

The eye is in specific environment to resist pharmaceutical approaches. Vitreoretinal diseases, including age-related macular degeneration (AMD) (Green & Enger, 1993; Sarks, 1976; van der Schaft et al., 1992), are refractory to both topical and systemic pharmacological approaches because of specific environment of the eye. More recently, a variety of pharmacological challenges to treat exudative age-related macular degeneration and macular edema are proceeding into clinical trials, as soon as antivascular endothelial growth factor (anti-VEGF) therapies have been proved to be effective by repeated intravitreal injections. Monthly injections of anti-VEGF therapies to maximize visual potential are a significant treatment burden on the patient. As a result, the need for better treatments for AMD remains (Brown et al., 2006; Geroski & Edelhauser, 2000; Hughes, 2005; Rosenfeld et al., 2006) (Figure 1).

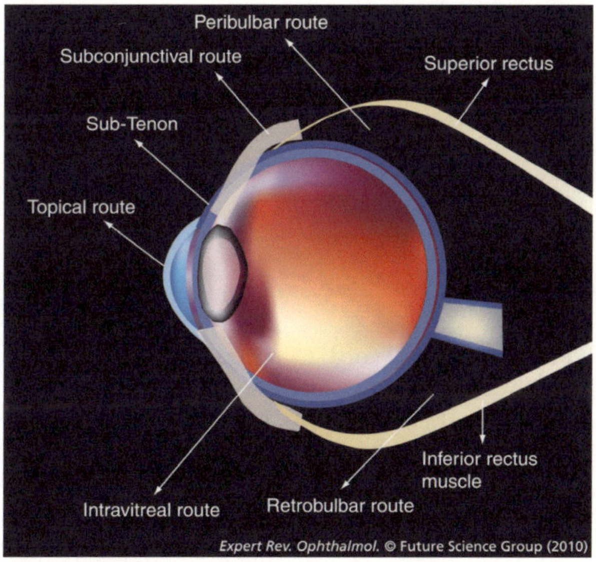

Fig. 1. Different methods of drug delivery

Opthalmic drug delivery is one of the most interesting and challenging endeavors facing the pharmaceutical scientist. A significant challenge to the formulator is to circumvent the protective barriers of the eye without causing permanent tissue damage. Development of newer, more sensitive diagnostic techniques and novel therapeutic agents continue to provide ocular delivery systems with high therapeutic efficacy. The goal of pharmacotherapeutics is to treat a disease in a consistent and predictable fashion. The efficacy of a compound is governed by its intrinsic effects on the target site (and any other sites with which it comes into contact), its distribution throughout and its elimination from the body. Alterations to the and elimination of a compound can thus radically alter its efficacy. For regions of the body with a significant barrier to drug permeation, such as the eye and brain, great care should be taken to deliver drugs appropriately (Figure 2).

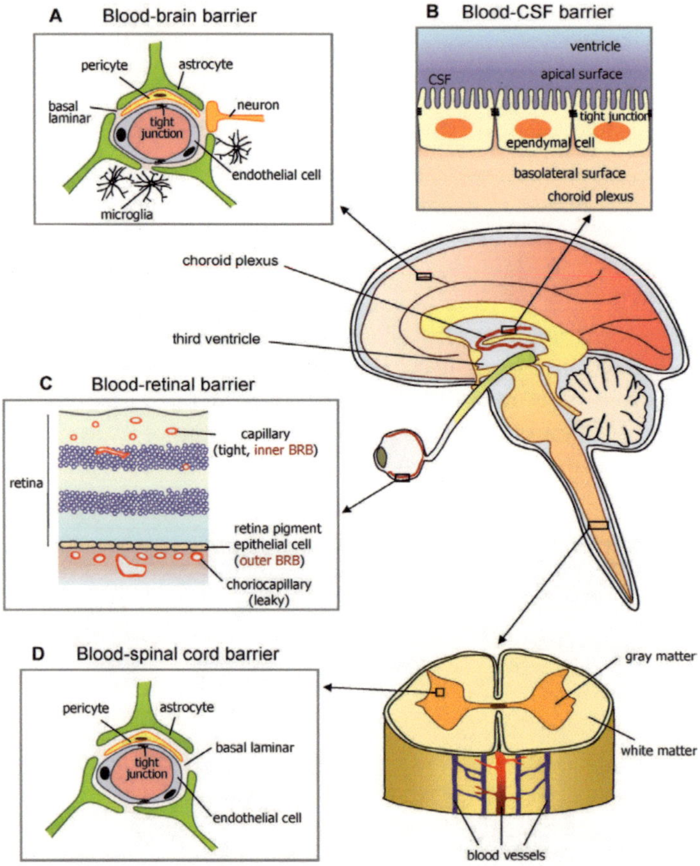

Fig. 2. Diagram of the brain and spinal cord. Diagram of the brain and spinal cord illustrating how the eye's inner and outer blood-retinal barriers (BRBs) fit into the overall scheme of blood-neural barriers (BNBs) Barriers between the blood and neural tissues are collectively referred to as BNBs and include the blood-brain barrier (A), the blood-CSF barrier (B), the BRB (C), and the blood-spinal cord barrier (D). Considering that several retinal disorders are accompanied by dysfunction or breakdown of this BRB and their associated cell-cell signaling mechanisms, elucidating the nature of the BRB is important for under standing normal health and disease (Choi & Kim, 2008).

In the design of a drug delivery system for the eye a balance must be struck between the limitations imposed by the physicochemical properties of the drugs, the limitations imposed by the anatomy and disease state of the eye, and the dosing requirements of the drug for that particular disease. In the recent past years review articles have focused on drug delivery to the eye (Acharya & Young 2004; Andreoli & Miller, 2007; Barar, Javadzadeh & Omidi, 2008; Barocas & Balachandran 2008; Bekeredjian, Katus & Kuecherer, 2006; Booth et al. 2007; Del Amo & Urtti, 2008; Gaudana et al. 2009; Hoffman, 2008; Hsu, 2007; Lee & Robinson, 2009; Lemley & Han, 2007; Liu & Regillo, 2004; Mitra, 2009; Novack, 2009; Sultana et al., 2006). The aim of this chapter is to emphasize recent advances in ocular drug delivery techniques most suitable for AMD.

2. Ocular delivery systems

2.1 Ocular barriers

The eye is in specific environment to resist pharmaceutical approaches (Maurice & Mishima, 1984). Systemically administered drug cannot easily reach the retina and vitreous cavity due to the blood-aqueous barrier, composed of ciliary non-pigmented epithelium and iridal vascular endothelium with tight junction (TJ) and the outer and inner BRB, which are formed by the retinal pigment epithelium (RPE) and retinal vascular endothelium, respectively. On the other hand, an eyeball is covered with collagenous walls (e.g. cornea and sclera) and epithelial and endothelial barriers (e.g. cornea and RPE). These barriers, continuous tear drainage, frontward flow of aqueous humor, and surrounding blood circulations limit the penetration of administered drug (e.g. eye drops and ointments) (Figure 3)

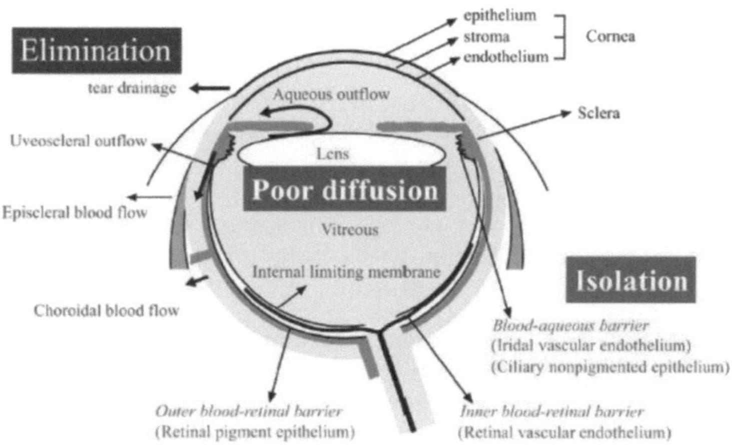

Fig. 3. Possible barriers interfering drug delivery into the eye (Tsutomu, Yasuhiko & Hideya et al. 2011)

Compliance is also problematic, particularly among patients who have chronic diseases such as glaucoma and refractory chorioretinal diseases, including uveitis, macular edema, neovascular (wet) and atrophic (dry) AMD, and retinitis pigmentosa. In this section, the function of ocular barrier systems is briefly described (Table 1).

Drug Delivery Mode	Intravitreal Injection	Sub-Tenon's Injection	Suprachoroidal/Intrascleral Hollow Microneedle Injection	Topical Drops	Systemic Oral Pills
Pathway to target posterior segment	Direct	Transscleral	Transchoroidal	Transconjunctival/ transscleral	Trans-RPE
Safety					
Risk	Highest injection risk	Highest injection risk, mild systemic exposure	Minimal injection risk, minimal systemic exposure	Safest, but moderate systemic exposure	Minimal local exposure; highest systemic exposure
Adverse Events	Vitreous hemorrhage, retinal detachment, endophthalmitis	Subconjunctival hemorrhage	Subconjunctival hemorrhage, suprachoroidal hemorrhage	Conjunctival redness and irritation	Gastrointestinal upset
Efficacy	Most direct and effective (only mode that directly penetrates BRB)	Much less bioavailable to the vitreous and retina	80-fold more bioavailable than sub-Tenon's injection	Worst bioavailability and second worst duration of action; convenient and can be self-administered at home	Second worst bioavailability and worst duration of action
Peak bioavailability					
Intravitreal	100%	0.01%–0.1%	0.8%–70%	0%–0.0004%	0%–2%
Intra-aqueous humor	3%	0.008%–0.8%	0.02%–2.1%	0.0007%–5%	1%–2%
Duration of action	21 Hours to 7 weeks	6 Hours to 1 month	18 Hours to 3 months	30 Minutes to 4 hours	<30 Minutes

Table 1. Drug delivery routes for Age-related macular de generation

2.2 Tear, cornea, conjunctiva and sclera

Tear: One of the precorneal barriers is tear film which reduces the effective concentration of the administrated drugs due to dilution by the tear turnover (approximately 1 μL/min), accelerated clearance, and binding of the drug molecule to the tear proteins (Craig, 2002).

Cornea: The cornea consists of three layers; epithelium, stroma and endothelium, with each one possessing a different polarity, rate-limiting structure for drug penetration and a mechanical barrier to inhibit transport of exogenous substances into the eye (Pederson, 2006). The corneal epithelium is characterized by tight junctions among cells; these are formed to restrict paracellular drug permeation from the tear film. The highly hydrated structure of the stroma (extracellular matrix of a lamellar arrangement of collagen fibrils) acts as a barrier to permeation of lipophilic drug molecules. Corneal endothelium acts as a separating barrier between the stroma and aqueous humor (Fischbarg, 2006). .

Conjunctiva: Conjunctiva or episclera has a rich supply of capillaries and lymphatics therefore, administrated drugs in the conjunctival or episcleral space may be cleared through blood and lymph (Gausas, Gonnering, Lemke, et al. 1999; Singh, 2003; Sugar, Riazi, & Schaffner, 1957). The conjunctival blood vessels do not form a TJ barrier which means drug molecules can enter into the blood circulation by pinocytosis and/or convective transport through paracellular pores in the vascular endothelial layer. The conjunctival lymphatics act as an efflux system for the efficient elimination from the conjunctival space. Drugs transported by lymphatics in conjunction with the elimination by blood circulation can contribute to systemic exposure, since the interstitial fluid is returned to the systemic circulation after filtration through lymph nodes (Lee, He, Robinson, et al. 2010).

Slera: Scleral permeability has been shown to have a strong dependence on the molecular radius (it consists of collagen fibers and proteoglycans embedded in an extracellular matrix); scleral permeability decreases roughly exponentially with molecular radius (Oyster, 1999). The ideal location for transscleral drug delivery is near the equator at 12–17 mm posterior to the corneoscleral limbus. Hydrophobicity of drugs affects scleral permeability; increase of lipophilicity shows lower permeability; and hydrophilic drugs may diffuse through the aqueous medium of proteoglycans in the fiber matrix pores more easily than lipophilic drugs.

2.3 Choroid/Bruch's membrane and retina

Choroid/Bruch's Membrane: Choroid is one of the most highly vascularized tissues of the body. The choroidal capillary endothelial cells are fenestrated and, are relatively large in diameter (20–40 μm). Previous histological studies have shown choroidal thickness changes from 200 μm at birth decreasing to about 80 μm by age 90 (Spaide, 2009). In contrast, Bruch's membrane (BM) causes thickening with age (Tout, Chan-Ling, Hollander, et al. 1993). These changes cause increased calcification of elastic fibers, increased cross-linkage of collagen fibers and increased turnover of glycosaminoglycans. Thickness changes of choroid and BM might affect drug permeability from subconjunctiva or episcleral space into the retina and the vitreous (Farboud, Aotaki-Keen, Miyata, et al. 1999; Handa, Verzijl, Matsunaga, et al. 1999; Hewitt, Nakazawa & Newsome, 1989; Hewitt & Newsome, 1985; Spraul, Lang, Grossniklaus, H.E. et al. 1999; Tout, Chan-Ling, Hollander, et al. 1993; Yamada, Ishibashi, Bhutto, et al. 2006).

Retina: in the vitreous drugs are eliminated by two main routes from anterior and posterior segments. Elimination via the posterior route takes place by permeation across the retina. In intact retina, the drugs in the subretinal fluid could either be absorbed by the sensory retinal blood vessels or transported across the RPE, where it may be absorbed into the choroidal vessels or pass through the sclera. Drug transport across the RPE takes place both by transcellular and paracellular routes. The driving forces of outward transport of molecules from the subretinal spaces are hydrostatic and osmotic, and small molecules might transport through the paracellular inter-RPE cellular clefts and by active transport through the transcellular route (Pederson, 2006).

2.4 Blood retinal barrier

The BRB controls the flux of fluid and blood-borne elements into the neural parenchyma, helping to establish the unique neural environment necessary for proper neural function.

BRB restricts drug transport from blood into the retina. BRB is composed of tight junctions (TJ) of retinal capillary endothelial cells and RPE, called iBRB for the inner and oBRB for the outer BRB, respectively. The function of iBRB is supported by Müller cells and astrocytes (Cunha-Vaz, 1979).

Müller cells are known to support neuronal activity and maintain the proper functioning of the iBRB under normal conditions.The astrocytes are closely associated with the retinal capillary vessels and help to maintain the capillary integrity (Zhang & Stone, 1997). Astrocytes are known to increase the barrier properties of the retinal vascular endothelium by enhancing the expression of the tight junction protein ZO-1 and modifying endothelial morphology (Gardner, Lieth, Khin, et al. 1997).

Following systemic drug administration, drugs can easily enter into the choroid since choroid is highly vascularized tissue compared to retina. The choriocapillaris are fenestrated resulting in rapid equilibration of drug molecules present in the bloodstream with the extravascular space of the choroid. Therefore, oBRB (RPE) restricts further entry of drugs from the choroid into the retina. RPE is a monolayer of highly specialized hexagonal-shaped cells, located between the sensory retina and the choroid. The TJ of the RPE efficiently restrict intercellular permeation into the sensory retina. Dysfunction of Müller cells may contribute to a breakdown of the iBRB in many pathological conditions (Tretiach, Madigan, Wen, et al. 2005). Müller cells enhance the secretion of VEGF under hypoxic and inflammatory conditions (Eichler, Kuhrt, Hoffmann, et al. 2000; Kaur, Sivakumar & Foulds, 2006). VEGF-induced occluding phosphorylation and ubiquitination causes trafficking of tight junction and leads to increased retinal vascular permeability (Murakami, Felinski & Antonetti, 2009).

3. Drug delivery systems to posterior segment of the eye and specific delivery systems

In drug delivery, a more common situation is one where the rate of change of concentration is directly proportional to the concentration of drug present, and drug's potential to diffuse from one region to another is directly proportional to its chemical potential, which can usually be approximated to its concentration. This situation is termed first order and can be expressed as (Higuchi, 1961)

$$- dc/dt = kc$$

where dc is the change in concentration, dt is the time interval over which that change occurs, k is a constant, also known as the rate constant, and it is in function of concentration.

Integrating this with respect to time gives (Peppas, 1995)

$$\ln C_t - \ln C_0 = - kt$$

where C_0 is the initial concentration and C_t is the concentration at time t.

A more common situation arises when drug release is both a function of its concentration within a vehicle and its ability to diffusion through it. When placed into a release medium, the drug closest to the surface is released the fastest. Over a period of time, the drug must diffuse from further and further back within the bulk of the device, which progressively slows the release.

Systems such as this can be described by solutions to Ficks's second law of diffusion (Knight, 1981)

$$\partial C/\partial t = D\partial^2 C/dx^2$$

where C is the concentration in a reservoir, t the time, x the distance and D the diffusion coefficient the diffusant through the media. Partial derivatives (∂) are used because C is a function of both t and x.

These formulae can be readily applied to drug release from ointments and gels typically used in eye drops, but an objective difficulty exist in finding a flawless technique to deliver drugs targeting diseases that directly affect the retina and vitreous humor, owing to the anatomic barriers and physiologic clearance mechanisms of the BRB. In this scenario a relevant implication have the importance of the transcellular and paracellular transport pathways across or between epithelial or endothelial BRBs. TJs are the most apical component of both the epithelial or endothelial intercellular junctional complexes. TJs are crucial for the formation and maintenance of epithelial and endothelial paracellular barriers since they semipermeably regulate intercellular passive diffusion of large or hydrophilic ions and solutes. Moreover, a complex network of TJ proteins have been identified, with the assembly and dynamic maintenance of various claudin proteins being the most crucial in regard to dictating the selectivity of this paracellular barrier. Using the transcellular route, drugs are delivered by simple passive diffusion to bind with cell surface membrane–bound transporters (cell surface receptors, pumps, channels, and transporters) where they can directly cross the cell via passive diffusion again or through active transport mechanisms. Various influx and efflux transporters have been found for small lipophilic peptides, organic anions, and cations. Transporter-mediated drug delivery is tissue-specific and has low toxicity since transmembrane concentration gradients are not required for it works. The transcellular pathway is not suitable for high-throughput production of drug candidates though, unlike the paracellular pathway, which is suitable for highthroughput production since drug modification is not needed and one method can be applied for various drugs. Knowing the rate-limiting tissue barrier based on the physiochemical properties of a drug helps when optimizing the absorption of passively penetrated drugs.

3.1 Intravitreal injections and intraocular drug delivery

Intraocular drug delivery is the only mode that currently directly broaches the BRB and thereby attains the highest peak intravitreal or intraretinal drug concentrations. However, intraocular drug delivery is the most invasive than other approaches, in that it involves penetrating the globe and thus is not free of injection-related complications. These complications may include trauma and increased risk of cataract, retinal detachment, hemorrhage and endophthalmitis (Jager, Aiello, Patel, et al. 2004).

Moreover, the presence of some moderate clearance mechanisms (posterior transretinal and anterior aqueous humor elimination pathways) cause the peak drug concentration levels achieved with intraocular administration to decline to non-therapeutic trough levels over time, unless the injections are given frequently and repeatedly. The disadvantage caused by the short to medium duration of action of intravitreal drug solutions has been partially alleviated through product formulation or drug device development. Currently, despite its shortcomings, intravitreal administration is the preferred drug delivery route to treat diseases of the posterior segment being the better approach achieving the highest intraocular bioavailability in posterior segment tissues such as the cone-containing macula or fovea.

Anti-VEGF drugs, such as pegaptanib, ranibizumab and bevacizumab are new intravitreal treatments for AMD. To understand the pharmacokinetics of intravitreal drug delivery a great attention should be made to understanding the molecular structure of the normal human vitreous gel and that normal vitreous gel undergoes age-related degenerative liquefaction. It was shown that immediately after intravitreal injection, drugs initially concentrate near the injection site or in the cisternae forming vitreous concentration gradients before distributing throughout the entire vitreous cavity and then reaching steady state equilibrium levels (Lee SS, et al. IOVS 2009;50:ARVO E-Abstract 5950). The location of implant placement in the vitreous (anterior placement behind lens versus posterior placement near the retina) influences drug levels in various tissues. When the implant was placed in the posterior region, drug levels were higher in the posterior retina, choroid-RPE and sclera and lower in the anterior retina, choroid-RPE, and sclera. Posterior placement of the implant is likely to support release of the drug to target tissues in case of retinal disorders. Although the posterior implant reduced drug levels in the lens, no such advantage was found with respect to corticosteroid levels in the trabecular meshwork, possibly due to the high affinity of the drug for this tissue.

After intravitreal placement of an implant, drug levels are not likely to achieve a uniform level throughout the vitreous. However, it is probable that a slow release system achieves zones of steady state concentration, with the contours dictated by the clearance mechanisms of a given therapeutic agent. The reason for such zones or contours of steady state concentration is not necessarily diffusion limitation, but rather the presence of continuous dynamic clearance mechanisms in the posterior segment. There are two main mechanisms of drug clearance for intravitreally administered drugs in the eye: the anterior elimination pathway via counterdirectional bulk aqueous flow and the posterior elimination pathway via vitreoretinochoroidal bulk flow due to hydrostatic and osmotic pressure gradients in the inner, middle, and outer coats of the posterior segment (Kim, Lutz, Wang, et al. 2007). An additional mechanism to consider is the transcellular carrier–mediated transporters found on the RPE. Influx transporters enhance the penetration of drugs and efflux transporters inhibit retention of drugs across the outer (o)BRB (Mannermaa, Vellonen & Urtti, 2006). The duration of action of an intravitreally administered drug may in part depend on the retention of the injected drug at the site of administration. The longer the intravitreal half-life, the greater the anticipated duration of therapeutic response. The half-lives of drugs that are eliminated through both the retina and the aqueous humor, such as small lipophilic drugs, tend to be shorter than the half-lives of drugs eliminated primarily via the anterior route, such as large hydrophilic drugs, and also intravitreal drug elimination depends on the molecular weight (MW) of the drug, with larger MW (> 70,000) drugs displaying longer half-lives. To overcoming the short to medium duration of action of intravitreal drug solutions is the use of one of several available sustained drug release systems. These systems may act through formulation modification to decrease the solubility of the drug via a suspension or to enhance the residence time in vitreous humor via a biodegradable implant, or through the use of a sustained release delivery device.

3.2 Non-biodegradable, biodegradable implants in AMD

Non-biodegradable implants are a reservoir type, which possesses a coating of non-biodegradable polymers such as poly (vinyl alcohol) (PVA), ethylene vinyl acetate (EVA), and silicone laminate, reserving drug in the inner space. This type exhibits the most stable and long-standing release profile of drug, as compared with other types of implants, because it can reserve a large amount of drug and regulate drug release just by surface area and thickness of PVA, a permeable polymer (Okabe, Kimura, Okabe, et al. 2003; Yasukawa, Ogura, Kimura, et al. 2006; Yasukawa, Ogura, Tabata, et al. 2004). However should be considered the weakness of this type of device involving relatively large size of the device requiring a large incision for implantation, which may increase the risk of retinal complications (vitreous hemorrhage, epiretinal membrane, and retinal detachment), and potential need of removal surgery to exchange the implant or treat possible complications such as retinal detachment and drug-induced adverse effects (Callanan, 2007). As compared with non-biodegradable implants, biodegradable implants have following merits: no need of removal surgery and the flexibility in shape. They can be processed into a variety of configurations involving microparticles, a rod, a disc, or tablet. Thus, the release profile of drug from this 2nd generation biodegradable implants may become as stable as non-biodegradable ones, while the duration of drug release may be shorter due to the limitation of drug contained. The drugs in the biodegradable implants are conjugated to a variety of polymers including poly(lactic acid) (PLA), poly(glycolic acid) (PGA), poly(lactic-co-glycolic acid) (PLGA), poly(caprolactone) and poly(methylene malonate) (table 2).

Active ingredient	Brand name	Dosage form	Release-controlling excipient	target indication
fluocinolone acetonide	illuvien ®	IVT, implant	Polyimide/PVA	wet AMD, DME
Brimonidina	-	IVT, implant	PLGA	Dry AMD, RP
CNTF (NT-501)	-	IVT, implant	semipermeabile membrane/ARPE-19	RP, dry AMD

Table 2. Current and future drugs in clinical trials for posterior disease (AMD)

The ongoing clinical trial clearly indicates that biodegradable polymers are biocompatible. In the near future, many types of biodegradable implants and microparticles will proceed for clinical trial.

An injectable, rod-shaped intravitreal implant with FA (Iluvien®, Alimera Sciences, Alpharetta, GA, U.S.) (length: 3.5 mm, diameter: 0.37 mm) has been developed for the treatment of diabetic macular edema (DME). Iluvien® is made of polyimide and PVA, small enough to be injected using an inserter with a 25-gauge needle and is expected to provide sustained delivery of FA to the back of the eye for up to three years. In addition to DME, Iluvien® is in Phase II for the treatment of wet AMD compared to Lucentis®

(ClinicalTrials.gov The MAP Study: Fluocinolone acetonide (FA)/MedidurTM for age related macular degeneration (AMD) Pilot. (2010). Available online: http://clinicaltrials.gov/ct2/show/ NCT00605423?term=Iluvien&rank=12), dry AMD (ClinicalTrials.gov Fluocinolone acetonide intravitreal inserts in geographic atrophy. (2010). Available online: http://clinicaltrials.gov/ct2/show/NCT00695318?term=Iluvien&rank=15.

Brimonidine is an a2 adrenergic agonist, which can release various neurotrophins including brain-derived neurotrophic factor (BDNF) and ciliary neurotrophic factor (CNTF) (Lonngren, Napankangas, Lafuente, et al. 2006; Kim, Chang, Kim, et al. 2007). These neurotrophins have a potential to prevent apoptosis of photoreceptors and/or RPE (Azadi, Johnson, Paquet-Durand, et al. 2007; Zhang, Mo, Fang, et al. 2009). PLGA intravitreal implant with two doses (200 mg, 400 mg) of brimonidine tartrate similar to Ozurdex® is now in Phase II clinical study for dry AMD (ClinicalTrials.gov Safety and efficacy of brimonidine intravitreal implant in patients with geographic atrophy due to age-related macular degeneration (AMD). (2010). Available online: http://clinicaltrials.gov/ct2/show/NCT00658619), and phase I/II clinical trials for RP (ClinicalTrials.gov An exploratory study to evaluate the safety of brimonidine intravitreal implant in patients with retinitis pigmentosa. (2010). Available online: http://clinicaltrials.gov/ct2/show/ NCT00661479) by Allergan, Inc. Neurotech Pharmaceuticals, Inc. (Lincoln, RI, U.S.) has been developing —"Encapsulated Cell Technology", this is an implantable intravitreal device that uses genetically modified ARPE-19 RPE cells (transfected with plasmid gene insertion techniques) to release a therapeutic growth factor protein, ciliary neurotrophic factor (CNTF), with zero-order kinetics. CNTF is a neurotrophic growth factor with profound antiapoptotic effects that prolong the lives of dying photoreceptor cells. The cells are encapsulated within a semipermeable, hollow-fiber membrane, intravitreal implant device so that the CNTF protein is released to ocular tissues but the modified RPE cells are immunologically isolated from the patient, avoiding immune rejection. Phase 2 trials showed that this delivery system was safe, and a dose-dependent biological effect on the retina was observed. Potential visual benefit was also shown in patients with geographic atrophy (US National Institutes of Health. ClinicalTrials.org. NCT00447954 CgI. A Study of an Encapsulated Cell Technology (ECT) Implant for Patients With Atrophic Macular Degeneration. Phase II study. (2009). http://clinicaltrials.gov/ct2/show/NCT00447954). The duration of action of this encapsulated cell therapy device was found to be up to 2 years. Next-phase clinical trials are under way to continue to evaluate encapsulated cell technology (ECT)-CNTF's effectiveness for the treatment of dry AMD and retinitis pigmentosa.

Anti-VEGF compounds are now required to be administered into the eye every 4 to 6 weeks. Moreover, vitrectomized eyes highly increase the clearance rate of injected drugs and are, therefore, refractory to these drugs. The companies are currently interested in new methods of prolongation of residence time of intravitreally-injected drugs such as ranibizumab and pegaptanib. Viscous medium such as hyaluronic acid or gelling solution are considered as an additive to prolong drug residence in the vitreous cavity (Table 3) (Lyons, Ma & Trogde, 2009; Giese, Kaufmann & Klippel-Giese, 2004; McSwiggen, Beigelman, Macejak, et al. 2003; Robinson, Blanda, Hughes, et al. 2010; Robinson, Blanda, Liu, et al. 2010; Robinson, Tsai, Almazan, et al. 2010).

Patent No.	Activity
WO2003070918	Technology of siRNA modification to improve biological stability
WO2004015107	Technology of siRNA modification to improve biological stability
US20100015158	Intraocular delivery of anti-angiogenic antibodies in a liquid or solid polymeric vehicle such as hyaluronic acid or PLGA
WO2010009034	Intraocular delivery of anti-angiogenic antibodies in a liquid or solid polymeric vehicle such as hyaluronic acid or PLGA
US20100098772	Delivery of anti-angiogenic agents with polymeric hyaluronic acid
US20100074957	Injectable intraocular drug delivery system by use of microspheres
US20090258924	Intraocular delivery of siRNA with a polymeric component

Table 3. List of Patents on Intraocular Drug Delivery Systems

3.3 Periocular dug derlivery route in AMD

Periocular delivery includes such avenues as subconjunctival, retrobulbar, peribulbar, sub-Tenon's and intrascleral delivery. This route requires drugs to pass through several layers of ocular tissue (episclera, sclera, choroid, Bruch's membrane, and RPE) to reach the retina or vitreous humor. Current knowledge shows that the combined effects of several static anatomic barriers and dynamic clearance mechanisms generally make periocular drug delivery one of the least effective ways of attaining high peak therapeutic intraocular drug concentrations in the retina or vitreous. These barriers are categorized into three major groups: static, dynamic and metabolic. Static barriers include the tissues that must be penetrated (e.g., sclera, Bruch's membrane-choroid and RPE). Dynamic barriers include blood flow, lymphatic drainage, transport proteins of the RPE, drug efflux pumps, organic ion transporters and bulk fluid flow from intraocular drainage systems. Metabolic barriers include enzyme systems such as cytochrome P450 and lysosomal enzymes, which have the ability to degrade or detoxify drugs. In addition to the static, dynamic and metabolic barriers, other factors must be considered in periocular delivery such the individual pharmacokinetic properties of the drug (molecular dimensions, molecular weight, atomic charge and chemical components of the drug). Taken together these factors result in low intraocular bioavailability of drug delivered by the various periocular drug techniques, compared with that of intravitreal injection.

Overall, when the safety and efficacy of this drug delivery route is compared with that of the others for the treatment of disease in the inner coat of the posterior segment, periocular injection is one of the best for safety, and it is in the middle to low end for efficacy, after intrinsic drug properties are factored in, such as potency and exposure-response relationships. With a few modifications, this route has the greatest potential to surpass intravitreal injection as the preferred treatment option for disease of the inner coat of the eye, since it deposits drug locally immediately adjacent to the targeted tissue without being overly invasive.

A major adjuvant used to overcome the short to medium duration of action of periocular drug solutions is the development of several sustained drug release systems, whether through formulation modifications or through various sustained release drug delivery devices. Many of these options include liposomes, microspheres, and microcapsules with diameters of 1–1000 µm, as well as nanospheres and nanocapsules with diameters of less than 1 µm, and biodegradable fibrin sealants (Bourges, Gautier, Delie, et al. 2003; Bu, Gukasyan, Goulet, et al. 2007; Guidetti, Azema, Malet-Martino, et al. 2008; Kearns & Williams, 2009). Polymeric microspheres have been used to target the RPE. Moritera et al. studied the use of surface-modified polymeric microspheres to localize drugs to the RPE (Moritera, Ogura, Yoshimura, et al. 1994). Phagocytosis by RPE was tracked by incorporating fluorescent dye into PLA microspheres with the rate of phagocytosis enhanced with gelatin-precoating as compared with bare microspheres. Intracellular dye release occurred following phagocytosis and could be controlled by varying the polymer formulation of the microspheres. Tuovinen et al. studied targeting drugs to the RPE using microparticles (11 µm in diameter) produced with starch acetate, which degrades more slowly than native starch (Tuovinen, Ruhanen, Kinnarinen, et al. 2004). These microparticles could be phagocytosed and degraded within the RPE.

Nanospheres have also been used to target the RPE for sustained drug delivery. Sakurai et al. studied the intraocular kinetics of nanospheres and found that polystyrene nanospheres containing fluorescein (2 µm in diameter) were detectable in the retina, vitreous and trabecular meshwork more than 1 month following an intravitreal injection in vivo in rabbits (Sakurai, Ozeki, Kunou, et al. 2001). Anionic nanoparticles traversed the collagen fibrils of the vitreous more readily than the cationic nanoparticles, showing potential as drug delivery vehicles for the subretinal space and the RPE. Muller cells take up the nanoparticles, possibly playing a key role in retinal penetration. Micro- and nanoparticles have potential in the field of gene therapy by functioning as nonviral vectors to enable cellular penetration, guard against degradation and maintain sustained delivery. Bejjani et al. explored the use of PLA and PLGA nanoparticles as vectors for gene transfer to a bovine and a human ARPE-19 cell line (Bejjani, BenEzra, Cohen, et al. 2005), concluding that PLGA could successfully sequester and internalize plasmids, resulting in gene expression in RPE detectable 48 h postinjection and maintained for 8 days. Another therapeutic approach is the inhibition of gene expression using antisense oligonucleotides, aptamers and siRNA (Fattal & Bochot, 2006; Fattal & Bochot, 2008; Tanito, Li, Elliott, et al. 2007). Aukunuru et al. showed that nanoparticles formulated using a PLGA (50:50) copolymer could deliver VEGF antisense oligonucleotide to the human ARPE-19 cell line, and inhibit VEGF secretion and mRNA expression (Aukunuru, Ayalasomayajula & Kompella, 2003). In a study performed by Carrasquillo et al. (Carrasquillo, Ricker, Rigas, et al. 2003) and summarized by Moshfeghi and Peyman (Moshfeghi & Peyman, 2005), the anti-VEGF RNA aptamer (EYE001, Macugen®, OSI Pharmaceuticals, NY, USA) was incorporated into PLGA microspheres to develop a sustainedrelease inhibition of VEGF for the treatment of neovascular AMD. Transport and drug efficacy studies of micro- and nanoparticles administered via periocular injection have been also published (Amrite, Edelhauser, Singh, et al. 2008; Amrite & Kompella, 2005; Ayalasomayajula & Kompella, 2003; Ayalasomayajula & Kompella, 2004; Ayalasomayajula & Kompella, 2005; Chiang, Tung & Lu, 2001; Saishin, Silva, Saishin, et al. 2003). In conclusion nano- and microparticles have shown great potential for expanding the arsenal of drug-delivery systems available for treating posterior segment disease. They provide sustained delivery and reduce complications that result from treatments requiring multiple injections. Transscleral delivery of anti-VEGF drugs loaded in PLA or PLGA nano- and microparticles is gaining much attention as a feasible and effective method of administration for the treatment of posterior segment disease.

3.4 Hybrid drug delivery in AMD

Minimally invasive hollow and solid microneedles (<1 mm diameter) have been developed to deliver drugs into the cornea, sclera, or suprachoroidal space to avoid some of the shortcomings in safety and bioavailability with intravitreal or periocular injection. Solid, drug-coated microneedles are used for intracorneal and intrascleral drug delivery, improved bioavailability, and duration of action. Hollow microneedles are used for intrascleral and suprachoroidal delivery of a sustained-release drug depot in a tissue layer, with clearance mechanisms that are minimal or less than those in the subconjunctival or sub-Tenon's space. Microneedles allow for better retinochoroidal targeting than periocular drug delivery, because it is closer to the target tissue (Jiang, Gill, Ghate, et al. 2007; Jiang, Moore, Edelhauser, et al. 2009). A hollow microcatheter cannulation drug delivery technique has also been developed for suprachoroidal drug delivery.

It is more directly invasive than the hollow microneedle approach, but microcatheter delivery may be promising for sustained drug delivery if it can be shown that continuous infusion of drugs into the suprachoroidal space can be tolerated better than a one-time injection with a microneedle. Overall, despite being relatively new and having few longterm data, the hybrid delivery route is arguably the second best for safety (tied with periocular and just behind topical) and second best for efficacy (the best being intraocular). This ranking has not been definitively proven in clinical trials. Another drawback that has not yet been calculated is the greater expense associated with this technology.

3.5 Topical drug delivery in AMD

Topical application to the anterior eye has been proven successful in the treatment of diseases owing to easy access to the target site. However, the adoption of mechanisms in ensuring topical drug penetration to the posterior eye presents numerous challenges. It is difficult to predict which drugs can achieve adequate therapeutic levels in the inner coat of the posterior segment after topical drug delivery and whether penetration can be enhanced by structural modifications or a particular formulation (Ghate & Edelhauser, 2006). Thus, experimental testing in animal models is critical. As this drug delivery route has two major shortcomings, extremely poor bioavailability to the inner coat of the posterior segment and a short duration of action, the main adjuvants are penetration enhancers and sustained-release drug delivery systems. Paracellular penetration by topical drugs can be improved by several mechanisms including: opening TJs by using preservatives in topical medications or by iatrogenic epithelial scraping; increasing drug lipophilicity through the use of prodrugs or other analogues, such as surfactants, and binding the drugs to dendrimers that use carrier-mediated influx transporters.

Recent research has focused on small-molecule penetration into the vitreous, with evidence that molecules with lower molecular weight have increased permeability into the posterior chamber. Molecules with higher molecular weights and superior water solubility (highly charged) may have longer half-lives than those with lower molecular weights. Thus, lower molecular-weight compounds have increased access to the posterior eye and may minimize the risk of toxicity compared with higher molecular-weight compounds, which degrade at slower rates. Therefore, each drug must be individually assessed and its uptake, efficiency and safety must be determined. As the list of drugs that achieve therapeutic levels in the retina and choroid after topical administration increases, it may be possible to identify structural characteristics that promote ocular penetration and to specifically design drugs and/or prodrugs accordingly. Another new technique is represented by Iontophoresis that is an old technology recently modified into a new innovative drug delivery platform. Recent clinical trials have demonstrated that iontophoresis is sufficiently safe and capable of delivering steroids to ocular tissue to some oculare disease (uveitis). It is performed by applying a small electrical current that has the same charge as the drug to create repulsive electromotive forces (Hayden, Jockovich, Murray, et al. 2006; Hughes, Olejnik, Chang-Lin, et al 2005; Myles, Neumann & Hill, 2005).

3.6 Systemic drug delivery routes

There have been advances in the use of systemic medications for the treatment of ophthalmic diseases, despite several limitations related to systemic penetration of many drugs, particularly large or hydrophilic ones, into the posterior segment of the eye. Further movement from the choroid into internal ocular structures such as the retina and vitreous humor, especially of large and/or hydrophilic drugs, is restricted by the RPE (oBRB) and TJs of the retinal vasculature (iBRB). Small lipophilic drugs, however, can penetrate the oBRB and iBRB, achieving appreciable concentrations in the retina and vitreous humor after systemic administration. The systemic application of drugs not only increases the quantity of a drug necessary to achieve therapeutic concentrations, but it also increases the risk of adverse effects due to the accumulation of a drug in other tissues throughout the body. Another limitation of systemic application includes potential reduced time of therapeutic effects and potency due to the dilution and degradation of the drug before reaching the target site. Despite these limitations, there have been advances in the use of systemic medications for the treatment of ophthalmic diseases.

To the wide sense, PDT with verteporfin is one of drug targeting systems. After intravenous administration, verteporfin, a relatively hydrophobic compound, is incorporated into lipoproteins. According to preferential accumulation of lipoproteins in and around choroidal neovascular membrane, verteporfin tends to be targeted into CNV. The photosensitizer targeted injures and closes new vessels in combination of laser irradiation to pathological lesion. However, most systemic drugs are now formulated with excipients that help overcome their tendency toward a brief duration of action and poor to medium bioavailability to the inner coat of the posterior segment.

One novel scheme to enhance the bioavailability of systemic drugs to the retina are penetration enhancers that help reversibly open up the BRB or improve transcellular penetration. Because TJ proteins are not very antigenic, it is difficult to develop antibodies against their extracellular domain, a fact that has severely hampered the development of TJ modulators. For example a novel approach to treat retinal disease by systemic drug delivery reviewed the role of the complement pathway in the pathogenesis of ARMD. Dysregulation of the alternate complement pathway, especially in the C3 amplification loop, may be a reasonable target for treating AMD and inflammatory retinal diseases by administering the intravenous fusion protein complement receptor 2 and factor H (CR2-fH), to recognize and inhibit complement- activation products (Holers, 2008; Rohrer, Long, Coughlin, et al. 2009; Thurman & Holers, 2006). Complement receptor 2 recognizes C3d, a tissue-bound activation product of complementmediated inflammation (e.g., drusen), whereas the fH component of the fusion molecule is the most potent inhibitor of the alternative complement pathway. Some experimental studies have shown how the oxidative stress sensitizes RPE cells to complement-mediated attack by decreasing regulatory cell surface membrane-bound complement inhibitors to the alternative pathway.

That oxidative stress also alters RPE cells in such a way that soluble fH in the serum is less functionally protective (Thurman, Renner, Kunchithapautham, et al. 2009). Complement-mediated attack of the RPE then results in sublytic activation of the membrane attack complex resulting in vascular endothelial growth factor VEGF release and breakdown of the oBRB (Thurman, Renner, Kunchithapautham, et al. 2009). In humans, this cascade of events can result in either dry geographic atrophy or wet AMD. Systemic CR2-fH therapy protects the retina using experimental mouse models of retinal degeneration and choroidal neovascularization.

4. Conclusion

Basic research and open clinical trials have provided breakthrough therapies for treatment of diseases of the posterior segment of the eye, such as the use of anti-VEGF agents for the treatment of AMD. More effective drugs and drug-delivery systems are needed to decrease the frequency of drug administration. Multiple drugs and drug delivery systems may be required to safely and successfully treat some conditions. However, effective treatment of posterior segment ophthalmic diseases represents a formidable challenge for scientists and clinicians in the ophthalmic pharmaceutical field. The challenges include the anatomic and physiologic barriers that can impede pharmacologically active levels of drug from reaching the targeted tissues inside the eye, immune reactions and clearance mechanisms to certain drugs and drug delivery materials, and the often irreversible nature of vision loss. A better understanding must be developed of the nature and effect of dynamic physiologic processes of the eye, such as clearance mechanisms and metabolism of drugs in specific tissue layers. Each static anatomic barrier encountered for each specific drug delivery technique must be better studied. Drug-protein or drug-pigment binding must be better characterized with needing of more research in formulation modifications that alter physicochemical properties of both new and old drugs, facilitating delivery through known paracellular and transcellular pathways. Ophthalmic drug delivery via nanotechnology-based products, development of ophthalmic gene delivery must be further explored, given the extensive potential of this technology. However a new "era" is coming, in which application of technological advances in vision science is progressing at a rapid rate. Advances in nanotechnology, gene therapy, and biomaterials, for example, hold promise for providing new solutions to the challenge of ocular drug delivery.

5. References

Acharya, N. & Young, L. (2004). Sustained-release drug implants for the treatment ofintraocular disease. Int. Ophthalmol. Clin. 44:33–39.

Amrite, A.C.; Edelhauser, H.F.; Singh, S.R. et al. (2008). Effect of circulation on thedisposition and ocular tissue distribution of 20 nm nanoparticles after periocular administration. Mol. Vis. 14:150–160.

Amrite, A.C. & Kompella, U.B. (2005). Size-dependent disposition of nanoparticles andmicroparticles following subconjunctival administration. J. Pharm. Pharmacol. 57:1555–1563.

Andreoli, C.M. & Miller, J.W. (2007). Anti-vascular endothelial growth factor therapy forocular neovascular disease. Curr. Opin. Ophthalmol. 18:502–508.

Aukunuru, J.V.; Ayalasomayajula, S.P. & Kompella, U.B. (2003). Nanoparticle formulation enhances the delivery and activity of a vascular endothelial growth factor antisense oligonucleotide in human retinal pigment epithelial cells. J. Pharm. Pharmacol. 55:1199–1206.

Azadi, S.; Johnson, L.E.; Paquet-Durand, F. et al. (2007). CNTF+BDNF treatment and neuroprotective pathways in the rd1 mouse retina. Brain Res. , 1129, 116-129.

Ayalasomayajula, S.P. & Kompella, U.B. (2003). Celecoxib, a selective cyclooxygenase-2 inhibitor, inhibits retinal vascular endothelial growth factor expression and vascular leakage in a streptozotocininduced diabetic rat model. Eur. J. Pharmacol. 458:283–289.

Ayalasomayajula, S.P. & Kompella, U.B. (2004). Retinal delivery of celecoxib is several-fold higher following subconjunctival administration compared to systemic administration. Pharm. Res. 21:1797–1804.

Ayalasomayajula, S.P. & Kompella, U.B. (2005). Subconjunctivally administered celecoxib–PLGA microparticles sustain retinal drug levels and alleviate diabetes-induced oxidative stress in a rat model. Eur. J. Pharmacol. 511:191–198.

Barar, J.; Javadzadeh, A.R. & Omidi. Y. (2008). Ocular novel drug delivery: impacts of membranes and barriers. Expert Opin. Drug Deliv. 5:567–581.

Barocas, V.H. & Balachandran, R.K. (2008). Sustained transscleral drug delivery. Expert Opin. Drug Deliv. 5:1–10.

Bejjani, R.A.; BenEzra, D.; Cohen, H. et al. (2005). Nanoparticles for gene delivery to retinal pigment epithelial cells. Mol. Vis. 11:124–132.

Bekeredjian, R.; Katus, H.A. & Kuecherer, H.F. (2006). Therapeutic use of ultrasound targeted microbubble destruction: a review of non-cardiac applications. Ultraschall. Med. 27:134–140.

Booth, B.A.; Denham, L.V.; Bouhanik, S.; et al. (2007). Sustained-release ophthalmic drug delivery systems for treatment of macular disorders: present and future applications. Drugs Aging. 24:581–602.

Bourges, J.L.; Gautier, S.E.; Delie, F. et al. (2003). Ocular drug delivery targeting the retina and retinal pigment epithelium using polylactide nanoparticles. Invest. Ophthalmol. Vis. Sci. 44:3562–3569.

Brown, D.M.; Kaiser, P.K.; Michels, M.; et al. (2006). ANCHOR Study Group. Ranibizumab versus verteporfin for neovascular age-related macular degeneration. N Engl J Med. 355:1432-44.

Bu, H.Z.; Gukasyan, H.J.; Goulet, L. et al. (2007). Ocular disposition, pharmacokinetics, efficacy and safety of nanoparticle-formulated ophthalmic drugs. Curr. Drug Metab .8:91–107.

Callanan, D.G. (2007). Novel intravitreal fluocinolone acetonide implant in the treatment of chronic noninfectious posterior uveitis. Expert Rev Ophthalmol . 2: 33-44.

Carrasquillo, K.G.; Ricker, J.A.; Rigas, I.K. et al. (2003). Controlled delivery of the anti-VEGF aptamer EYE001 with poly(lactic-co-glycolic) acid microspheres. Invest. Ophthalmol. Vis. Sci. 44:290–299.

Chiang, C.H.; Tung, S.M. & Lu, D.W. (2001). In vitro and in vivo evaluation of an ocular delivery system of 5-fluorouracil microspheres. J. Ocul. Pharmacol. Ther. 17:545–553.

Choi, Y.K. & Kim, K.W. (2008). Blood-neural barrier: its diversity and coordinated cell-to-cell communication. BMB Rep. 41:345–352.

ClinicalTrials.gov An exploratory study to evaluate the safety of brimonidine intravitreal implant in patients with retinitis pigmentosa. Available online: http://clinicaltrials.gov/ct2/show/ NCT00661479 (accessed on 18 October 2010).

ClinicalTrials.gov Fluocinolone acetonide intravitreal inserts in geographic atrophy.
Available online: http://clinicaltrials.gov/ct2/show/NCT00695318?term=Iluvien&rank=15 (accessed on 18 October 2010).

ClinicalTrials.gov Safety and efficacy of brimonidine intravitreal implant in patients with geographic atrophy due to age-related macular degeneration (AMD). Available online: http://clinicaltrials.gov/ct2/show/NCT00658619 (accessed on 18 October 2010).

ClinicalTrials.gov The MAP Study: Fluocinolone acetonide (FA)/MedidurTM for age related macular degeneration (AMD) Pilot. Available online: http://clinicaltrials.gov/ct2/show/NCT00605423?term=Iluvien&rank=12 (accessed on 18 October 2010).

Craig, J. (2002). Structure and function of the preocular tear film. In The tear film; Korb, D.R., Craig, J., Doughty, M., Guillon, J., Smith, G., Tomlinson, A., Eds.; Butterworth-Heinemann: Oxford, UK. pp. 18-50Hoffman, A.S. (2008) The origins and evolution of 'controlled' drug delivery systems. J. Control. Release. 132:153–163.

Cunha-Vaz, J. (1979). The blood-ocular barriers. Surv. Ophthalmol. 23, 279-296.

Del Amo, E.M. & Urtti, A. (2008). Current and future ophthalmic drug delivery systems. A shift to the posterior segment. Drug Discov. Today. 13:135–143.

Eichler, W.; Kuhrt, H.; Hoffmann, S. et al. (2000). VEGF release by retinal glia depends on both oxygen and glucose supply. Neuroreport . 11, 3533-3537.

Farboud, B.; Aotaki-Keen, A.; Miyata, T. et al. (1999). Development of a polyclonal antibody with broad epitope specificity for advanced glycation endproducts and localization of these epitopes in Bruch's membrane of the aging eye. Mol. Vis. ; 5, 11.

Fattal, E. & Bochot, A. (2006). Antisense oligonucleotides, aptamers and SiRNA: promises for the treatment of ocular diseases. Arch. Soc. Esp. Oftalmol. 81:3–6.

Fattal, E. & Bochot, A. (2008). State of the art and perspectives for the delivery of antisense oligonucleotides and siRNA by polymeric nanocarriers. Int. J. Pharm. 364:237–248.

Fischbarg, J. (2006). The corneal endothelium. In The Biology of Eye; Fischbarg. J., Ed.; Academic Press: New York, NY, USA, pp. 113-125.

Gardner, T.W.; Lieth, E.; Khin, S.A. et al. (1997). Astrocytes increase barrier properties and ZO-1 expression in retinal vascular endothelial cells. Invest. Ophthalmol. Vis. Sci. 38, 2423-2427.

Gaudana, R.; Jwala, J.; Boddu, S.H.; et al. (2009) Recent perspectives in ocular drug delivery. Pharm. Res. 26:1197–1216.

Gausas,R.E.; Gonnering, R.S.; Lemke, B.N. et al. (1999). Identification of human orbital lymphatics. Ophthal. Plast. Reconstr. Surg. 15, 252-259.

Geroski, D.H & Edelhauser, H.F. (2000). Drug delivery for posterior segment diseases. Invest Ophthalmol Vis Sci. 41:961–964.

Ghate, D. & Edelhauser, H.F. (2006). Ocular drug delivery. Expert Opin. Drug Deliv. 3:275–287.

Giese, K.; Kaufmann, J. & Klippel-Giese, A. (2004) Future novel forms of interfering RNA molecules. WO2004015107.

Green, W.R. & Enger, C. (1993). Age-related macular de generation histopathologic studies: the 1992 Lorenz E. Zimmerman Lecture. Ophthalmology. 100:1519–39.

Guidetti, B.; Azema, J.; Malet-Martino, M. et al. (2008). Delivery systems for the treatment of proliferative vitreoretinopathy: materials, devices and colloidal carriers. Curr. Drug Deliv . 5:7–19.

Handa, J.T.; Verzijl, N.; Matsunaga, H. et al. (1999). Increase in the advanced glycation end product pentosidine in Bruch's membrane with age. Invest. Ophthalmol. Vis. Sci. 40, 775-779.

Hayden, B.; Jockovich, M.E.; Murray, T.G. et al. (2006). Iontophoretic delivery of carboplatin in a murine model of retinoblastoma. Invest. Ophthalmol. Vis. Sci. 47:3713–3721.

Hewitt, A.T. & Newsome, D.A. (1985). Altered synthesis of Bruch's membrane proteoglycans associated with dominant retinitis pigmentosa. Curr. Eye Res. 4, 169-174.

Hewitt, A.T.; Nakazawa, K. & Newsome, D.A. (1989). Analysis of newly synthesized Bruch's membrane proteoglycans. Invest. Ophthalmol. Vis. Sci. 30, 478-486.

Higuchi, T. (1961). Release of medicaments from ointment bases containing drugs in suspension. J Pharm Sci . 50:874–875.

Holers, V.M. (2008). The spectrum of complement alternative pathwaymediated diseases. Immunol Rev. 223:300–316.

Hughes, P.M. Olejnik, O.; Chang-Lin, J.E. et al (2005). Topical and systemic drug delivery to the posterior segments. Adv. Drug Deliv. Rev. 57:2010–2032.

Hsu, J. (2007) Drug delivery methods for posterior segment disease. Curr. Opin. Ophthalmol. 18:235–239.

Jager, R.D.; Aiello, L.P.; Patel, S.C. et al. (2004). Risks of intravitreous injection: a comprehensive review. Retina. 24:676–698.

Jiang, J.; Gill, H.S.; Ghate, D. et al. (2007). Coated microneedles for drug delivery to the eye. Invest Ophthalmol Vis Sci. 48:4038–4043.

Jiang, J.; Moore, J.S.; Edelhauser, H.F. et al. (2009). Instrsclera drug delivery to the eye using hollow microneedles. Pharm Res. ; 26:395–403.

Kaur, C.; Sivakumar, V. & Foulds, W.S. (2006). Early response of neurons and glial cells to hypoxia in the retina. Invest. Ophthalmol. Vis. Sci. 47, 1126-1141.

Kearns, V.R. & Williams, R.L. (2009). Drug delivery systems for the eye. Expert Rev. Med. Devices. 6(3): 277–290.

Kim, S.H.; Lutz, R.J.; Wang, N.S. et al. (2007). Transport barriers in transscleral drug delivery for retinal diseases. Ophthalmic Res. 39:244–254.

Kim, H.S.; Chang, Y.I.; Kim, J.H. et al. (2007). Alteration of retinal intrinsic survival signal and effect of alpha2-adrenergic receptor agonist in the retina of the chronic ocular hypertension rat. Vis. Neurosci. 24, 127-139.

Knight, C.G, ed. Liposomes: From Physical Structure to Therapeutic applications. Amsterdam: Elsevier/North Holland Biomedical Press, 1981.

Lee, S.J.; He, W.; Robinson, S.B. et al. (2010). Evaluation of clearance mechanisms with trans-scleral drug delivery. Invest. Ophthalmol. Vis. Sci. 51, 5205-5212.

Lee, S.S. & Robinson, M.R. (2009). Novel drug delivery systems for retinal diseases. A review. Ophthalmic Res. 41:124–135.

Lemley, C.A. & Han, D.P. (2007) Endophthalmitis: a review of current evaluation and management. Retina. 27:662–680.

Liu, M. & Regillo, C.D. (2004). A review of treatments for macular degeneration: a synopsis of currently approved treatments and ongoing clinical trials. Curr. Opin. Ophthalmol. 15:221–226.

Lonngren, U.; Napankangas, U.; Lafuente, M. et al. (2006). The growth factor response in ischemic rat retina and superior colliculus after brimonidine pre-treatment. Brain Res. Bull. 71, 208-218.

Lyons, R.T.; Ma, H. & Trogde, J.T. (2009). Methods, compositions and drug delivery systems for intraocular delivery of siRNA molecules. US20090258924.

Mannermaa, E.; Vellonen, K.S. & Urtti, A. (2006). Drug transport in corneal epithelium and blood retina barrier: emerging role of transporters in ocular pharmacokinetics. Adv Drug Deliv Rev. 58:1136- 1163.

Maurice, D.M. & Mishima, S. (1984). Ocular Pharmacokinetics. In: Pharmacology of the Eye. In: Sears ML, Ed. New York: Springer. 116-9.

McSwiggen, J.; Beigelman, L.; Macejak, D. et al. (2003) RNA interference by modified short interfering nucleic acid. WO2003070918 .

Mitra, A.K. (2009). Role of transporters in ocular drug delivery system. Pharm. Res. 26:1192–1196.

Moritera, T.; Ogura, Y.; Yoshimura, N. et al. (1994). Feasibility of drug targeting to the retinal pigment epithelium with biodegradable microspheres. Curr. Eye Res. 13:171–176.

Moshfeghi, A.A. & Peyman, G.A. (2005). Micro- and nanoparticulates. Adv. Drug Deliv. Rev. 57:2047– 2052.

Murakami, T.; Felinski, E.A. & Antonetti, D.A. (2009). Occludin phosphorylation and ubiquitination regulate tight junction trafficking and vascular endothelial growth factor-induced permeability. J Biol. Chem. 284: 21036-21046.

Myles, M.E.; Neumann, D.M. & Hill, J.M. (2005). Recent progress in ocular drug delivery for posterior segment disease: emphasis on transscleral iontophoresis. Adv. Drug Deliv. Rev. 57:2063–2079.

Novack, G.D. (2009). Ophthalmic drug delivery: development and regulatory considerations. Clin. Pharmacol. Ther. 85:539–543.

Okabe, K.; Kimura, H.; Okabe, J. et al. (2003). Intraocular tissue distribution of betamethasone after intrascleral administration using a non-biodegradable sustained drug delivery device. Invest Ophthalmol Vis Sci . 44: 2702-7.

Oyster, CW. (1999). The cornea and sclera. In The Human Eye; Oyster. C.W., Ed.; Sinauer Associates, Inc.: Sunderland, UK. pp. 325-378.

Pederson, J.E. (2006). Fluid physiology of the subretinal space. In Retina, Fourth edition; Ryan, S.J., Ed.; Elsevier Inc.: Philadelphia, PA, USA, Volume III, pp. 1909-1920.

Peppas, N.A. (1995). Controlling protein diffusion in hydrolgels. In: Lee VH-L, Hashida M, Misushima Y, eds. Trends and Future Perspectives in Peptide and Protein Delivery. Chur, Switzerland: Harwood Academic Publishers. :23–38.

Robinson, M.R.; Blanda, W.M.; Hughes, P.M. et al. (2010) Method for treating atrophic age related macular degeneration. US20100015158 & WO2010009034 .

Robinson, M.R.; Blanda, W.M.; Liu, H. et al. (2010). Intraocular formulation. US20100074957.

Robinson, M.R.; Tsai, S.Y.; Almazan, A.S. et al. (2010). Drug delivery systems and methods for treating neovascularization. US20100098772 & WO2010048086 .

Rohrer, B.; Long, Q.; Coughlin, B. et al. (2009). A targeted inhibitor of the alternative complement pathway reduces angiogenesis in a mouse model of age-related macular degeneration. Invest Ophthalmol Vis Sci. 50:3056–3064.

Rosenfeld, P.J.; Brown, D.M.; Heier, J.S.; et al. (2006). MARINA Study Group. Ranibizumab for neovascular age-related macular degeneration. N Engl J Med. 355: 1419-31.

Saishin, Y.; Silva, R.L.; Saishin, Y. et al. (2003). Periocular injection of microspheres containing PKC412 inhibits choroidal neovascularization in a porcine model. Invest. Ophthalmol. Vis. Sci. 44:4989–4993.

Sakurai, E.; Ozeki, H.; Kunou, N. et al. (2001). Effect of particle size of polymeric nanospheres on intravitreal kinetics. Ophthalmic Res. 3:31–36.Tanito, M.; Li, F.; Elliott, M.H. (2007). Protective effect of TEMPOL derivatives against light-induced retinal damage in rats. Invest. Ophthalmol. Vis. Sci. 48:1900–1905.

Sarks, SH. (1976). Ageing and degeneration in macular region: a clinicopathological study. Br J Ophthalmol. 60:324–41.

Singh, D. (2003). Conjunctival lymphatic system. J. Cataract. Refract. Surg. 29, 632-633.

Spaide, RF. (2009). Enhanced depth imaging optical coherence tomography of retinal pigment epithelial detachment in age-related macular degeneration. Am. J. Ophthalmol. 147, 644-652.

Spraul, C.W.; Lang, G.E.; Grossniklaus, H.E. et al. (1999). Histologic and morphometric analysis of the choroid, Bruch's membrane, and retinal pigment epithelium in postmortem eyes with age-related macular degeneration and histologic examination of surgically excised choroidal neovascular membranes. Surv. Ophthalmol. 44 Suppl 1, S10-32.

Sugar, H.S.; Riazi, A. & Schaffner, R. (1957). The bulbar conjunctival lymphatics and their clinical significance. Trans. Am. Acad. Ophthalmol. Otolaryngol., 61, 212-223.

Sultana, Y.; Jain, R.; Aqil, M.; et al. (2006) Review of ocular drug delivery. Curr. Drug Deliv. 3:207–217.

Thurman, J.M. & Holers, V.M. (2006). The central role of the alternative complement pathway in human disease. J Immunol. 176:1305–1310.

Thurman, J.M.; Renner, B.; Kunchithapautham, K. et al. (2009). Oxidative stress renders retinal pigment epithelial cells susceptible to complement-mediated injury. J Biol Chem. 284:16939-16947.

Tout, S.; Chan-Ling, T.; Hollander, H. et al. (1993). The role of Muller cells in the formation of the blood-retinal barrier. Neuroscience. 55, 291-301.

Tretiach, M.; Madigan, M.C.; Wen, L. et al. (2005). Effect of Muller cell co-culture on in vitro permeability of bovine retinal vascular endothelium in normoxic and hypoxic conditions. Neurosci. Lett. 378, 160-165.

Tsutomu, Y.; Yasuhiko, T.; Hideya, K. et al. (2011). Recent Advances in Intraocular Drug Delivery Systems. Recent Patents on Drug Delivery & Formulation. 5(1): 1-10.

Tuovinen, L.; Ruhanen, E.; Kinnarinen, T. et al. (2004). Starch acetate microparticles for drug delivery into retinal pigment epithelium–in vitro study. J. Control. Release ;98:407–413.

Van der Schaft, T.L.; de Bruijn, W.C.; Mooy, C.M.; et al. (1992). Histologic features of the early stages of age-related macular degeneration: a statistical analysis. Ophthalmology. 99:278–86.

US National Institutes of Health. ClinicalTrials.org. NCT00447954 CgI. A Study of an Encapsulated Cell Technology (ECT) Implant for Patients With Atrophic Macular Degeneration. Phase II study. 2009.
http://clinicaltrials.gov/ct2/show/NCT00447954.
Accessed December 24,2009.

Zhang, M.; Mo, X; Fang, Y. et al. (2009). Rescue of photoreceptors by BDNF gene transfer using in vivo electroporation in the RCS rat of retinitis pigmentosa. Curr. Eye Res. 34, 791-799.

Zhang, Y. & Stone, J. (1997). Role of astrocytes in the control of developing retinal vessels. Invest. Ophthalmol. Vis. Sci. 38, 1653-1666.

Yamada, Y.; Ishibashi, K.; Bhutto, I.A. et al. (2006). The expression of advanced glycation endproduct receptors in rpe cells associated with basal deposits in human maculas. Exp. Eye Res. 82, 840-848.

Yasukawa, T.; Ogura, Y.; Kimura, H. et al. (2006). Drug delivery from ocular implants. Expert Opin Drug Deliv . 3: 261-73.

Yasukawa, T.; Ogura, Y.; Tabata, Y. et al. (2004). Drug delivery systems for vitreoretinal diseases. Prog Retin Eye Res . 23: 253-81.

Part 2

Clinical Research

7

Treatment of Neovascular Age Related Macular Degeneration

Ratimir Lazić and Nikica Gabrić
University Eye Clinic Svjetlost Zagreb
Croatia

1. Introduction

Neovascular Age Related Macular Degeneration (nAMD) has been a therapeutic challenge until recently. The natural course of the disease leads to a great deterioration of visual acuity and is considered to be the leading cause of legal blindness in people 50 years of age or older, especially in the Western countries.

Until the end of the last century, no intervention could alter the natural history of the disease. Only in the last few decades, the retina specialists began to intervene in order to minimize the visual loss in those patients. Last ten years have been especially exciting as the new treatment modalities emerged and for the first time we could not only halt the progression of the deterioration, but rather improve vision in some patients.

In this chapter we will present therapeutic modalities which were applied chronologically and then we will present the up to date treatment options. Finally we will briefly summarize new emerging drugs which are still under clinical evaluation.

2. Past treatments

2.1 Laser photocoagulation

The first major clinical trial evaluating laser photocoagulation in treatment of nAMD was performed in the 1980-ies, at times when no treatment modality could change natural course of this disease. However, the Macular Photocoagulation Study (MPS) (1), which took 5 years to complete, demonstrated that argon laser photocoagulation could postpone or even prevent significant visual loss in patients with juxtafoveol and extrafoveol choroidal neovascular membranes (CNV).

It was later shown that some benefits of reducing the damage generated by the natural course of the disease could be achieved by performing laser treatment on subfoveol CNV as well (2). As the reduction of visual acuity occurred immediately after the laser treatment, patients' dissatisfaction became a major issue.

2.2 Photodynamic therapy

Photodynamic therapy (PDT) represented the first specific treatment option in treating nAMD and the treatment protocol consisted of intravenous application of a photosensitive drug verteporfin, which was then activated by a 693-nanometer-long, verteporfin-sensitive laser beam light.

Verterporfin activation was followed by a series of photochemical reactions, resulting in destruction and thrombosis of endothelial cells in the neovascular membrane complex (3). The PDT had a double selectivity mechanism:

1. Verteporfin was utilized only by cells with accelerated metabolism (neovascular membrane),
2. Laser beam was applied only to the area of CNV.

With verteporfin accumulating itself selectively within the neovascular complex, the collateral damage to surrounding healthy tissue was minimal. Verteporfin was in circulation carried by plasma lipoproteins, which were utilized by endothelial cells due to accelerated metabolism of neovascular complex. Within the area illuminated by the laser beam, short-acting free oxygen radicals induced endothelial cell damage, which process occurred through lipo and cyclooxigenase modulated pathways, the final result being trombocyte aggregation and vasoconstriction of neovascular complex vessels (4). The slow metabolism of normal blood vessels made the utilization of verteporfin-carrying lipoproteins in normal vessels slow as well. Verterporfin was utilized by neovascular complex vessels within 15 minutes. It took 30 minutes for normal blood vessels to utilize verteporfin. Therefore, the laser beam of 90 seconds duration must had been applied to the neovascular membrane no later than 30 minutes after the infusion was started, in order to prevent damage to normal blood vessels. The exact size and location of neovascular complex was determined by fluorescein angiography, which was a precondition to laser application.

Treatment of AMD with Photodynamic Therapy (TAP) study (5) was a double blind placebo controlled randomized clinical trial evaluating the efficacy of PDT in treatment of minimally classic CNV. 609 patients were enrolled (402 in the verteporfin group and 207 in the placebo group). The treatment was repeated every 3 months in case of relapse of leakage or continuous leakage, which was confirmed by fluorescein angiography. At 12 month follow-up 61.2% of patients from the verteporfin group, compared to 46.4% patients from the placebo group lost less than 3 logMar lines (minimal angle resolution logarithm) or 15 letters which was statistically significant. At 24 months follow-up, 213 (53%) patients from the verteporfin group, compared to 78 (38%) patients from the placebo group lost fewer than 3 lines (6). The mean visual acuity was 1.3 lines better in the verteporfin group. The eyes treated with verteporfin had a 16% better chance for visual improvement by 1 or more lines, compared to the placebo group. The benefits of the verteporfin treatment were higher in case of the predominantly CNV (at least 50% of the neovascular complex has a classic component): 33% of patients from the verteporfin group lost 3 or more lines, compared to 61% of patients from the placebo group after 12 months. If CNV was completely classic, the results were even better: 23% of patients from the verteporfin group lost fewer than 3 lines, whereas in the placebo group, 73% of patients lost 3 or more lines.

In case of the minimally classic type of the CNV, results were however modest - positive effects of the treatment were noticed only if the maximal diameter of neovascular lesion was smaller than 4 disc diameters. The efficacy of the PDT for the minimally classic CNV with the greatest diameter of lesion up to 6 discs was later confirmed by the VIM study (Verteporfin Therapy of Subfoveal Minimally Classic CNV in AMD) (7).

The VIP study (Verteporfin in Photodynamic Therapy) evaluated PDT in patients with occult CNV and showed that 121 (54%) patients from the verteporfin group lost fewer than 15 letters during 24 months of the follow-up, compared to 76 (67%) patients from the control group (8), whereby the best results were displayed by the patients with lesions smaller than 4 disc diameters or with the initial visual acuity better than 20/50 (9).

The mentioned studies demonstrated the efficacy of the PDT with verteporfin in maintaining the visual acuity or slowing down visual loss. It was the very first time that we could positively interfere with the natural course of the disease using PDT.

2.3 Surgical treatment

Surgical techniques in treatment of nAMD included submacular surgery, macular translocation, and submacular hemorrhage displacement.

Macular translocation was a surgical procedure involving the detachment of the retina along with macula in order to move or translocate fovea from the diseased RPE onto healthy RPE. Although there had been reports of case series with quite good visual outcomes after the surgery, severe complications could arise during the process of retinal displacement (10,11). Therefore nowadays macular translocation may not be considered for most patients with nAMD given the treatment options already available. In the anti-VEGF era macular translocation may be employed in patients either with very advanced AMD or in those patients with disease recalcitrant to anti-VEGF therapy.

Unfortunately the surgery undertaken in a very advanced cases wouldn't result in significant improvement of vision as the degenerative process had already damaged the retinal macular tissue along with the diseased underlying RPE: but retina specialist are reluctant to recommend macular translocation at the stage of the disease while macular retina is still viable at which point macular translocation would result in better functional outcome.

The full macular translocation surgery involved a detachment of the entire retina from the RPE by subretinal infusion of balanced saline solution fluid via 40 gauge needle with 360 degrees circumferential retinotomy followed by the retinal rotation under perflorocarbon liquid during which process macula was displaced onto healthy RPE. The site of the 360 retinotomy and the holes artificially created for detaching retina were sealed by endolaser photocoagulation. Then an exchange between perflorocarbon liquid with silicone oil was performed. After 3 months silicone oil was removed.

3. Current treatment options

3.1 Anti-VEGF drugs

3.1.1 Pegaptanib sodium

An additional step forward was made by introducing the anti-VEGF drugs as a treatment option for nAMD. Pegaptanib sodium (Macugen) was actually a synthetically derived polyonucleotide ligand binding specifically to VEGF-A 165 isoform. The affinity to only one isoform of VEGF cluster explained pegaptanib sodium inferior therapeutic effect, compared to non-selective infibitors of all VEGF isoforms.

Data from VISION trial indicated that 70% of the treated patients with intravitreal pegaptanib sodium given on a 6-week basis lost fewer than 15 letters during a 24 month follow-up, compared to 55% of patients from the placebo group. The mean visual acuity decreased by 8 letters during the follow-up period in the patients treated with intravitreal pegaptanib sodium in this study (12).

3.1.2 Ranibizumab

Ranibizumab is a humanized antigen-binding FAB fragment monoclonal antibody towards human VEGF-A, derived from rodents. It is produced by recombinant technology from Escherichiae coli, with molecular weight of 48 kilodaltons. Ranibizumab inhibits all VEGF-A isoforms. Furthermore, it penetrates well through all layers of retina up to choroidea. The binding affinity of ranibizumab is 5-20 times higher comparing to bevacizumab(13). Ranibizumab was approved for intravitreal application in 2006.

A large multicentric randomized clinical trial MARINA (Ranibizumab in Treatment of Occult and Minimally Classic CNV)(14) and ANCHOR (Ranibizumab in Treatment of Predominantly Classic CNV)(15) confirmed that ranibizumab, given on a monthly basis substantially improved visual acuity compared to placebo. The MARINA study enrolled 716 patients and evaluated the efficacy of monthly ranibizumab (0.3mg and 0.5 mg), versus placebo given for 24 months. In the ranibizumab groups over 90% of patients lost fewer than 15 letters (or 3 lines) compared to 62% patients from the placebo group. One third of patients from the ranibizumab group (0.5mg) gained 15 letters or more, while in the placebo group only 5% of patients achieved this effect. This was a significant breakthrough compared to all previous treatment options. Mean visual acuity improved by 7.2 letters (about 1 line of logMAR) at 12 month follow-up in the ranibizumab group (0.5mg), while in the placebo group, the visual acuity deteriorated by more than 10 letters. The benefit in visual acuity was maintained at 24 months. During 24 months, presumed endophthalmitis was identified in five patients (1.0%) and serious uveitis in six patients (1.3%).

The ANCHOR study enrolled 423 patients and compared the efficacy and safety of ranibizumab given on a monthly basis with standard PDT with verteporfin. The follow-up period was 24 months. At the end of the study, over 90% of patients from the ranibizumab group and 65% of patients from the photodynamic group lost fewer than 15 letters. Furthermore, over one third of patients from the ranibizumab group gained 15 letters or more, compared to 5.6% of patients from the PDT group. Mean visual acuity improved by 11.3 letters in the ranibizumab group (0.5mg), whereas patients from the photodynamic group had mean decrease of 9.5 letters. Reduction in central retinal thickness, measured by OCT, was also observed through the follow-up.

Endophthalmitis or serious uveitis occurred in around 2% of patients from the ranibizumab group (0.5 mg). Even though visual results were good, it took 24 injections over 2 year period to achieve it. Several studies were conducted in order to see whether a number of retreatments could be reduced with sustained visual results.

PIER study (16) analyzed a treatment protocol of three consecutive monthly injections of ranibizumab, followed by injections every three months. The results of this study were inferior when compared to the results achieved by the MARINA and ANCHOR trials, in particular between 3rd and 12th month when injections were given quarterly.

In PRONTO study (17) patients received 3 injections of ranibizumab on a monthly basis and thereafter as needed, based on strictly defined criteria, which included visual acuity decline, reoccurrence of fluid and central retinal thickness increase measured by OCT and clinical manifestation of macular hemorrhage. The results obtained by the PRONTO study were comparable to those of the MARINA and ANCHOR studies, but the number of injections required was lower: 5 injection of ranibizumab in the PRONTO versus 12 injections in the MARINA and the ANCHOR per year.

SAILOR study (18) was designed with the purpose of confirming the results obtained by the PRONTO study. The SAILOR study lasted for 12 months. After three monthly injections of ranibizumab the additional injections were given based on predefined criteria, similar to those applied in the PRONTO study. The results of the SAILOR study were better than the ones of the PIER study, but not as good as those of the MARINA and ANCHOR, where injections were given on a monthly basis. The rate of the systemic side effects indicated a satisfactory safety profile.

SUSTAIN study (19) confirmed the results given by the SAILOR study. The SUSTAIN study achieved better results than the PIER study, but inferior to those of the MARINA and ANCHOR and the PRONTO studies. During a 1-year follow-up period, mean number of injections applied was around 5 and visual acuity improved by 3.6 letters. Central retinal thickness was reduced by 92 microns.

The HORIZON study (20) was a sequel to the MARINA and ANCHOR studies, its main purpose was to analyze the long term follow-up results and furthermore, to switch from monthly dosing to dosing as needed and to observe an impact on visual acuity. Additional treatment was required in more than 60% of patients during the 2 year follow-up period. Visual gain achieved after two years of monthly injections of ranibizumab was not maintained with less frequent dosing of ranibizumab.

The monthly dosing remained, however, the best way to preserve the visual acuity. Any reduction in number of injections led to inferior visual outcome. Due to frequent dosing and other paramedical factors, regular monthly drug application presented a great burden to substantial number of patients.

3.1.3 Bevacizumab

Bevacizumab (Avastin) is a humanized recombinant monoclonal mouse antibody. A molecular weight of bevacizumab is 149 kilodaltons. It is active against all VEGF-A isoforms. Bevacizumab has been approved as an intravenous drug in the treatment of metastatic colon cancer (21), along with chemotherapy. It helps to induce the reduction of the tumor volume by deprivation of tumor vascularization (22).

In 2005, bevacizumab was administered as ocular treatment for the first time. First bevacizumab trial included 9 patients with nAMD. Bevacizumab was given intravenously (5mg/kg) at two week intervals resulting in 12-letters gain with a significant reduction of intraretinal macular edema at the 12 week follow-up period (23). 7 patients experienced mild hypertension as a side-effect.

Due to systemic side-effects (hypertension, gastrointestinal bleeding, thromboembolic events), bevacizumab was then applied intravitrealy in a concentration of 1 mg/0.1 ml, which was a significantly lower dose compared to the systemic one, while the good visual outcome was maintained (24). Despite its large molecular weight, bevacizumab showed satisfying penetration into subretinal space, without any harmful neurophysiologic effects (25). Many clinical trials confirmed later the efficacy of bevacizumab in improving the visual acuity, reducing the retinal exudation and the acceptable safety profile (26,27,28,29,30).

Bevacizumab and ranibizumab exhibit differences and similarities in the treatment of nAMD:

- Both drugs inhibit all VEGF-A isoforms.
- Bevacizumab has weaker affinity towards the VEGF factor than ranibizumab.
- Bevacizumab has larger molecular weight, which could interfere with the penetration ability.
- Given that the bevacizumab is a full antibody with the Fc fragment, whereas ranibizumab is only an antibody fragment, it might be more immunogenic.

Several studies showed no difference in efficiency between ranibizumab and bevacizumab(31,32,33). Interesting results came from a study which concluded that functional result were alike, however bevacizumab needed a longer period of time to achieve resolution of retinal edema than ranibizumab: 60 versus 90 days. The period of the drug potency was 110 days for bevacizumab, and 70 days for ranibizumab, suggesting a longer interval of bevacizumab dosing(34).

Comparison of AMD Treatment Trials (CATT) study (35) was designed to compare ranibizumab and bevacizumab in treatment of nAMD. 1208 patients were enrolled. Patients were randomized into four study arms: ranibizumab monthly or as needed and bevacizumab monthly or as needed. Ranibizumab and bevacizumab showed equivalent results in terms of efficiency. Patients treated with monthly bevacizumab gained 8 letters, while patients treated with monthly ranibizumab gained 8.5 letters after 12 month follow-up period. In as-needed arms bevacizumab was equivalent to ranibizumab with 5.9 and 6.8 letters gained.

Ranibizumab as needed was equivalent to monthly ranibizumab, while comparison between bevacizumab as needed and bevacizumab monthly showed inconclusive results. Rates of death, myocardial infarction, and stroke were similar for patients receiving either ranibizumab or bevacizumab. The proportion of patients with serious systemic adverse events (SSAE) requiring hospitalization was higher with bevacizumab than with ranibizumab arms (24.1% vs.19.0%). The importance of the CATT trial was in reporting the same efficacy of bevacizumab in a major randomized clinical trial. The raised concern with higher incidence of SSAE in bevacizumab is worth of noting but still inconclusive and needs to be further analyzed.

4. Drugs under investigation

4.1 VEGF Trap Eye (aflibercept)

To initiate molecular mechanism of neovascularization, it is essential for the VEGF to bind to endothelial cell receptors VEGFR1 and VEGFR2, which act as transmembrane tyrosine kinases.

By binding VEGF to their outer subunit, tyrosine kinase is activated which then triggers intracellular signaling pathways. The VEGF Trap Eye is a fusion protein containing VEGFR1 and VEGFR2 similar domains combined with Fc immunoglobulin segment (36). This means that VEGF Trap Eye has antibody inhibiting characteristics for all VEGF-A isoforms and binding affinity 800 times greater than bevacizumab. A clinical trial with 25 patients has shown good tolerability and increased visual acuity 6 weeks after single intravitreal injection (37).

VIEW 1 and VIEW 2 were phase III, randomized, double- masked, clinical trials (38,39) evaluating VEGF Trap Eye effect on maintaining and improving vision as compared to ranibizumab.The studies have been completed in 2011. VIEW 1 was conducted in USA and VIEW 2 was conducted in Asia, Europe, Japan and Latin America. In both studies patients were randomized evenly to one of four treatment groups:0.5 mg ranibizumab monthly, VEGF trap 0.5 mg monthly, VEGF trap 2 mg monthly or VEGF trap 2 mg dosed every 8 weeks following a tree-injection loading dose.

VIEW 1 enrolled 1217 patients. Prevention of moderate vision loss was achieved in 94-96% of patients from all four groups showing VEGF Trap Eye non inferior to ranibizumab. Mean gain in visual acuity in all four groups was as follow: VEGF Trap 0.5 mg group achieved a mean gain of seven letter, the 2 mg VEGF Trap montly group a mean gain of 11 letters, the 2 mg VEGF Trap dosed every two months after initial loading dose gained a mean of 8 letters while ranibizumab monthly group gained a mean of 8 letters. The only statistically significant difference in visual gain was between patients receiving VEGF Trap Eye 2mg monthly compared to ranibizumab monthly with $p<0.01$ (11 letter vs. 8 letter gain at week 52) showing superiority of VEGF Trap Eye dosed 2mg monthly.

International VIEW 2 study enrolled 1240. As in VIEW 1 study, prevention of moderate vision loss was achieved in 94- 96 percent of patients from all four groups confirming non inferiority of VEGF Trap Eye at all doses compared to monthly ranibizumab.

A generally favorable safety profile was observed for both VEGF Trap Eye and ranibizumab. The most frequent ocular adverse events were conjunctival hemorrhage, macular degeneration, eye pain, retinal hemorrhage, and vitreous floaters.

In conclusion both VIEW 1 and VIEW 2 studies showed VEGF-Trap-Eye being non inferior to monthly ranibizumab in prevention of moderate vision loss with good safety profile and potential for VEGF-Trap to achieve equally superior visual results as monthly ranibizumab with less frequent dosing. When dosed 2 mg monthly VEGF Trap Eye even showed superior in terms of vision gain compared to ranibizumab monthly

4.2 Interfering RNA

Small interfering RNAs (siRNA) are synthetic nucleotide chains, containing 20 nucleotides.

While VEGF antibodies neutralize the already produced VEGF, siRNA interferes with VEGF -A messenger RNA (mRNA)(40,41), inhibiting thereby the production of all VEGF-A isoforms.

As a result, the already produced VEGF persists within the eye for a couple of the first treatment weeks, leading to delayed therapeutic effect.

SiRNA 027 interferes with the VEGF-R1 mRNA production. As demonstrated by CNV models, intravitreal and periocular injection of siRNA resulted in a significant CNV lesion reduction (42).

Other siRNA target hypoxia-induced transcription factor (HIF-1). This factor is important not only in tumor angiogenesis but also in normal vessel formation. HIF-1 is composed of the constitutively expressed HIF-1 beta subunit and the 3-alfa subunit. In non-hypoxia conditions, HIF-1 alpha dissolves rapidly, whereas in the hypoxic environment, HIF-1 alpha becomes stable and acts as a hypoxia-provoked inducible gene regulator (43). Currently there are no ongoing clinical trials investigating this compound in treatment of nAMD but data from previous studies showed the compound to have a potential for VEGF inhibition.

4.3 Tyrosine kinase inhibitors

One of the most important biochemical mechanisms of intracellular signaling mediation is reverse phosphorilation. This reaction is catalysed by kinase proteins, which transfer g-phosphate ATP group to hydroxyl group of targeted proteins (44). There are 518 of such proteins in human genome, 90 of which are selective hydroxyl group tyrosine phosphorilation catalysts(45).

Cytosol tyrosine kinases are intracellular, while the receptor tyrosine kinase (RTK) have intracellular and extracellular domain and function as membrane receptors. The RTKs modulate cellular responses as such to signalling from the environment and act as various cell processes boosters of cellular proliferation, migration and survival. Otherwise the RTK signal mechanisms are well regulated, while their excessive activation can stimulate growth, survival and tumor cell metastasis development (46). Members of the VEGF and PDGF receptor group, which belong to the RTK family, promote tumor progression through various mechanisms: angiogenesis, limphangenesis and vascular permeability.

PTK 787 is a RTK inhibitor with binding affinity to VEGF receptor tyrosine kinase and thus inhibits all VEGF-A isoforms. PTK 787 displayed functional improvement of ischemic retinopathy induced in mice. A single intravitreal injection of PTK reduced angiproliferative changes compared to the control eye of each animal (n=37) when retinopathy scores were compared (47). Currently there are no clinical trials of PTK 787 in treatment of nAMD, but the compound has a potential for VEGF inhibition.

4.4 Cytokine PEDF

Pigment Epithelial Derived Factor (PEDF), produced by retinal pigment epithelial cells is one of the most important endogenous angiogenesis inhibitors (48). The exact location of the PEDF production is on the apical side of pigment epithelial cells and contrary to VEGF it is inhibited by hypoxia.

A high PEDF concentration can be found in extracellular photoreceptor matter, vitreous and cornea, indicating its major role in maintaining the tissues avascularity (49). The PEDF's anti-angiogenic capacity has been proven in laser-stimulated CNV animal model (50). The PEDF concentrations are lower in the eyes suffering from CNVs, which is consistent with its anti-angiogenic properties. Therefore gene transferring adenovirus coding over-expression of PEDF could suppress the angiogenesis process.

4.5 Epimacular brachytherapy

Previously used, radiation therapy from external radiation source produced inconsistent results with high rate of side-effects. It was therefore abandoned from everyday clinical practice. Localized radiation treatment, on contrary has an ability to prevent proliferation of vascular tissue by inhibiting neovascularization (51,52). After low-dose radiation, vascular endothelium demonstrates morphologic and DNA changes, inhibition of replication, increased cell permeability, and apoptosis. Fibroblast proliferation and subsequent scar formation, a hallmark of end-stage nAMD are also inhibited.

CNVs which contain proliferating endothelial cells due to the hypoxic environment and the produced chemokines are more sensitive to radiation treatment than the retinal vasculature and non-proliferating capillary endothelial cells and larger vessels. Therefore to reduce complication rate and to improve visual outcome epimacular brachytherapy was introduced. It uses strontium-90 beta radiation as radiation source (NeoVista, Fremont, CA.). Total radiation dose is 24 gy. Epimacular brachytherapy is designed to deliver precisely controlled dose of beta radiation to CNV lesion. Compared to previously used radiation therapy strontium-90 beta radiation is ideal for treating retina because its delivery system ensues no collateral damage to surrounding retinal tissues (53,54). After pars plana vitrectomy is done, radiation applicator is placed directly above CNV lesion and held for 2-4 minutes. This has a dual effect: vitrectomy increases retinal oxygen saturation and in contrast to external beam radiotherapy a larger dose of radiation can be delivered to the macula with less irradiation of normal ocular structures and surrounding tissues. This novel device is currently being evaluated in two prospective, randomized, controlled trials in treatment-naive subjects: the CNV Secondary AMD Treated with Beta Radiation Epretinal Therapy (CABERNET) and in subjects already treated with anti-vascular endothelial growth factor therapy: Macular Epiretinal Brachytherapy versus Lucentis Only Treatment (MERLOT).

4.6 Combination treatment

Having in mind the multiplicity of signaling mechanisms which are crucial for the development of nAMD as well as multistage evolution of the disease, combination treatments could have synergistic effect in halting the progression of disease.

The anti-VEGF and PDT with verterpofin have up to now been the only available options mostly used in everyday clinical practice. The introduction of the PDT in treatment of nAMD in 2001 for the very first time affected natural course of the disease. This was achieved by acting on the last arm in pathophysiologic cascade of neovascularisation process: destruction of already formed neovascular membrane.

The second major breakthrough in the therapy of nAMD was the introduction of anti-VEGF drugs.

The anti-VEGF drugs act one step earlier in pathogenesis of the disease opposite to PDT, by preventing neovascularization and inducing regression of the newly formed neovascular blood vessels still dependent on VEGF support. Unlike PDT, which could only slow down the disease progression and reduce the visual acuity decline, patients treated with anti-VEGF could expect their visual acuity to be maintained and even improved in significant number of patients.

Although the anti-VEGF drugs are for the time being the best treatment option in managing nAMD, there are a few setbacks that caused the initial enthusiasm to drop. Regardless of anti-VEGF frequent dosing, a significant number of patients suffer further visual acuity deterioration throughout the course of the disease. Frequent intravitreal applications raise a risk for local complications such as: endophthalmitis, uveitis, vitreous hemorrhage, retinal detachment, posterior vitreous detachment etc. Despite continuous anti-VEGF blockage, active signaling pathways and expression of VEGF genes lead to continuous VEGF production, so continuous and regular treatment over a longer period of time is required as anti-VEGF drugs block only already produced VEGF.

Besides already mentioned increased complication risks, another problem is cost of anti-VEGF drugs as well as discomfort caused by intravitreal mode of application which ultimately leads to poor patient compliance. Having this in mind, new treatment options should be investigated. A potential new therapy regimen should actually have the following characteristics:

1. Increased treatment efficacy.
2. Prolonged remission period.
3. Low reapplication rate.
4. Low complications rate.
5. Acceptable cost.
6. Comfortable mode of administration.

In pursuit of better treatment modality in 2006 we proposed a combination of PDT and anti-VEGF with an idea to address two different steps of CNV formation: VEGF induced neovascularization and destruction of already formed CNV. In future a third potential drug acting on gene transcription could also be included thus preventing revascularization even earlier in the cascade of events. Further experimental and clinical trials are needed to support this hypothesis.

Clinical studies conducted between 2001 and 2006, i.e. before the introduction of anti-VEGF drugs, investigated a possibility of a combination treatment for nAMD using PDT and trimacinolone. Trimacinolone is a long-acting corticosteroid, otherwise employed in treatment of rheumatic diseases of locomotor system. In ophthalmology trimacinolone was used intravitreally for diabetic macular edema. A significant number of studies demonstrated the same functional outcome of triamcinolone and PDT combined versus the PDT alone, with longer remission interval and a reduced need for additional reapplications of PDT when combined with triamcinolone(55,56,57,58). Since the combination therapy of triamcinolone and PDT proved to have synergistic effect, we hypothesized that combination of anti-VEGF drugs and PDT could either improve functional outcome or extend treatment intervals in patients with nAMD. We suggested a possible synergistic effect due to different target-points of choroidal neovascularization process: PDT inducing vascular occlusion to already formed neovascular vessels while anti-VEGF drugs preventing formation of new neovascular tissue, inducing regression of the newly formed VEGF-dependent vessels and reducing permeability of neovascular tissue. Additional production of VEGF after PDT-induced hypoxia of choriocapilaris and inflammatory reaction due to neovascular tissue destruction could also be targeted with anti-VEGF drugs. In 2006, we concluded a pilot study on a small number of patients, divided into three groups - one treated with PDT, one with bevacizumab and the last one with bevacizumab and PDT together. The achieved results indicated possible synergistic effect: the visual acuity was better in patients who underwent combination therapy than in monotherapy groups, whereas the remission period was longer in combination group (59).

Other studies also indicated possible amplifying effect of the combination treatment with PDT and anti-VEGF. Also some studies included addition of intravitreal corticosteroid to address the inflammatory component of the disease (60-70).

The RADICAL was a phase II, multicentric, randomized, single-masked study of 162 patients with nAMD. The purpose of the study was to determine whether the PDT combined with ranibizumab reduced re-treatment rate compared with ranibizumab monotherapy. Patients were randomized into 4 groups: ranibizumab monotherapy, triple therapy with quarter-fluence verteporfin followed by ranibizumab and then dexamethasone, triple therapy with half-fluence verteporfin followed by ranibizumab and then dexamethasone and double therapy with half-fluence verteporfin followed by ranibizumab. The 24-month results showed significantly fewer retreatments in combination groups than in ranibizumab monotherapy group. Mean visual acuity change was not statistically different among the treatment groups. Through 24 months, patients in the triple therapy half-fluence group had a mean of 4.2 retreatment visits compared with 8.9 for patients who received ranibizumab monotherapy. At the month 24, mean VA in the triple therapy half-fluence group improved 1.8 letters fewer compared with the ranibizumab monotherapy group which was not significantly inferior. This results show a potential of combination therapy in reducing the retreatment rate while sustaining the same visual outcome. The concept of combination therapy with new emerging drugs could further show a synergistic effect when those drugs would be combined.

The displayed figures depict 2 patients from an extension of our pilot study throughout the period of 3 years. Both patients were treatment naïve. First patient N.U. was randomized to bevacizumab monotherapy treatment group and was treated with bevacizumab only and second patient R.K. was randomized to combination treatment group and was treated with combination treatment initially and then bevacizumab as needed. The second patient treated with combination treatment required less intravitreal bevacizumab injections during a 3 year follow-up period.

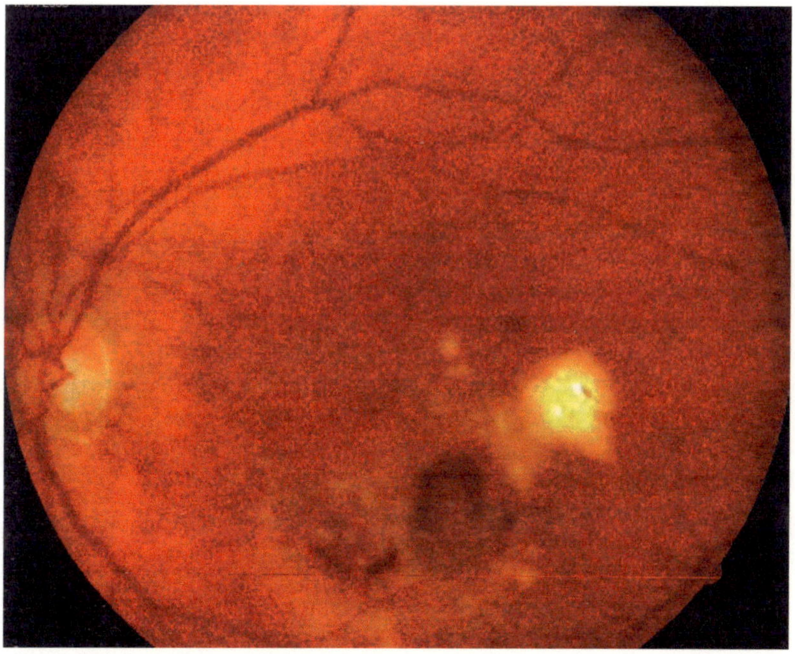

Fig. 1. Patient N.U. 76 yrs., fundus photography at baseline before bevacizumab treatment showing exudation and hemorrhage.

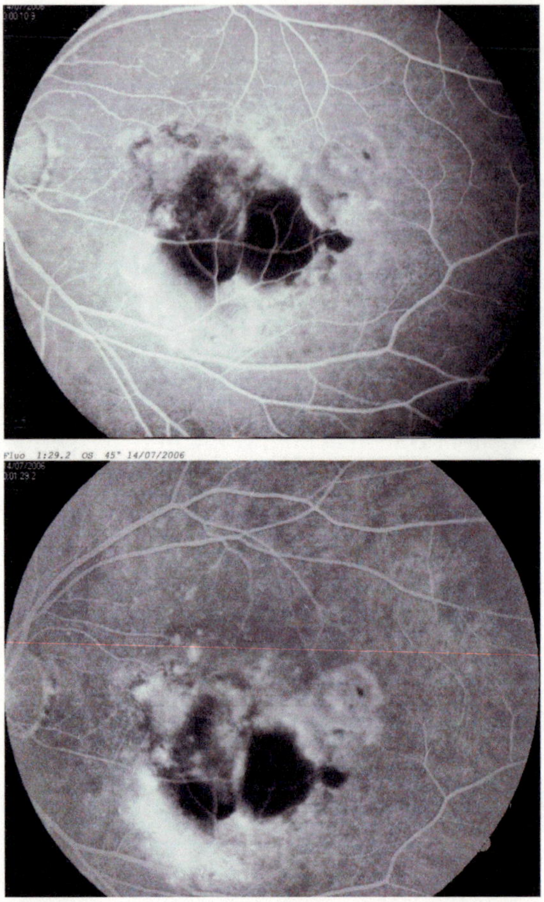

Fig. 2. Patient N.U. 76 yrs, early and late phase fluorescein angiography pictures at baseline before bevacizumab treatment showing blockage of retrofluorescence by hemorrhage, and a leakage of dye from the CNV.

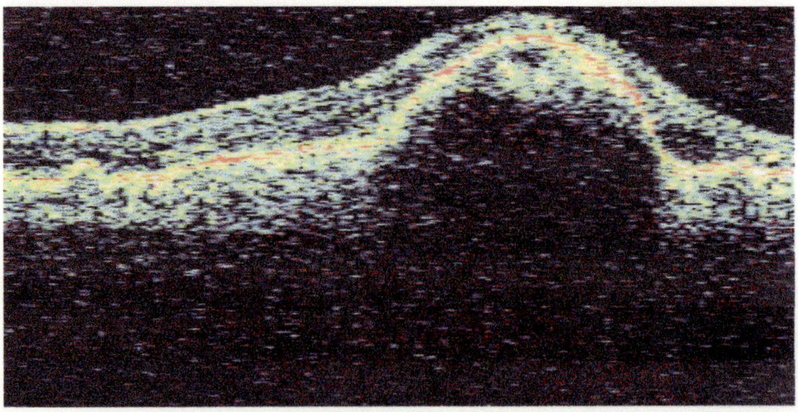

Fig. 3. Patient N.U. 76 yrs OCT scan (Zeiss Stratus II device) at baseline before bevacizumab treatment. It shows accumulation of intraretinal and subepithelial fluid.

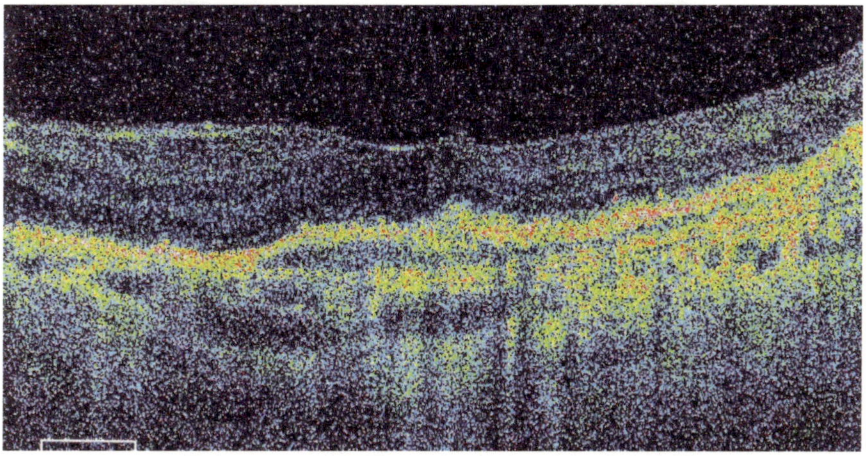

Fig. 4. Patient N.U. 76 yrs, OCT scan (Optopol SD device). It shows the resolution of fluid 3 years after repeated intravitreal bevacizumab treatment.

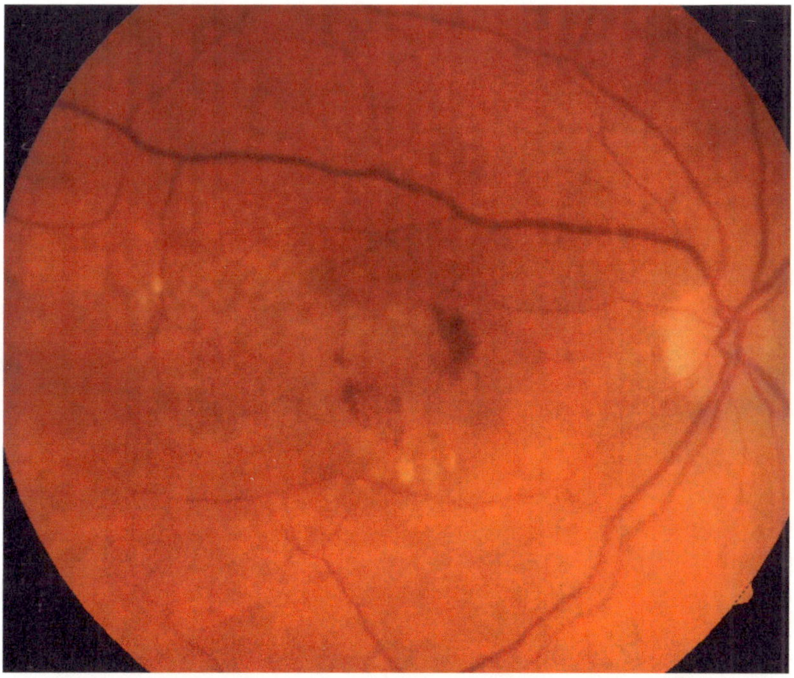

Fig. 5. Patient R.K. 74 yrs., fundus photography at baseline before combination treatment (bevacizumab + PDT) showing exudation and hemorrhage.

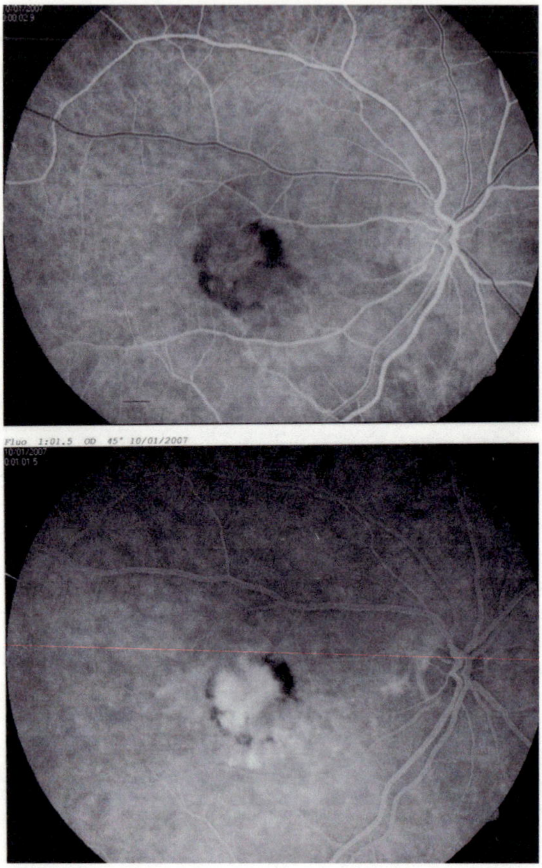

Fig. 6. Patient R.K. 74 yrs, early and late phase of fluorescein angiography at baseline before combination treatment (bevacizumab+PDT). It shows marginal hemorrhage and leakage of dye from the CNV.

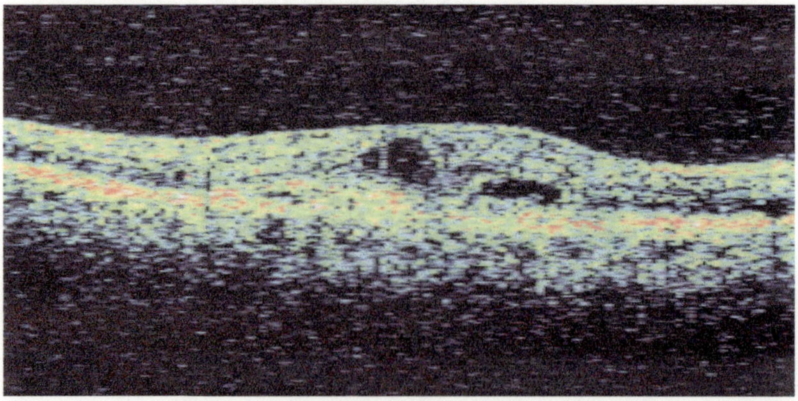

Fig. 7. Patient R.K. 74 yrs OCT scan (Zeiss Stratus II device) at baseline before combination treatment. It shows accumulation of intraretinal and subretinal fluid.

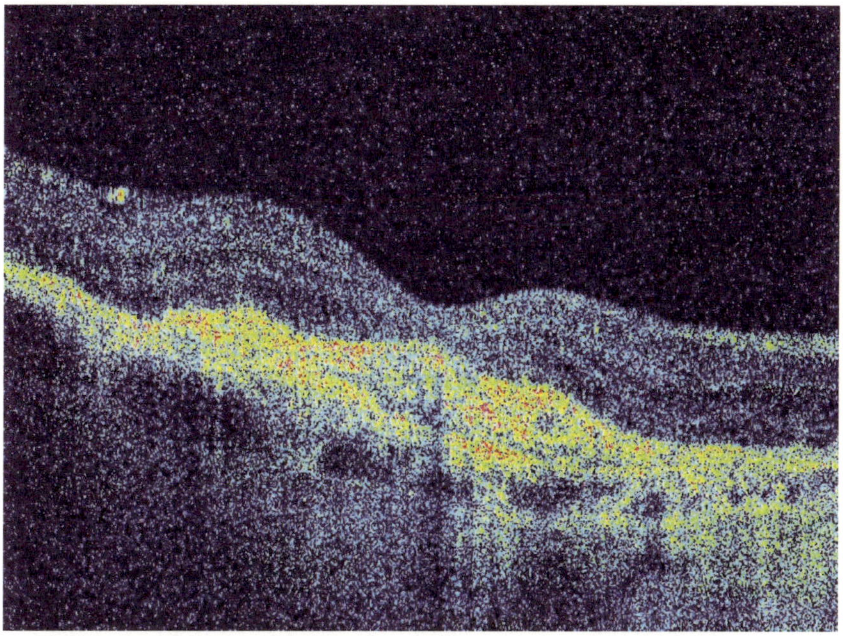

Fig. 8. Patient R.K. 74 yrs OCT scan (Optopol SD device). It shows resolution of fluid 3 years after initial combination treatment of intravitreal bevacizumab and photodynamic therapy followed by repeated bevacizumab treatment.

In summary we can conclude that new emerging therapies for nAMD for the first time in history managed to revert the natural history of disease. In significant number of patients some improvement could be achieved while in a majority of patients the treatment resulted in maintenance of visual acuity. However the significant burden of repeated intravitreal injections, increased risks of ocular and possibly systemic side effects and decreased patients' compliance lead to further visual loss over time. Also some patients do not respond to the available treatments favorably. So the need for new and more efficient drugs in terms of better functional outcome and reduced need for retreatment is fully justified. VEGF-Trap-Eye is pending approval and it may show to be more potent and requiring less treatment. Also combination of present treatment modalities should further be evaluated. Hopefully with better understanding of the genes responsible for different variants of nAMD we could either employ some form of genetic therapy or we can adjust already available treatments according to a certain genotype in order to achieve most favorable results.

5. References

[1] Macular Photocoagulation Study Group. Argon laser photocoagulation for neovascular maculopathy. Five-year results from randomized clinical trials. Arch Ophthalmol 1991;109(8):1109-14.

[2] Macular Photocoagulation Study Group. Subfoveal neovascular lesions in age-related macular degeneration. Guidelines for evaluation and treatment in the macular photocoagulation study. Arch Ophthalmol 1991;109(9):1242-57.

[3] Schmidt-Erfurth U, Laqua H, Schlotzer-Schrehard U, Viestenz A, Naumann GO. Histopathological changes following photodynamic therapy in human eyes. Arch Ophthalmol 2002;120:835-44.
[4] Fingar VH, Wieman TJ, Wiehle SA, Cerrito PB.The role of microvascular damage in photodynamic therapy: the effect of treatment on vessel constriction, permeability, and leukocyte adhesion.Cancer Res 1992;52(18):4914-21.
[5] Treatment of age-related macular degeneration with photodynamic therapy (TAP) Study Group. Photodynamic therapy of subfoveal choroidal neovascularization in age-related macular degeneration with verteporfin: one-year results of 2 randomized clinical trials--TAP report.Arch Ophthalmol 1999;117:1329-45.
[6] Treatment of Age-Related Macular Degeneration with Photodynamic Therapy Study Group. Photodynamic therapy of subfoveal choroidal neovascularization in age-related macular degeneration with verteporfin: two-year results of 2 randomized clinical trials--TAP report 2. Arch Ophthalmol 2001;119:198-207.
[7] Azab M, Boyer DS, Bressler NM et al. Verteporfin therapy of subfoveal minimally classic choroidal neovascularization in age-related macular degeneration: 2-year results of a randomized clinical trial. Arch Ophthalmol 2005;123(4): 448-57.
[8] Bressler NM. Verteporfin therapy of subfoveal choroidal neovascularization in age-related macular degeneration: two-year results of a randomized clinical trial including lesions with occult with no classic choroidal neovascularization-verteporfin in photodynamic therapy report 2. Am J Ophthalmol 2002;133:168-9.
[9] Barbazetto I, Burdan A, Bressler NM et al. Photodynamic therapy of subfoveal choroidal neovascularization with verteporfin: fluorescein angiographic guidelines for evaluation and treatment--TAP and VIP report No. 2. Arch Ophthalmol 2003;121:1253-68.
[10] McLeod D. Foveal translocation for exudative age related macular degeneration. Br J Ophthalmol. 2000;84:344–345.
[11] Akduman L, Karavellas MP, MacDonald JC, Olk RJ, Freeman WR.Macular translocation with retinotomy and retinal rotation for exudative age-related macular degeneration. Retina. 1999;19:418–423.
[12] Graroudas ES, Adamis AP, Cunningham ET Jr et al. Pegaptanib for neovascular age-related macular degeneration. N Engl J Med 2004;351(27):2805-16.
[13] Ferrara N, Damico L, Shams N et al. Development of ranibizumab, an anti-vascular endothelial growth factor antigen binding fragment, as therapy for neovascular age-related macular degeneration. Retina 2006;26:859-70.
[14] Rosenfeld PJ, Brown DM, Heier JS et al. MARINA Study Group. Ranibizumab for neovascular age-related macular degeneration. N Engl J Med 2006;355:1419-31.
[15] Brown DM, Kaiser PK, Michels M et al. ANCHOR Study Group. Ranibizumab versus verteporfin for neovascular age-related macular degeneration. N Engl J Med 2006;355:1432-44.
[16] Regillo CD, Brown DM, Abraham P et al. Randomized, double-masked, sham-controlled trial of ranibizumab for neovascular age-related macular degeneration: PIER Study year 1. Am J Ophthalmol 2008;145(2): 239-48.
[17] Lalwani GA, Rosenfeld PJ, Fung AE et al. A variable-dosing regimen with intravitreal ranibizumab for neovascular age-related macular degeneration: year 2 of the PrONTO study. Am J Ophthalmol 2009;148(1):43-58.

[18] Boyer DS, Heier JS, Brown DM et al. A Phase IIIb study to evaluate the safety of ranibizumab in subjects with neovascular age-related macular degeneration. Ophthalmology 2009;116(9):1731-9.
[19] Meyer CH, Eter N, Holz FD. SUSTAIN Study Group. Ranibizumab in Patients With Subfoveal Choroidal Neovascularization Secondary to Age-Related Macular Degeneration. Interim Results From the Sustain Trial. Invest Ophthalmol Vis Sci 2008;49: E-Abstract 273.
[20] Brown DM, Wang OW, Scott LC. HORIZON extension trial of Ranibizumab for wet AMD: subanalysis of year 1 results. AAO/SOE Joint Annual Meeting 2008, Atlanta, Georgia, USA.
[21] Kabbinavare F, Hurwitz HI, Fehrenbacher L et al. Phase II, randomized trial comparing bevacizumab plus fluorouracil (FU)/leucovorin (LV) with FU/LV alone in patients with metastatic colorectal cancer. J Clin Oncol 2003; 21:60-5.
[22] Hurwitz H, Fehrenbacher L, Novotny W et al. Bevacizumab plus irinotecan, fluorouracil, and leucovorin for metastatic colorectal cancer. N Engl J Med 2004;350:2335-42.
[23] Michels S S, Rosenfeld PJ, Puliafito CA et al. Systemic bevacizumab (Avastin) therapy for neovascular age-related macular degeneration. Twelve-week results of an uncontrolled open-label clinical study. Ophthalmology 2005;112(6):1035-47.
[24] Rosenfeld PJ, Moshfeghi AA, Puliafito CA. Optical coherence tomography findings after an intravitreal injection of bevacizumab (avastin) for neovascular age-related macular degeneration. Ophthalmic Surg Lasers Imaging 2005;36(4):331-5.
[25] Shahar J, Avery RL, Heilwell G et al. Electrophysiologic and retinal penetration studies following intravitreal injection of bevacizumab (Avastin). Retina 2006;26(3):262-9.
[26] AveryRL, Pieramici DJ, Rabena MD et al. Intravitreal bevacizumab (Avastin) for neovascular age-related macular degeneration. Ophthalmology 2006;113:363-72.
[27] Spaide RF, Laud K, Fine HF et al. Intravitreal bevacizumab treatment of choroidal neovascularization secondary to age-related macular degeneration. Retina 2006;26:383-90.
[28] Aisenbrey S, Ziemssen F, Volker M et al. Intravitreal bevacizumab (Avastin) for occult choroidal neovascularisation in age-related macular degeneration. Graefes Arch Clin Exp Ophthalmol 2007;245(7):941-8.
[29] Lazic R, Gabric N. Intravitreally administered bevacizumab (Avastin) in minimally classic and occult choroidal neovascularization secondary to age-related macular degeneration. Graefes Arch Clin Exp Ophthalmol 2007;245(1):68-73.
[30] Arevalo JF, Sánchez JG, Wu L et al. Intravitreal Bevacizumab for Subfoveal Choroidal Neovascularization in Age-Related Macular Degeneration at Twenty-four Months: The Pan-American Collaborative Retina Study Group.Ophthalmology 2010;Članak u tisku.
[31] Gamulescu MA, Radeck V, Lustinger B, Fink B, Helbig H. Bevacizumab versus ranibizumab in the treatment of exudative age-related macular degeneration. Int Ophthalmol 2010;30(3):261-6.
[32] Landa G, Made W, Doshi BV at al. Comparative study of intravitreal bevacizumab (Avastin) versus ranibizumab (Lucentis) in the treatment of neovascular age-related macular degeneration. Ophthalmologica 2009;223(6):370-5.

[33] Fong DS, Custis P, Howes J, Hsu JW. Intravitreal Bevacizumab and Ranibizumab for Age-Related Macular Degeneration: A Multicenter, Retrospective Study. Ophthalmology 2010;117(2):298-302.
[34] Shaha AR, Del Priore LV. Duration of action of intravitreal ranibizumab and bevacizumab in exudative AMD eyes based on macular volume measurements. Br J Ophthalmol 2009;93(8):1027-32.
[35] CATT Research Group, Martin DF, Maguire MG, Ying GS, Grunwald JE, Fine SL, Jaffe GJ. Ranibizumab and bevacizumab for neovascular age-related macular degeneration.N Engl J Med. 2011; 364(20):1897-908.
[36] Holash J, Davis S, PapadopoulosN et al. VEGF-Trap: a VEGF blocker with potent antitumor effects. Proc Natl Acad Sci USA 2002;99(17):11393-8.
[37] Nguyen QD, Shah SM, Hafiz G et al. A phase I trial of an IV-administered vascular endothelial growth factor trap for treatment in patients with choroidal neovascularization due to age-related macular degeneration. Ophthalmology 2006;113(9):1522.
[38] Heiner JS. VEGF Trap Eye Phase III Trial Results. VIEW 1 results.Paper presented at:Angiogenesis, Exudation and Degeneration 2011; Miami, Florida.
[39] Schmidt-Erfurt U. VEGF Trap Eye Phase III Trial Results. VIEW 2 results.Paper presented at: Angiogenesis, Exudation and Degeneration 2011; Miami, Florida.
[40] Reich S, Fosnot J, Akiko K et al. Small interfering RNA (siRNA) targeting VEGF effectively inhibits ocular neovascularization in a mouse model. Molecular Vision 2003;9:210-6.
[41] Tolentino MJ, Brucker AJ, Fosnot J et al. Intravitreal injection of vascular endothelial growth factor small interfering RNA inhibits growth and leakage in a nonhuman primate, laser-induced model of choroidal neovascularization. Retina 2004;24(4):660.
[42] Shen J, Samul R, Silva RL et al. Suppression of ocular neovascularization with siRNA targeting VEGF receptor 1. Gene Ther 2006;13(3):225-34.
[43] Mabjeesh NJ, Amir S. Hypoxia-inducible factor (HIF) in human tumorigenesis. Histol Histopathol 2007;22(5):559-72.
[44] Hunter T. Signaling: 2000 and beyond. Cell 2000;100:113–27.
[45] Robinsnon DR, Wu YM, Lin SF. The protein tyrosine kinase family of the human genome. Oncogene 2000;19:5548–57.
[46] Blume-Jensen P, Hunter T. Oncogenic kinase signalling. Nature 2001;411:355–65.
[47] Maier P, Unsoeld AS, Junker B at al. Intravitreal injection of specific receptor kinase inhibitor PTK787/ZK222584 improves ischemia-induced retinopathy in mice. Graefes Arch Clin Exp Ophthalmol 2005;243(6):593-600.
[48] Dawson DW, Volpret OV, Gillis P at al. Vascular permeability factor/vascular endothelial growth factor and the significance of microvascular hyperpermeability in angiogenesis. Curr Top Microbiol Immunol 1999;237:97-132.
[49] StellmachV, Crawford SE, Zhou W, Bouck N. Prevention of ischemia-induced retinopathy by the natural ocular antiangiogenic agent pigment epithelium-derived factor. Proc Natl Acad Sci USA 2001;98:2593-7.
[50] Mori K., Gehlbach P, Yamamoto S at al. AAV-mediated gene transfer of pigment epithelium-derived growth factor inhibits choroidal neovascularization. Invest Ophthalmol Vis Sci 2002;43:1994-2000.

[51] Jaakkola A, Heikkonen J, Tommila P et al. Strontium plaque brachyterapy for exudative age related macular degeneration: 3 year results of a randomized study. Ophthalmology 112 (4), 2005;567-573.

[52] Finger PT, Berson A, Ng T, Szechter A. Ophthalmic plaque radiotherapy for age-related macular degeneration associated with subretinal neovascularization. Am J Ophthalmol 1999; 127:170-177.

[53] Avila MP, Farah ME, Duprat JP et al. Twelve month short-term safety and visual acuity results from a multicentre prospective study of epiretinal strontium-90 brachytherapy with bevacizumab for the treatment of subfoveal choroidal neovascularization secondary to age-related macular degeneration. Br J Ophthalmol. 2009; 93: 305-309.

[54] Kuppermann BD. Epimacular brachytherapy for the treatment of choroidal neovascularization associated with age related macular degeneration. Presented at the Retina sub-specialty meeting, AAO, 2008.

[55] Augustin AJ, Schmidt-Erfurth U. Verteporfin therapy combined with intravitreal triamcinolone in all types of choroidal neovascularization due to age-related macular degeneration.Ophthalmology 2006;113:14 –22.

[56] Spaide RF, Sorenson J, Maranan L. Photodynamic therapy with verteporfin combined with intravitreal injection of triamcinolone acetonide for choroidal neovascularization. Ophthalmology 2005;112(2):301-4.

[57] Chan WM, Lai TY, Wong AL, Tong JP, Liu DT, Lam DS.Combined photodynamic therapy and intravitreal triamcinolone injection for the treatment of subfoveal choroidal neovascularisation in age related macular degeneration: a comparative study. Br J Ophthalmol 2006;90(3):337-41.

[58] Schadlu R, Kymes SM, Apte RS. Combined photodynamic therapy and intravitreal triamcinolone for neovascular age-related macular degeneration: effect of initial visual acuity on treatment response..Graefes Arch Clin Exp Ophthalmol 2007;245(11):1667-72.

[59] Lazic R, Gabric N.Verteporfin therapy and intravitreal bevacizumab combined and alone in choroidal neovascularization due to age-related macular degeneration. Ophthalmology 2007;114(6):1179-85.

[60] Bakri SJ, Couch SM, McCannel CA, Edwards AO. Same-day triple therapy with photodynamic therapy, intravitreal dexamethasone, and bevacizumab in wet age-related macular degeneration Retina 2009;29(5):573-8.

[61] Kaiser PK, Boyer DS, Garcia R et al. Verteporfin photodynamic therapy combined with intravitreal bevacizumab for neovascular age-related macular degeneration. Ophthalmology 2009;116(4):747-55.

[62] Shah GK, Sang DN, Hughes MS. Verteporfin combination regimens in the treatment of neovascular age-related macular degeneration. Retina 2009;29(2):133-48.

[63] Maier M, Haas K, Feucht N et al. Photodynamic therapy with verteporfin combined with intravitreal injection of bevacizumab for occult and classic CNV in AMD. Klin Monatsbl Augenheilkd 2008;225(7):653-9.

[64] Ahmadieh H, Taei R, Soheilian M, Riazi-Esfahani M, Ahadi H. Single-session photodynamic therapy combined with intravitreal bevacizumab for neovascular age-related macular degeneration. Eur J Ophthalmol 2008;18(2):297-300.

[65] Ladewig MS, Karl SE, Hamelmann V et al. Combined intravitreal bevacizumab and photodynamic therapy for neovascular age-related macular degeneration. Graefes Arch Clin Exp Ophthalmol 2008;246(1):17-25.
[66] Oner A, Gumus K, Arda H, Yuce Y, Karakucuk S, Mirza E. Pattern electroretinographic results after photodynamic therapy alone and photodynamic therapy in combination with intravitreal bevacizumab for choroidal neovascularization in age-related macular degeneration. Doc Ophthalmol 2009;119(1):37-42.
[67] Rudnisky, C.J.Liu, C.,Ng, M. Weis, E. Tennant, M.T.S. Intravitreal bevacizumab alone versus combined verteporfin photodynamic therapy and intravitreal bevacizumab for choroidal neovascularization in age-related macular degeneration: Visual acuity after 1 year of follow-up. Retina 2010;30:548-54.
[68] Mataix J, Palacios E, Carmen DM, Garcia-Pous M, Navea A .Combined ranibizumab and photodynamic therapy to treat exudative age-related macular degeneration. An Option For Improving Treatment Efficiency. Retina 2010;Članak u tisku.
[69] Costagliola C, Romano MR, Rinaldi M et al. Low fluence rate photodynamic therapy combined with intravitreal bevacizumab for neovascular age-related macular degeneration.Br J Ophthalmol 2010;94(2):180-4.
[70] Debefve E, Pegaz B, Ballini JP, van den Bergh H.Combination therapy using verteporfin and ranibizumab; optimizing the timing in the CAM model. Photochem Photobiol 2009;85(6):1400-8.

Re-Treatment Strategies for Neovascular AMD: When to Treat? When to Stop?

Sengul Ozdek[1] and Mehmet Cuneyt Ozmen[2]
[1]*Gazi University, School of Medicine, Department of Ophthalmology, Ankara*
[2]*Yenisehir State Hospital, Department of Ophthalmology, Kahramanmaras*
Turkey

1. Introduction

Age-related macular degeneration (AMD) is a leading cause of severe, irreversible vision impairment in developed countries (Friedman et al., 2004; Klein et al., 1992). Although an estimated 80% of patients with AMD have the non-neovascular form, the neovascular form is responsible for almost 90% of severe visual loss (visual acuity 20/200 or worse) resulting from AMD (Ferris et al., 1984). There was no effective treatment for most of the neovascular AMD lesions till 2004. By this time, the role of vascular endothelial growth factor (VEGF) in neovascular AMD became obvious and anti-VEGF agents emerged for this purpose. Pegaptanib sodium intravitreal injection (Macugen; [OSI] Eyetech, New York, NY, 2004), ranibizumab intravitreal injection (Lucentis, Genentech, Inc., South San Francisco, CA, 2006) were the FDA approved treatments for AMD. The first report of intravitreal bevacizumab (Avastin; Genentech, Inc., South San Francisco, CA) administration for neovascular AMD was published in 2005 (Rosenfeld et al., 2005). By early 2006, off-label intravitreal bevacizumab was used by many retina specialists as a first-line therapy for neovascular AMD because of the low cost of this drug. Wholesale prices of the medications range from $1950 per dose for ranibizumab and $995 per dose for pegaptanib, to approximately $50 per dose for bevacizumab (Champan & Beckey, 2006; Web, 2008).

MARINA and ANCHOR were the first studies showing level 1 evidence for the effect of ranibizumab for the treatment of neovascular ARMD (Brown et al., 2009; Rosenfeld et al., 2006a; Rosenfeld et al., 2006b). These studies have shown that 33-40% of the eyes with neovascular AMD treated with ranibizumab gained 15 letters or more (Brown et al., 2009; Rosenfeld et al., 2006a). However these studies used monthly injections of the drug for 24 months. This is the most effective treatment but almost impossible to apply in routine applications both for patients and doctors. Additionally monthly injections will cost so much that treatment cannot be afforded neither by patients nor the social security systems.

2. How to decrease the number of injections without compromising visual acuity?

PIER study was the first study investigating the results of less frequent dosing regimens with ranibizumab (3-monthly) for the treatment of AMD (Regillo et al., 2008). However

PIER study revealed disappointing results showing loss of early gained vision during 3-monthly injection period. Other prospective studies, PrONTO and SUSTAIN, investigated the efficacy of PRN (pro re nata; as needed) treatment regimen. Results from these studies suggested that fewer injections by using a variable dosing regimen with OCT will most likely result in visual acuity improvements similar to the results from the phase III trials which used monthly injections (Holz et al., 2011; Lalwani et al., 2009; Rosenfeld et al., 2006b)

2.1 What is "PRN" treatment regimen and what are the most reliable criteria for treatment decision?

PRN treatment regimen is a treatment schedule which allows treatment only if the lesion is active. The aim of the PRN treatment is to avoid monthly injections and to decrease the number of injections as much as possible while preserving the vision gained in the loading period (first three months).

The key point in PRN treatment is assessment of the activity of the lesion to decide for additional treatments. It is obvious that a totally fibrotic yellow scarring lesion without any hemorrhage around, only late staining of the scar tissue in fluorescein angiography (FA), and no subretinal or intraretinal fluid in optical coherence tomography (OCT) with stable vision for a long time does not need any treatment. On the other side of the spectrum, a lesion with subretinal hemorrhages all around, significant late leakage in FA and a considerable subretinal or intraretinal fluid in OCT and deteriorating vision recently needs treatment with no doubt. However most of the lesions are in between these two ends of the spectrum especially during the course of anti-VEGF treatments and may be difficult to decide if any further treatment is necessary or not.

Until recently, the presence or absence of fluorescein leakage and the angiographic appearance of the lesion were the main criteria for the decision to treat neovascular ARMD and re-treat using PDT or anti-VEGF therapy (Schmidt-Erfurth et al., 2007). Within the last decade OCT has emerged and enhanced our understanding in many central retinal diseases. For AMD, OCT appears to be useful for evaluating the responses of the retina and retinal pigment epithelium (RPE) to the treatment (Cohen et al., 2007; Eter & Spaide, 2005; Fung et al., 2007; Krebs et al., 2008; Lalwani et al., 2009; Salinas-Alamán et al., 2005; Schmidt-Erfurth et al., 2007; van Velthoven et al., 2006;). Clinical trials have shown that in the two thirds of patients requiring ranibizumab therapy because of recurrent neovascularization, OCT seemed to detect early anatomic changes in the macula before any vision loss (observation during the extension trials of phase I-II studies by P. Rosenfeld: unpublished data). The PrONTO study was initiated to explore the use of OCT as the basis for a less frequent variable dosing regimen with ranibizumab (Fung et al., 2007; Lalwani et al., 2009). This study used some criteria for retreatment including an OCT based parameter (an increase in central OCT thickness of at least 100 mm) during the first year. However they made an amendment to their OCT based criteria in the second year. They changed the retreatment criteria to include any qualitative change in the appearance of the OCT images that suggested recurrent fluid in the macula. These qualitative changes included the appearance of retinal cysts or subretinal fluid or an enlargement of a PED. Any of these qualitative changes alone was sufficient to permit retreatment (Lalwani et al., 2009).

2.2 Treatment regimens other than PRN

Although PRN treatment regimen may reduce the number of intravitreal injections and allow the treatment plan to be individualized, it may still require monthly visits to specialized centers. In contrast to mandated monthly injections, patients treated with PRN strategies may develop multiple recurrences of CNV activity over time. Recurrent intra- or subretinal fluid could potentially induce progressive, cumulative dysfunction of the neural retina, resulting in a decreased ability of the retina to recover despite further treatment. There are some other treatment regimens like "treat and extend" and "individualized injection intervals" regimens which aim to individualize the treatment plan and decrease the number of injections per year, but at the same time attempts to achieve a fluid-free macula and decrease the number of visits (Brown & Regillo, 2007; Gupta et al., 2010; Hörster et al., 2011; Oubraham et al., 2011; Spaide, 2007).

2.2.1 Treat & extend dosing regimen

In an attempt to minimize the number of intravitreal injections, office visits, and ancillary testing, a "treat and extend" regimen (TER) was first put forth by Bailey Freund, (unpublished data, February 2006) and then adopted by others (Gupta et al., 2010; Oubraham et al., 2011). A typical TER starts with monthly injections until the signs of exudation have resolved with confirmation by OCT. The treatment interval is then sequentially lengthened by 1 to 2 weeks as long as there are no signs of recurrent exudation. When recurrent exudation is detected on a follow-up visit, the treatment interval is reduced to the prior interval. Treatment is rendered at every visit but the time between visits is individualized based on a given patient's response to treatment. As with traditional PRN regimens, the goal is to maintain an exudation-free macula with the fewest number of injections. This approach also may allow for a significant reduction in office visits and tests.

In a study by Gupta et al., eyes with neovascular AMD experienced significant visual improvement when managed with intravitreal ranibizumab using a TER. This treatment approach also was associated with significantly fewer patient visits, injections, and direct annual medical cost compared with monthly injections such as in the phase III clinical trials (Gupta et al., 2010). The interval was individualized for each patient in an attempt to maintain an exudation-free macula. In another study comparing the results of this treatment regimen with the standard PRN regimen, patients reinjected by the TER had a far better visual outcome than PRN regimen but needed more injections (Oubraham et al., 2011).

2.2.2 Individualized injection intervals

Another individualized treatment strategy that aims to avoid recurrent CNV activity in addition to reducing the number of injections and visits may be to perform the injection immediately prior to the next recurrence. This would require the ability to determine or predict the recurrence interval for an individual patient. A treatment schedule can be obtained for some of the cases after a couple of years of experience with PRN regimen (Hörster et al., 2011). Knowledge of individual recurrence interval times may allow for the development of an individualized treatment plan (Figure 1).

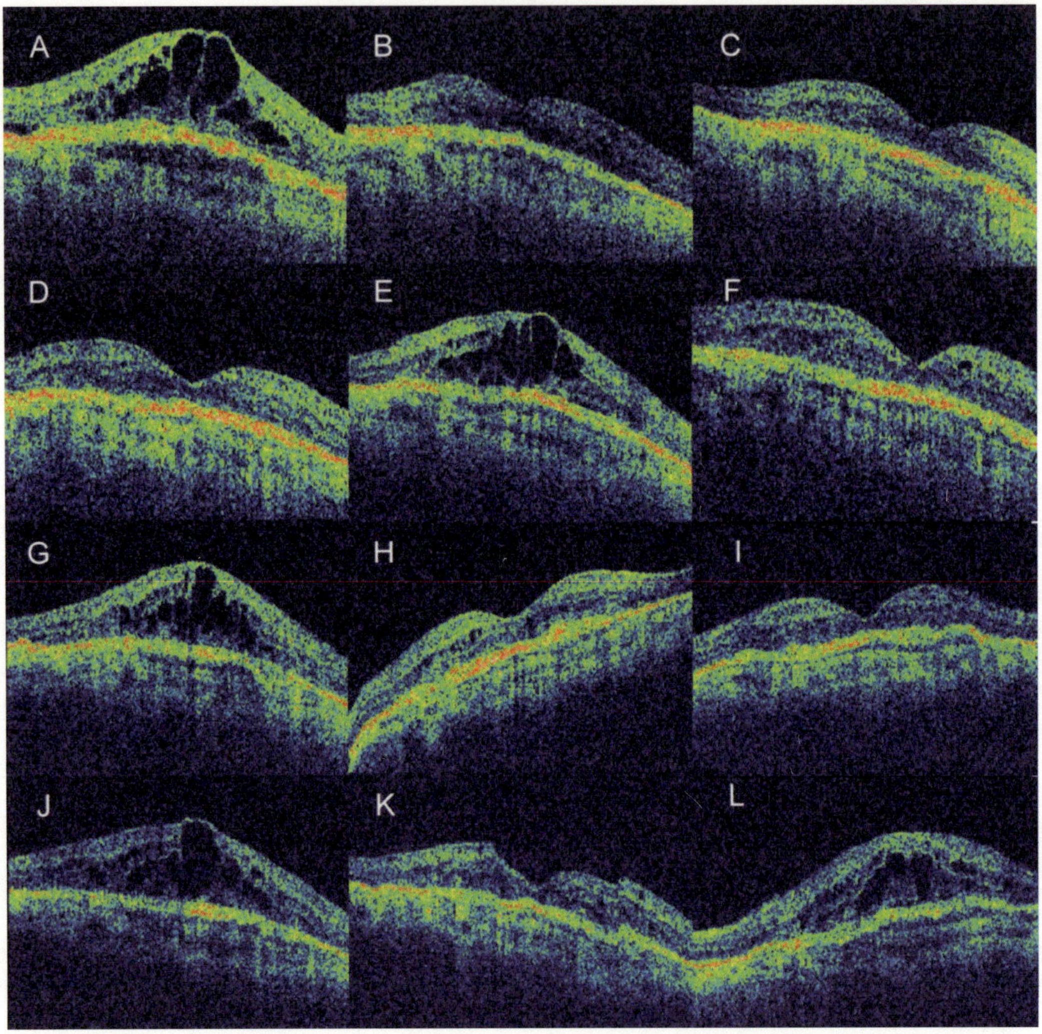

Fig. 1. A, Baseline, VA: 44 letters, 1st injection. B, 1st month, 53 letters, 2nd injection. C, 2nd month, 54 letters, 3rd injection. D, 51 letters, no treatment. E, 4th month, 46 letters, 4th injection. F, 5th month, 47 letters, no treatment. G, 6th month, 46 letters, 5th injection. H, 7th month, 42 letters, 6th injection. I, 8th month, 50 letters, no treatment. J, 8th month, 44 letters, 7th injection. K, 9th month, 48 letters, no treatment. L, 10th month, 38 letters, 8th injection. According to the data, this patient has a recurrence pattern of 8 weeks, thus needs re-treatment every 7 weeks.

A retrospective study in University of Cologne analyzed the recurrence intervals of patients undergoing anti-VEGF therapy for neovascular AMD to determine whether predictable, regular recurrence patterns were present for individual patients (Hörster et al., 2011). The paper reported that, all recurrences occurred at regular intervals in 41% of the eyes and the recurrence interval time may vary between individuals (Hörster et al., 2011).

In conclusion, re-injections of ranibizumab shortly prior to a recurrence may avoid recurrent leakage and fluid accumulation, as well as further growth of the CNV lesion size. Therefore, avoiding recurrent CNV activity with prophylactic injections may protect the neural retina from additional damage and improve the long-term prognosis. However, this approach requires the ability to determine individual recurrence intervals with a couple of years of experience with PRN regimen.

2.3 The need for an activity scoring for re-treatment of exudative AMD

All treatment regimens mentioned above aims to reduce injection numbers without compromising the patients visual acuity. Yet there is not a consensus about the objective criteria of an active neovascular CNV lesion.

Definition of an active lesion should not be done only with the OCT based criteria. We believe that, other parameters like visual acuity, presence of hemorrhage associated with the lesion, lesion size and FA staining pattern (when needed) are all also important for assessment of neovascular AMD activity. The PrONTO study put some of these parameters together and created their criteria for retreatment. Retreatment with ranibizumab was performed only if one of the following occurred in PrONTO study (Fung et al., 2007):

1. An increase in central OCT thickness of at least 100 mm,
2. A loss of five letters in conjunction with recurrent fluid by OCT,
3. New-onset classic neovascularization,
4. New macular hemorrhage.

SUSTAIN study used only VA and OCT criteria for retreatment decision. We believe that these are very well prepared criteria, however, some of the items could be changed and some new criteria could be added to make it more reliable.

3. A clinical activity scoring for re-treatment of exudative AMD

A new clinical activity scoring (AS) is proposed to assess activity of lesions, to quantify the activity for statistical purposes in clinical studies and to standardize the re-treatment protocols during the course of anti-VEGF treatments of neovascular AMD lesions. This may be a basis for treatment regimens.

3.1 Methods

The proposed AS is based on the well known and widely used signs and findings of active neovascular AMD (Table 1):

1. Presence of subretinal or intraretinal fluid in OCT,
2. Presence of hemorrhage associated with the lesion,
3. Change in vision;
    a. Objective measured visual acuity (VA)
    b. Subjective vision (what patient feels about his vision)
4. Change in size of the lesion,
5. FA staining pattern (when needed).

PARAMETER	GRADING	SCORE
Hemorrhage Amount of hemorrhage associated with the lesion	No hemorrhage	0
	decreased	1
	Same amount	2
	increased	3
OCT Subretinal fluid / retinal thickening / PED	None	0
	Decreased	1
	Any amount at beginning / Stable	2
	Increased	3
Visual assessment Objective	Increased	0
	No change	1
	Decreased	2
Visual assessment Subjective	Increased	0
	No change	1
	Decreased	2
FA Staining pattern	No staining/window defect	0
	Staining of scar tissue/PED	1
	Late leakage	2
Size of the lesion Lesion area in FA	Decreased	0
	Beginning size / Stable	1
	Increased	2

Table 1. Clinical Activity Scoring for neovascular AMD lesions

Apart from FA staining pattern, all of the other assessments are based on the changes (same-baseline/increased/decreased) in each parameter and given a number to define the activity. At the end of the assessment, given numbers are summed and an activity score is calculated.

This scoring has been used in a group of neovascular AMD patients all of which have been involved in a prospective study for intravitreal bevacizumab (IVB) in our clinic (Şekeryapan et al., 2011). All of them received IVB monotherapy. The reports of the patients were reviewed retrospectively and demographic features as well as lesion characteristics of the patients were noted. AS of all of the lesions were calculated according to the following criteria:

1. **OCT:** OCT was performed using the Humphrey model 3000 (Zeiss-Humphrey Instruments, San Leandro, CA). After pupil dilatation, six consecutive 6mm long scans containing 128 axial profiles (A-scans) at equally spaced angular orientations in a radial spoke pattern centered on the fovea (known as Fast Macular Thickness Protocol) were obtained for each eye. Using Retinal Thickness Mapping Software mean retinal thickness value which was measured in the central disc with a diameter of 1000µm in the center of the macula was used as central foveal thickness (CFT). The fluid pattern (subretinal / intraretinal diffuse / cystoid / pigment epithelial detachment - PED) was also noted. Only the CFT was used as an activity parameter in AS and at least 10% increase or decrease in CFT was accepted as a decrease or increase. The amount of fluid at the beginning was scored as 2. It was scored as "0" if there is no fluid, "1" if there is a decrease and "3 if there is an increase in CFT.

2. **Amount of hemorrhage**: The amount of hemorrhage associated with the lesion (in ophthalmoscopy, colored fundus photography or FA) was noted and if there is any hemorrhage at the beginning it was scored as 2. If there is no hemorrhage it was scored as 0, if it was decreased it was scored as 1, if it was the same, scored as 2, and if it was increased scored as 3.
3. Visual assessment:
   a. *Objective VA* is measured with ETDRS and noted as a baseline and scored as 1. If there is a decrease in vision (any line or ≥5 letters loss) it was scored as 2 and if there is any increase in vision (any line or ≥5 letters gain) it was scored as 0.
   b. *Subjective vision* (what patient feels about his vision): Patient's feeling about any change in his vision was also asked and noted as subjective vision which was scored as 0 if he feels better, 2 if he feels worse and 1 if he did not feel any change (baseline).
4. **FA staining pattern**: No staining or window defect (0), staining of scar tissue or PED (1) and late leakage (2) were noted.
5. **The area of the lesion** (mm^2): It was measured in FA and the baseline area (or no change) was scored as 1, at least 10% (of the original area) increase was scored as 2 and at least 10% decrease was scored as 0.

Records of the patients at the 1st month visit after the treatment were also noted and all of the above parameters were again noted, so that an AS is calculated both before and after the treatment. AS could range between 0 and 14. Change in AS after the treatment was analyzed by using Wilcoxon signed rank test.

It can be hypothesized that, the more active the lesion the more it may respond to the anti-VEGF therapy. A possible correlation between pretreatment AS and posttreatment decrease in AS was investigated by using Pearson correlation test to test this hypothesis.

Eyes with favorable treatment response (two or more units of decrease in AS) and unfavorable treatment response (one unit or no decrease in AS) were separated and the mean pre and posttreatment AS were calculated for both groups. The mean AS of these two groups were compared by using Mann-Whitney U test. At this stage, a cut off point for AS was searched to determine the eyes that need treatment. Sensitivity, specificity, negative and positive predictive values of the AS were calculated to determine the cut off point for AS which will be used to decide on re-treatments.

3.2 Results

In this section, the results of an ongoing study is presented to better understand the activity scoring.

A total of 52 eyes with neovascular AMD were involved in the study. Mean age of the patients was 72.7 (52-89), mean visual acuity (logMAR) was 0.68 (0-1.6) and mean lesion area was 8.9 mm^2 (0.6-33mm^2) before treatment.

Pretreatment mean AS of eyes was 7.4 (ranged between 3 and 10) which decreased significantly to 4.2 after treatment ($p<0.001$, Wilcoxon). There was a significant positive correlation between the pretreatment AS of eyes and the posttreatment decrease in AS (Pearson correlation coefficient: 0.534, $p<0.001$, Figure 2).

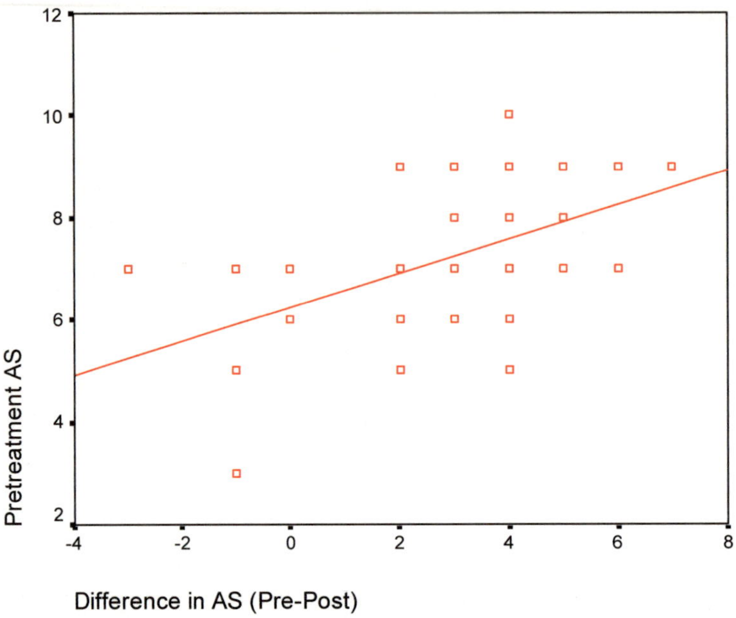

Fig. 2. Correlation between the pretreatment AS of eyes and the post-treatment decrease in AS (Pearson correlation coefficient: 0.534, $p<0.001$)

To define a cut-off point a group of eyes with favorable treatment responses is formed by separating those who had at least 2 point decrease in AS and named the favorable response group. The remaining eyes formed the unfavorable response group. The pretreatment mean AS was 7.5 (6-10) in favorable response group and 6 (3-7) in unfavorable response group. The pretreatment AS in favorable treatment response group was statistically significantly higher than those of unfavorable treatment response groups ($p=0.003$, Figure 3).

The sensitivity, specificity, negative and positive predictive values of the AS with different cut off points were calculated (table 2) and an AS of 7 was found to be most suitable as a cut-off point for further analysis.

	Pretreatment AS≥ 6	Pretreatment AS≥ 7	Pretreatment AS≥ 8
Positive predictive value	85,10%	90,20%	100,00%
Negative predictive value	40,00%	45,50%	25,70%
Sensitivity	93,00%	86,00%	39,50%
Specificity	22,20%	55,60%	100,00%

Table 2. Predictive values, sensitivity and specificity of AS for detecting favorable treatment response (2 or more decrease in AS)

Eyes with an AS of 7 or more (group 1, highly active group, n=41) were separated from those less than 7 (group 2, less active group, n=11) and a subgroup analysis was done. The mean AS in group 1 was 7.8 (7-10) before treatment and 4.3 (1-10) after treatment. The decrease was statistically significant (p<0.001, Figure 4). The mean pretreatment AS was 5.4 (3-6) in group 2 which decreased to 4 (1-6) after treatment. Although the decrease was less than that in group 1, it was still statistically significant (p=0.034, Figure 4). The mean decrease in AS was 3.5 in group one and 1.4 in group two (p=0.003, Figure 5).

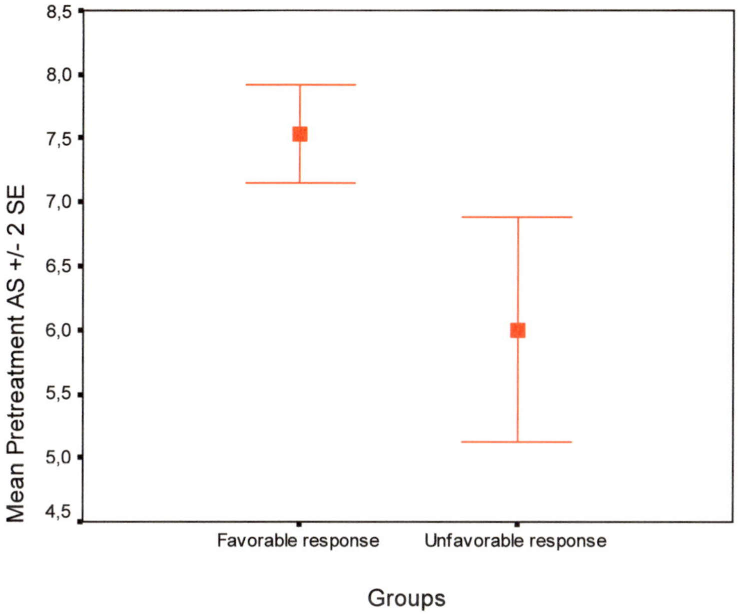

Fig. 3. The pretreatment AS was statistically significantly higher in favorable treatment response group than unfavorable treatment response group (Mann Whitney U test p=0.003).

Sensitivity of AS (ratio of eyes with a favorable response and an AS of 7 or more to the total number of eyes with favorable response) was 86% and, specificity of AS (ratio of eyes with an unfavorable response and an AS of less than 7 to the total number of eyes with unfavorable response) was 56% with a cut-off point of 7 (table 3). Positive predictive value (ratio of eyes with AS of 7 or more and a favorable response to the total number of eyes with AS of 7 or more) of AS was 90% and negative predictive value (ratio of eyes with AS of less than 7 and an unfavorable response to the total number of eyes with AS of less than 7) of AS was 45% (table 3). These may be assumed as indicators for accuracy of AS.

	Favorable Response	Unfavorable Response	Total
AS ≥7	37	4	41
AS <7	6	5	11
Total	43	9	52

Positive predictive value, 37 of 41 = 90%; negative predictive value, 5 of 11 = 45%, sensitivity, 37 of 43 = 86%, specificity, 5 of 9 = 56%.

Table 3. Accuracy of activity score (AS) in predicting therapeutic outcome of treatment in neovascular AMD.

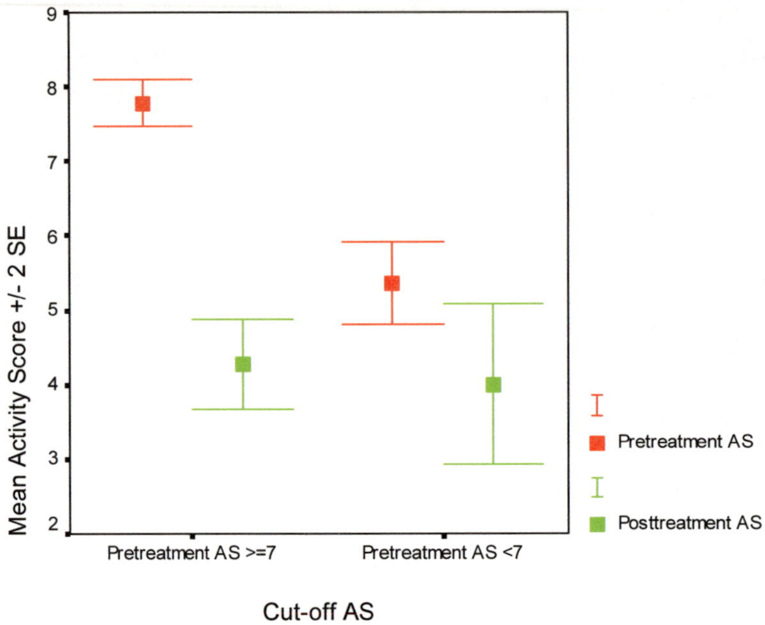

Fig. 4. Pretreatment and posttreatment mean AS of eyes in group 1 (with an AS of 7 or more, highly active group) and in group 2 (with an AS of less than 7, less active group).

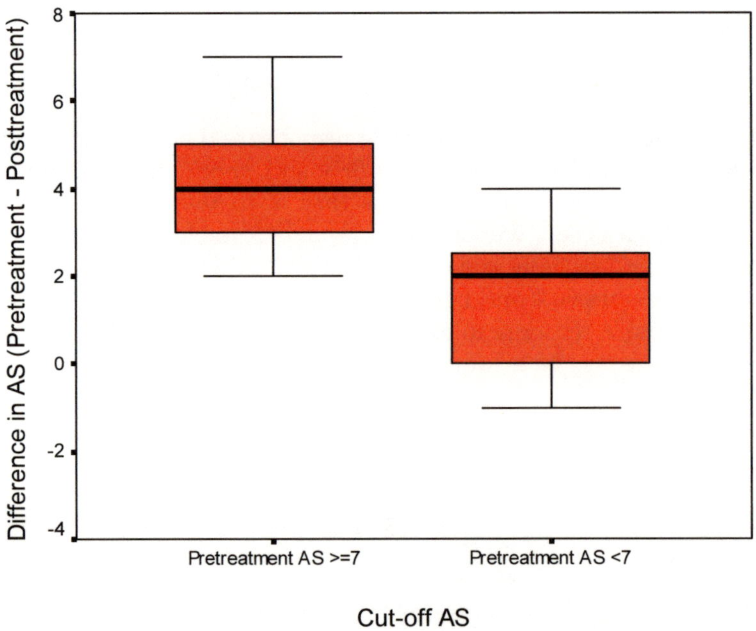

Fig. 5. Pre and post treatment difference in AS of highly active group and less active group. Decrease in AS was significantly more in highly active group (pretreatment AS≥7) (p=0.003).

4. Discussion

Neovascular AMD activity is an important factor to determine if it should be treated or not. It is important not to over-treat these eyes to avoid from injection and drug related complications as well as high cost of the treatment. There is no standard protocol for the treatment and retreatment schedule of these eyes and most ophthalmologists use their clinical experience to decide. Following the disappointing results from the quarterly regimen of the PIER study, which showed us loss of early gained vision during 3-monthly injection period (Regillo et al., 2008), new prospective studies like PrONTO, and SUSTAIN are under way investigating less frequent dosing regimens and preliminary results from these studies suggest that fewer injections (mean: 9.9 injections within 24 months in PrONTO, 5.7 injections within 12 months in SUSTAIN) will most likely result in visual acuity improvements similar to the results from the phase III trials by using a variable dosing regimen with OCT (Fung et al., 2007; Lalwani et al., 2009; Rosenfeld et al., 2006b).

Although most of the studies used OCT findings and VA changes to determine the need for additional therapy (Holz et al., 2011), we believe that, some other parameters like, subjective feeling of patients about their vision, presence of hemorrhage associated with the lesion, lesion size, FA staining pattern and are also important for assessment of neovascular AMD activity especially in those undetermined cases. AS is defined to standardize the understanding of findings and definition of active lesion. We are studying on this system since 2002 and have used it in our practice as well as in some of our studies (Ozdek et al.,2005; Ozdek et al.,2007).

It is obvious that ophthalmoscopic appearance of a lesion is very important during interpretation of OCT and FA findings. This is to see new subretinal hemorrhages, exudates and fibrotic scar tissues so that FA and OCT findings can correctly be interpreted. OCT is a very important indicator of neovascular AMD activity and may be assumed as the main determinant for deciding the need for re-treatment in patients with AMD. Recently, there is a tendency to assess the activity of neovascular AMD lesions with only OCT without performing FA after the initial assessment (Brown & Regillo, 2007; Cohen et al., 2007; Rosenfeld et al., 2006b; Salinas-Alamán et al., 2005). This approach has emerged especially after anti-VEGF treatments of neovascular AMD lesions to avoid from monthly FA. Once the diagnosis of neovascular AMD was established with FA before treatment, OCT was reported to have a sensitivity of 96% for detecting lesion activity and a diagnostic efficiency (proportion of correct results) of 83% (Salinas-Alamán et al., 2005). However, OCT cannot detect other features including blood, lipid, and vascular patterns so effectively. When a subretinal new hemorrhage associated with the lesion appears in an eye with a dry OCT and FA (without any late leakage) most of the retina specialists assume it as an active lesion and treat it. This is the case when activation takes place on a far edge of the subfoveal neovascular AMD lesion. Salinas et al reported that, OCT may be complementary to FA, especially in cases in which FA was inconclusive. They have found that OCT was considered as positive (presence of sub-retinal fluid and/or intraretinal fluid) in 14.2% of the cases in which FA did not show clear leakage. On the other hand, most of the cases with positive OCT findings without any leakage on FA (false positives) had a disciform scar with persistent cystic cavities on OCT (Salinas-Alamán et al., 2005). It can be concluded that if there is no fibrotic scar visible during the fundus examination, the presence of remaining fluid on the OCT scan may indicate residual lesion activity. It is also valid to assume that a hyperreflective structure on OCT could be misinterpreted without a fundus examination. Therefore, we believe that OCT, FA, and a fundus examination are complementary examinations that should be interpreted together in those undetermined cases.

Although we used FA as a parameter in AS, we do not mean to say that we have to perform FA at every visit. Actually, we need to score the lesion only if it is not so clear that the lesion is active or not what we call as "undetermined cases"(Figure 6) . In other words, if we are not sure that a patient should be retreated or not, we can apply to the AS just to bring all the parameters together. If we still do not want to perform a FA, we can add only 1 point for FA which is neutral for activity scoring for FA.

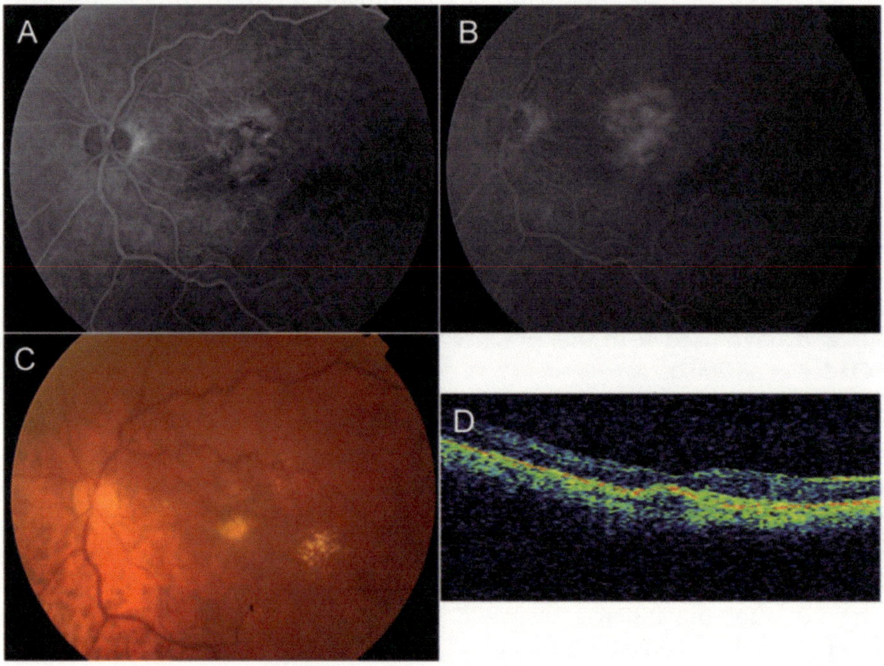

Fig. 6. 85 year old woman with a neovascular AMD on the left eye received four doses of intravitreal bevacizumab. On the last visit she had lost 5 letters with a subjective visual impairment. A, early phase of the angiogram. B, late phase of the angiogram. C, fundus photograph. D, OCT image of fovea. This would be an undetermined case without FA. Although the OCT has no sign of active lesion, there are late leakage in FA and objective and subjective visual loss. According to table 1 the patient has an activity score of 8 and assessed as an active lesion.

Change in VA is another very important determinant factor in assessment of treatment effect on neovascular AMD. Usually worsening of VA is a sign of bad response to the treatment and, a stable or increased VA is supposed as a favorable treatment response. It is possible to see patients with a dry OCT and silent ophthalmoscopy without any hemorrhage having a decreased VA both objectively and subjectively. Those patients may have a late leakage in FA indicating activity and treatment need or that VA decrease may be a sign of progression of dry component of AMD.

Vision is not only the central VA and it has many other components like scotomas in visual field, contrast sensitivity, color vision etc. So snellen or ETDRS visual acuity measurement may not be enough to assess vision especially in macular diseases. The simplest measure may be to ask the patient his feelings about his vision; if it is the same, decreased or increased. The subjective change in vision may also give important clues about the effect of treatment. However, it is highly dependent on the patients' personality and on the eye (in the better eye or in the worse eye). Patient may feel always worse if he is pessimistic and depressive or vice versa. Patient may feel the changes more precisely if the problem is in the better eye, on the other hand, may not feel the significant changes if the disease is in the worse eye. To overcome such shortcomings of subjective assessment of vision, more objective measures for the assessment of the other components of the central vision may be used. VFQ25 may be an option but takes a long time for these cases and is not so practical. Unver et al have developed a new tool for the automated assessment of functional central vision called central field acuity perimetry to solve such problems (Unver et al., 2009). However there is no clinical study with central field acuity perimetry for this purpose up till now. Microperimetry and functional magnetic resonance imaging are other new tools to measure objective measure of topographic visual function (Baseler et al., 2011; Uppal et al., 2011). On the other hand, deterioration of vision is not always an indication of lesion activity itself. Progression of the dry component of the disease (atrophic changes), fibrosis and cicatrisation of the lesion during healing period following treatment may also cause deterioration of vision. Vision cannot be a sole criterion (just like other parameters) but may add to other factors indicating lesion activity.

Change in lesion area is another important determinant of the activity of the lesion. It is not seldom to see a central inactive lesion without any fluid in OCT or any change in objective measured VA may enlarge with a pseudo-pod like extension from one side indicating an active lesion. They usually feel this difference as a subjective worsening of the vision. On the other side, the lesion area may become smaller after treatment indicating a decreased activity of the lesion. This is also an important complementary parameter for assessment of lesion activity and the response to treatment that needs to be taken into account during assessment especially in those gray cases.

The major problem that we faced during the assessment of the reliability of this scoring system was the absence of a gold standard to define an active lesion which can be used for comparison. Rosenfeld et al were the first to define some criteria to identify an active lesion which needs retreatment with anti-VEGF agents in PrONTO study (Ozdek et al., 2005; Rosenfeld et al., 2006b). However, these criteria were not tested for reliability or sensitivity. Our scoring system has some differences from the criteria used in PrONTO study. Firstly, we used a 10% change in CFT in OCT to be significant instead of 100 micron increase for all cases. Sometimes only 30 microns of increase in CFT may be an important change (especially in minimally edematous fovea) on the other hand, even 100 microns of increase in OCT may be meaningless (especially in highly edematous/elevated fovea). Secondly, we have added change in size of the lesion as another criterion. Thirdly, we used subjective changes in vision as another criterion to decide on retreatments. This is because most of the patients feel some very early changes in lesion activity before any change become apparent in FA, OCT or ETDRS visual acuity testing. We strongly believe that this should be taken into account during assessment of lesion activity.

We would like to emphasize on the unequal distribution of points between different parameters of the AS. We have purposefully given higher scores for hemorrhage (3 points), OCT (3 points) and VA (2+2 points) which are more powerful indicators of the lesion activity than the FA and lesion size.

When we take all of these parameters into account and score it, we observed that pretreatment mean AS was 7.4 which decreased significantly to 4.2 after treatment. Which means that AS really indicates the activity of the lesion. We also observed that a lesion with a higher AS is more likely to give more dramatic response to the anti-VEGF treatment with a more significant decrease in AS (Figure 4).

Transferring these data to the clinical applications, it seems logical to treat lesions with an AS of 7 or more with anti-VEGF therapy. The high sensitivity (86%) and positive predictive values (90%) of the AS strongly suggest retreatment of lesions with an AS of 7 or more. However the lower sensitivity and negative predictive values of AS weakly supports observation of the ones with lower AS without treatment. The lower rates are most possibly because of the lower number of the eyes with less AS who had still been treated with anti-VEGF. When the number of such eyes had been equal to the treated eyes with higher AS, the specificity and negative predictive values of AS might have been higher which would make the AS a more reliable measure.

In addition to routine clinical practice, AS may be used as a standard way of assessment of lesion activity especially in clinical studies for the statistical comparison of the results. AS may be a valuable tool to see the picture (both the lesion and the response to the treatment) as a whole.

5. Conclusions

In conclusion, assessment of the lesion activity is important for PRN treatment approaches and AS seems to be a standardized measure to assess the activity of the lesion at the beginning as well as the treatment effect after anti-VEGF therapy. It may be modified with use of some other tools like central field acuity perimetry to be more objective. A lesion with an AS of 7 or more seems to be an active lesion which needs treatment and it most possibly will give a favorable response to anti-VEGF treatment as a decrease in activity. However, the sensitivity and specificity of AS needs to be tested with further studies with larger number of patients to be conclusive. Additionally scoring of the lesion activity quantifies the lesion activity allowing for statistical comparisons between different treatment methods in clinical studies.

Individualized approaches, on the other side, may be a good option in suitable cases. Re-injections shortly prior to a recurrence may avoid further growth of the CNV lesion size, protecting the neural retina from additional damage and improve the long-term prognosis. This may be a better option than PRN approaches preventing recurrences other than treating the recurrence. However, this approach requires the ability to determine individual recurrence intervals with a couple of years of experience with PRN regimen and some lesions do not obey any rule of periodical recurrence in long term. The results of these approaches need to be proven with further randomized controlled studies to be conclusive.

6. References

Baseler HA, Gouws A, Crossland MD, Leung C, Tufail A, Rubin GS & Morland AB, (2011). Objective Visual Assessment of Antiangiogenic Treatment for Wet Age-Related Macular Degeneration. In: *Optom Vis Sci.*, e-pub, June 2011, Available from: <http://www.ncbi.nlm.nih.gov/pubmed/21705938>

Brown DM & Regillo CD, (2007). Anti-VEGF agents in the treatment of neovascular age-related macular degeneration: applying clinical trial results to the treatment of everyday patients. *Am J Ophthalmol.*, Vol.144, No.4, (October 2007), pp.627-37, ISSN 0002-9394

Brown DM & Regillo CD, (2007). Anti-VEGF agents in the treatment of neovascular age-related macular degeneration: applying clinical trial results to the treatment of everyday patients. *Am J Ophthalmol.*, Vol.144, No.4, (October 2007), pp.627–37, ISSN 0002-9394

Brown DM, Michels M, Kaiser PK, Heier JS, Sy JP & Ianchulev T, ANCHOR Study Group, (2009). Ranibizumab versus verteporfin photodynamic therapy for neovascular age-related macular degeneration: Two-year results of the ANCHOR study. *Ophthalmology.* Vol.116, No.1, (January 2009), pp.57-65.e5, ISSN 0161-6420

Chapman JA & Beckey C, (2006). Pegaptanib: a novel approach to ocular neovascularization. *Ann Pharmacother.*, Vol.40, No.7-8, (July-August 2006), pp.1322–6, ISSN 1060-0280

Cohen SY, Korobelnik JF, Tadayoni R, Coscas G, Creuzot-Garcher C, Devin F, Gaudric A, Mauget-Faysse M, Sahel JA, Souied E, Weber M & Soubrane G, (2007). Monitoring anti-VEGF drugs for treatment of exudative AMD. *J Fr Ophtalmol*, Vol.30, No.4, (April 2007), pp.330-4, ISSN 0181-5512

Eter N & Spaide RF, (2005). Comparison of fluorescein angiography and optical coherence tomography for patients with choroidal neovascularization after photodynamic therapy. *Retina*, Vol.25, No.6, (September 2005), pp.691-6, ISSN 0275-004X

Ferris FL III, Fine SL & Hyman L, (1984). Age-related macular degeneration and blindness due to neovascular maculopathy. *Arch Ophthalmol.*, Vol.102, No. 11, (November 1984), pp.1640–2, ISSN 0003-9950

Friedman DS, O'Colmain BJ, Muñoz B, Tomany SC, McCarty C, de Jong PT, Nemesure B, Mitchell P & Kempen J, Eye Diseases Prevalence Research Group, (2004). Prevalence of agerelated macular degeneration in the United States. *Arch Ophthalmol.*, Vol.122, No.4, (April 2004), pp.564 –72, ISSN 0003-9950 Friedman et al., 2004

Fung AE, Lalwani GA, Rosenfeld PJ, Dubovy SR, Michels S, Feuer WJ, Puliafito CA, Davis JL, Flynn HW Jr & Esquiabro M, (2007). An optical coherence tomography-guided, variable-dosing regimen with intravitreal ranibizumab (Lucentis) for neovascular age-related macular degeneration. *Am J Ophthalmol.* Vol.143, No.4, (April 2007), pp.566–583, ISSN 0002-9394

Gupta OP, Shienbaum G, Patel AH, Fecarotta C, Kaiser RS & Regillo CD, (2010). A treat and extend regimen using ranibizumab for neovascular age-related macular degeneration clinical and economic impact. *Ophthalmology,* Vol.117, No.11, (November 2010), pp.2134-40, ISSN 0161-6420

Holz FG, Amoaku W, Donate J, Guymer RH, Kellner U, Schlingemann RO, Weichselberger A & Staurenghi G, SUSTAIN Study Group, (2011). Safety and efficacy of a flexible dosing regimen of ranibizumab in neovascular age-related macular degeneration: the SUSTAIN study. *Ophthalmology,* Vol.118, No.4, (April 2011), pp.663-71, ISSN 0161-6420

Hörster R, Ristau T, Sadda SR & Liakopoulos S, (2011). Individual recurrence intervals after anti-VEGF therapy for age-related macular degeneration. *Graefes Arch Clin Exp Ophthalmol.,* Vol.249, No.5, (May 2011), pp.645-52, ISSN 0721-832X

Klein R, Klein BE & Linton KL, (1992). Prevalence of age-related maculopathy: the Beaver Dam Eye Study. *Ophthalmology,* Vol.99, No.6, (June 1992), pp.933–43, ISSN 0161-6420

Krebs I, Ansari-Shahrezaei S, Goll A & Binder S, (2008). Activity of neovascular lesions treated with bevacizumab: comparison between optical coherence tomography and fluorescein angiography. *Graefes Arch Clin Exp Ophthalmol.,* Vol.246, No.6, (June 2008), pp.811-5, ISSN 0721-832X

Lalwani GA, Rosenfeld PJ, Fung AE, Dubovy SR, Michels S, Feuer W, Davis JL, Flynn HW Jr & Esquiabro M, (2009). A variable-dosing regimen with intravitreal ranibizumab for neovascular age-related macular degeneration: year 2 of the PrONTO Study. *Am J Ophthalmol.,* Vol.148, No.1, (July 2009), pp.43-58.e1, ISSN 0002-9394

Oubraham H, Cohen SY, Samimi S, Marotte D, Bouzaher I, Bonicel P, Fajnkuchen F & Tadayoni R, (2011). Inject and extend dosing versus dosing as needed: a comparative retrospective study of ranibizumab in exudative age-related macular degeneration. *Retina,* Vol.31, No.1, (January 2011), pp.26-30, ISSN 0275-004X

Ozdek S, Bozan E, Gurelik G & Hasanreisoglu B, (2007). Transpupillary thermotherapy for the treatment of choroidal neovascularization secondary to angioid streaks. *Can J Ophthalmol.,* Vol.42, No.1, (February 2007), pp.95-100, ISSN 0008-4182

Ozdek S, Hondur A, Gurelik G & Hasanreisoglu B, (2005). Transpupillary t hermotherapy for myopic choroidal neovascularization: 1-year follow-up: TTT for myopic CNV. *Int Ophthalmol.,* Vol.26, No.4-5, (August-October 2005), pp.127-33, ISSN 0165-5701

Regillo CD, Brown DM, Abraham P, Yue H, Ianchulev T, Schneider S & Shams N (2008). Randomized, double-masked, sham-controlled trial of ranibizumab for neovascular age-related macular degeneration: PIER Study year 1. *Am J Ophthalmol.,* Vol.145, No.2, (February 2008), pp.239-48, ISSN 0002-9394

Rosenfeld PJ, Brown DM, Heier JS, Boyer DS, Kaiser PK, Chung CY & Kim RY, MARINA Study Group, (2006). Ranibizumab for neovascular age-related macular degeneration. *New England Journal of Medicine,* Vol.355, No.14, (October 2006), pp.1419-31, ISSN 0028-4793

Rosenfeld PJ, Moshfeghi AA & Puliafito CA, (2005). Optical coherence tomography findings after an intravitreal injection of bevacizumab (Avastin) for neovascular age-related macular degeneration. *Ophthalmic Surg Lasers Imaging.*, Vol.36, No.4, (July-August 2005), pp.331-5, ISSN 1542-8877

Rosenfeld PJ, Rich RM & Lalwani GA, (2006). Ranibizumab: Phase III clinical trial results. *Ophthalmol Clin North Am.*, Vol.19, No.3, (September 2006), pp.361-72, ISSN 0896-1549

Salinas-Alamán A, García-Layana A, Maldonado MJ, Sainz-Gómez C & Alvárez-Vidal A, (2005). Using optical coherence tomography to monitor photodynamic therapy in age related macular degeneration. *Am J Ophthalmol.*, Vol.140, No.1, (July 2005), pp.23-8, ISSN 0002-9394

Schmidt-Erfurth UM, Richard G, Augustin A, Aylward WG, Bandello F, Corcòstegui B, Cunha-Vaz J, Gaudric A, Leys A, Schlingemann RO; European Society for Retina Specialists' Guidelines Committee (EURETINA), (2007). Guidance for the treatment of neovascular age-related macular degeneration. *Acta Ophthalmologica Scandinavica,* Vol.85, No.5, (August, 2007), pp.486-94, ISSN 1395-3907

Spaide R. Ranibizumab according to need: a treatment for age-related macular degeneration. *Am J Ophthalmol.* Vol.143, No.4, (April 2007), pp.679–80, ISSN 0002-9394

Şekeryapan B, Özdek Ş, Özmen MC, Gürelik G & Hasanreisoğlu B, (2011). Yaşa Bağlı Maküla Dejenerasyonuna Bağlı Koroidal Neovaskülarizasyon Tedavisinde Tek Başına Bevacizumab veya Fotodinamik Tedavi ile Kombinasyon: 12 Ay Sonuçları. *Retina-Vitreus,* Vol.19, No.2, (June 2011), pp.97-102, ISSN 1300-1256

Unver YB, Yavuz GA, Bekiroğlu N, Presti P, Li W & Sinclair SH, (2009). Relationships between clinical measures of visual function and anatomic changes associated with bevacizumab treatment for choroidal neovascularization in age-related macular degeneration. *Eye,* Vol.23, No.2, (February 2009), pp.453-60, ISSN 0950-222X

Uppal G, Feely M, Crossland M, Membrey L, Lee J, da Cruz L & Rubin GS, (2011). Assessment of Reading Behaviour with an Infrared Eyetracker after 360 Degree Macular Translocation for Age Related Macular Degeneration. *Invest Ophthalmol Vis Sci.*, Vol.52, No.9, (August 2011), pp.6486-96, ISSN 1552-5783

van Velthoven ME, de Smet MD, Schlingemann RO, Magnani M & Verbraak FD, (2006). Added value of OCT in evaluating the presence of leakage in patients with age-related macular degeneration treated with PDT. *Graefes Arch Clin Exp Ophthalmol.*, Vol.244, No.9, (September 2006), pp.1119-23, ISSN 0721-832X

Web JA. (January 2008). Genentech decision expands access to bevacizumab. In: *Ophthalmology Times,* 2011, Available from: <http://ophthalmologytimes.modernmedicine.com/ophthalmologytimes/issue/issueDetail.jsp?id=13920>.

9

Combined Therapies to Treat CNV in AMD: PDT + Anti-VEGF

Jorge Mataix, M. Carmen Desco, Elena Palacios and Amparo Navea
Fundacion Oftalmologica Mediterraneo, Valencia
Spain

1. Introduction

Age-related macular degeneration (AMD) causes a high incidence of morbility in the elderly. The dry forms of the disease are the most usual, but wet forms (15% of the total of cases) are responsible for 80% of AMD-related cases of severe vision loss. Age-related macular degeneration is essentially a choroidal/retinal pigment epithelium (RPE) disease which affects the overlying neurosensory retina. Formation of choroidal neovessels that penetrate the subretinal space is the main cause of vision loss. Knowing what role the vascular endothelial growth factor (VEGF) plays in angiogenesis of the formation of these neovessels is a determining factor. Ferrara's studies describe the four main biological functions in VEGF agents (Ferrara & Gerber, 2001):

1. Increase in vascular permeability
2. Growth and proliferation of vascular endothelial cells
3. Migration of vascular endothelial cells
4. Survival of immature endothelial cells by preventing apoptosis

Since the formation of choroidal neovascularization (CNV) is a determining factor in vision loss in wet AMD, it is reasonable to expect a reduction in the risk of vision loss by inhibiting new vessel formation and preventing their growth. The efficacy of antiangiogenesis agents for this purpose has provided proof of the concept of therapy targeted at a specific molecular step in the process, namely the inhibition of VEGF (Gragouas et al. 2004). Therefore the appearance of antibodies against VEGF (anti-VEGF) brought about a considerable advance in the treatment of exudative forms of AMD. The most important effects are **regression** of existing vessels, **normalization** of surviving vessels, and **inhibition** of vessel growth.

Antiangiogenesis agents have proved to be beneficial but are often administered late in the process when the aim of the treatment is to salvage vision rather than to prevent vision loss. One obstacle in developing a single approach to treatment stems from the possibility that AMD is the product of multiple pathologic processes. A more exciting goal is halting the process at a subclinical stage or preventing the disease in patients identified as being at risk for vision loss. Progress in isolating multiple processes responsible for disease progression is creating new opportunities for combination therapies.

2. Composition of neovessels

Histopathologic examination of CNV shows granulation-like tissue, with the invasion of not only blood vessels, but also inflammatory and mesenchymal cells embedded in a loosely formed extracellular matrix. Although the majority of damage attributed to CNV is due to neovessel bleeding or leakage, there are other components and factors associated with CNV that influence the visual prognosis decisively.

A two-component model of CNV has been developed to offer a conceptual framework to structure combination treatments. One is the *vascular component*, which is composed of vascular endothelial cells and associated pericytes. The other is the *nonvascular component* which is made up of the remaining cells, such as the inflammatory cells, glial cells, myofibroblasts, and fibrocytes (Spaide, 2006a, 2009). Inhibiting one has the potential to inhibit, at least partially, the other due to mutual interactions between the two components and each component can potentially cause damage. Inhibiting either one would seem to offer some hope in slowing down or arresting the process, but inhibition of both would intuitively lead to the best theoretical outcome.

Blocking the vascular component is achieved mainly by administering anti-VEGF agents, although in advanced lesions with mature neovessels covered by pericytes, anti-VEGF on their own cannot make these neovessels regress. In these cases, a combination of other therapies has to be resorted to which act by means of selective mechanisms, such as blocking the platelet-derived growth factor (PDGF) to target the pericytes, or a non-selective attack mechanism, such as ionizing radiation which is explained further on (Jain RK, 2005) in this chapter.

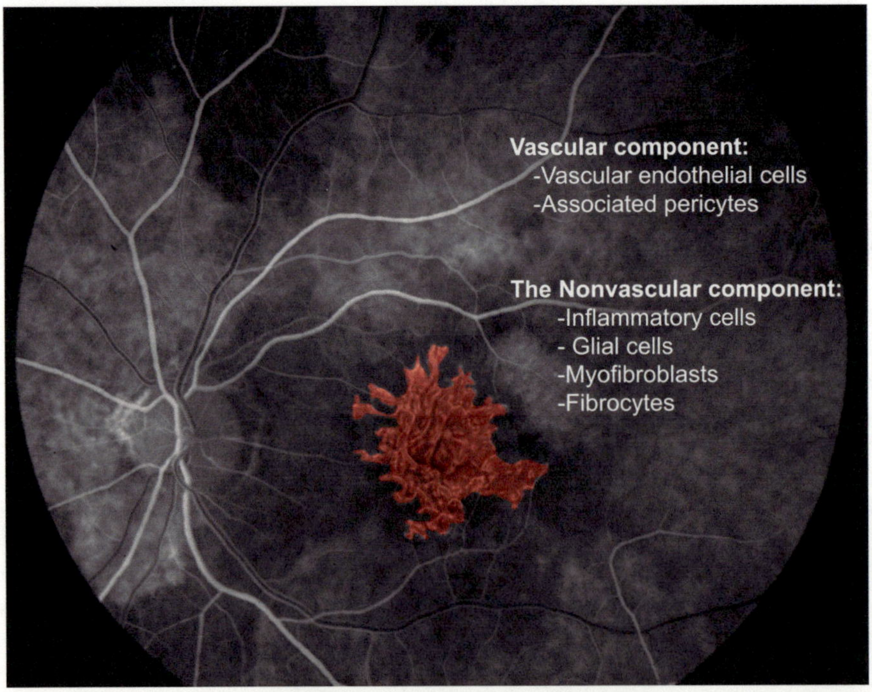

Fig. 1. CNV components: vascular and nonvascular components

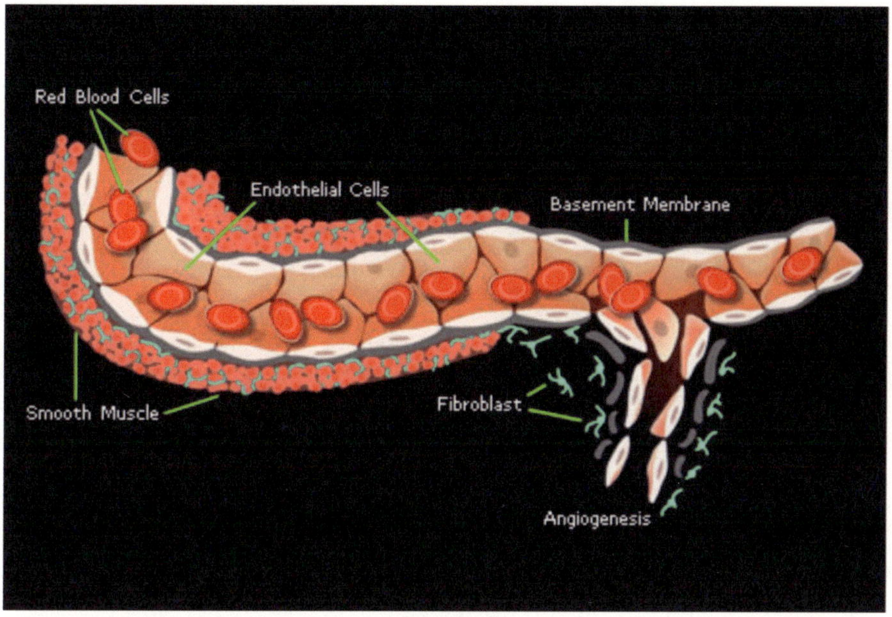

Fig. 2. Phases in angiogenesis in which the formation of a neovessel guided by the extracellular matrix is shown (Genentech image).

Blocking the extravascular component, like inhibiting subretinal fibrosis, can considerably reduce the morbility of the disease. Biological therapies mediated by cytokines, such as the tumor necrosis factor, ionizing radiation which does not only act on the vascular component but also on the extravascular component, corticosteroid drugs combined with anti-VEGF can improve the therapeutic response, inhibiting the development of the extracellular matrix which, in the long term, often plays a determining role in vision loss.

Currently, the most relevant therapy available is VEGF inhibition. Possibly, greater success could be achieved if other key factors in pathogenesis were also inhibited. It would be more advantageous if angiogenesis, scarring, and inflammation were targeted simultaneously. Combination approaches may not only increase overall efficacy but also reduce the potential for side effects by allowing relatively low doses to yield a greater level of efficacy than higher doses of a single agent.

3. Limitations of anti-VEGF in CNV treatment

The appearance of anti-VEGF is a revolutionary treatment in wet AMD as, for the first time, the progression of the disease can be stopped. Nevertheless, it cannot restore vision and there are still many cases that progress in spite of repeated treatment with anti-VEGF. Listed below are several limitations of anti-VEGF that make the quest for other therapies, or a combination of therapies, necessary.

3.1 Anti-VEGF agents do not affect mature vessels

As described above, one of the functions of VEGF is favoring the survival of endothelial cells, but this function is just restricted to immature vessels in which angiogenesis necessarily requires the activation of survival pathways to maintain the condition of the vessels (Gerber et al., 1998). Nonetheless, the mechanisms involved in the maturing process of the vessels, such as pericyte coverage and the formation of interaction between endothelial and periendotherlial cells with the basal membrane, free the endothelial cell from the requirement of the survival function of VEGF.

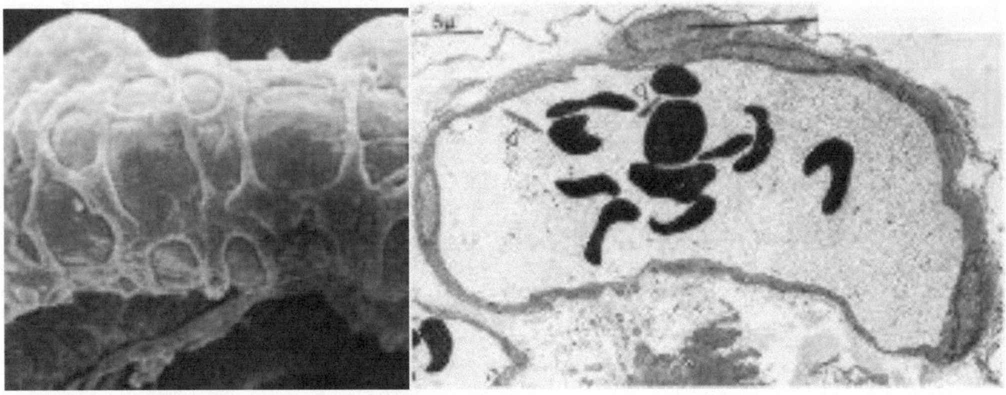

Fig. 3. Composition of a mature blood vessel, made up of endothelial cells, pericyte coverage, and the interactions between them.

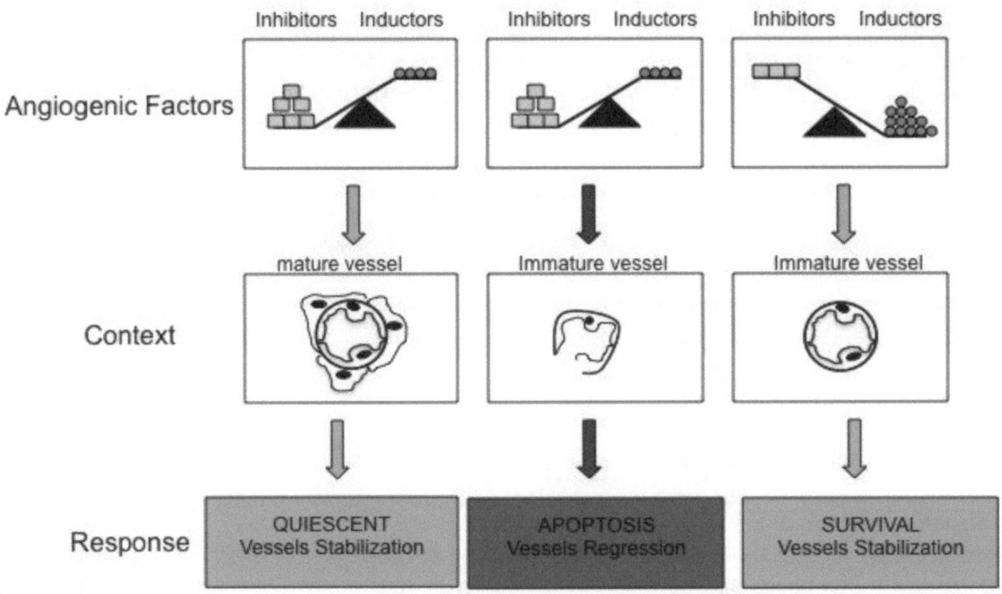

Fig. 4. When the factors that inhibit angiogenesis predominate over those that induce it, two things can occur, depending on the context. If the vessel is mature, it will show no response as it is quiescent and is not affected by the effect of the antiangiogenic drugs. However, if the vessels are immature, with no pericyte coverage, the angiogenesis inhibitors will favor apoptosis and the regression of the vessel. When proangiogenic factors predominate the immature vessel survives and stabilizes.

In this way, the angiogenic factors basically act as survival factors, while antiangiogenic factors act as apoptosis-inducing factors in the context of endothelial expansion, which is an immature endothelium. Thus the balance between the inducing and inhibiting factors determines the destiny of immature vessels, but they do not bear an influence on mature vessels that are in a quiescent state due to the interaction between endothelial cells, pericytes, and the extracellular matrix (Jimenez Cuenca B, 2003). Therefore, if the neovessels are already mature, they will not react to VEGF, nor will they respond to anti-VEGF (Benjamin et. al., 1999). This fact underpins the value of combined therapies like photodynamic therapy (PDT) with verteporfin, which is necessary to destroy the architecture of different mature components of the neovascular membrane that do not respond to anti-VEGF.

3.2 Anti-VEGF agents do not decrease the CNV size

Despite their beneficial clinical effects in AMD, anti-VEGF therapies are ineffective in regressing existing lesions. Endothelial cells and pericytes that form the structure of new vascular tissue typically do not regress with VEGF inhibition alone. This limitation is confirmed by data from the key prospective, randomized clinical trials with Ranibizumab, such as PIER, ANCHOR, and MARINA (Regillo et al., 2008; Brown et al., 2006; Rosenfeld et al., 2006) which did not produce any significant evidence of neovascular regression despite improvement in visual acuity. There are no changes from baseline in the CNV area. This lack of regression is also consistent with experimental models in which monotherapy with anti-VEGF agents inhibits new vascular formation but has little effect on existing capillaries.

Despite the importance of VEGF agents in the cascade of events that stimulates and sustains new vascular formation, VEGF inhibition may have limited effects on existing neovascular tissue once subsequent molecular events are triggered, making inhibition of additional molecular steps essential to build on the benefits of anti-VEGF therapies.

3.3 Tachyphylaxis

Recent publications refer to the possible existence of tachyphylaxis after use of intravitreal Bevacizumab. Forooghian and co-workers describe a decrease in the duration of the beneficial effect, and even a lack of response, after a mean of eight intravitreal injections (Forooghian et al., 2009) in six (n = 59) patients with AMD treated with Bevacizumab in monotherapy.

Currently, the existence of tachyphylaxis is under discussion and its mechanism is unknown. This author poses the possibility of an autoimmune mechanism after a patient, suffering from uveitis, presented tachyphylaxis immediately after intravitreal injection. It must be remembered that Bevacizumab, in spite of being a "humanized" antibody for decreasing immunogenicity, could trigger the formation of new anti-Bevacizumab antibodies after repeated treatments; this hypothesis has yet to be studied.

In addition, it should be considered that always inhibiting the same vascular pathway may potentiate other pathogenic pathways, such as the inflammatory pathway, or that it may increase other cytokines involved in wet AMD. Certainly, a greater inflammatory activity and a proliferation of macrophages in the membranes that were surgically extracted with prior Bevacizumab treatment were observed compared with those extracted without prior intravitreal treatment (Tatar et al., 2009).

Furthermore a better response to intravitreal corticoids has been observed in patients who stop responding to anti-VEGF intravitreal injections (Schaal et al., 2008). Therefore we pose a future problem regarding the use of anti-VEGF, i.e., how to avoid this occurrence. One of the most appropriate options would be to find the way to reduce the number of intravitreal injections in the treatment of AMD and, to date, the only way is with combined therapies.

3.4 Anti-VEGF agents do not act on fibrosis and atrophy

Long-term follow-up of patients who participated in the initial studies of anti-VEGF therapies suggests that late visual loss is often caused by processes that seem to be independent of neovascularization, particularly fibrosis and atrophy. Although more effective antiangiogenesis treatments, including combination strategies, for better blockade of new vessel formation are likely to improve outcome, it is appropriate to expand targets to other pathophysiologic processes associated with AMD. It is necessary to incorporate therapies that block fibrosis and inhibit atrophy or other pathophysiologic processes not directly related to neovascularization.

In Ranibizumab trials (Rosenfeld et al., 2006; Brown et al., 2006), protection against visual loss was highly significant relative to controls during a follow-up of twelve and 24 months. Gains in visual acuity were much smaller: only 34% achieved >15 letter gain at twelve months or 24 months on the most effective dose of Ranibizumab and 65% of patients with very modest gains, no gains, or visual loss over the course of these studies. The subgroup of patients with a loss of three or more lines of visual acuity tended to have better visual acuity than average at baseline, but a larger area of CNV and a larger area of CNV leakage. Over the course of treatment, these patients had a greater growth in total lesion area and more retinal pigment epithelium abnormalities.

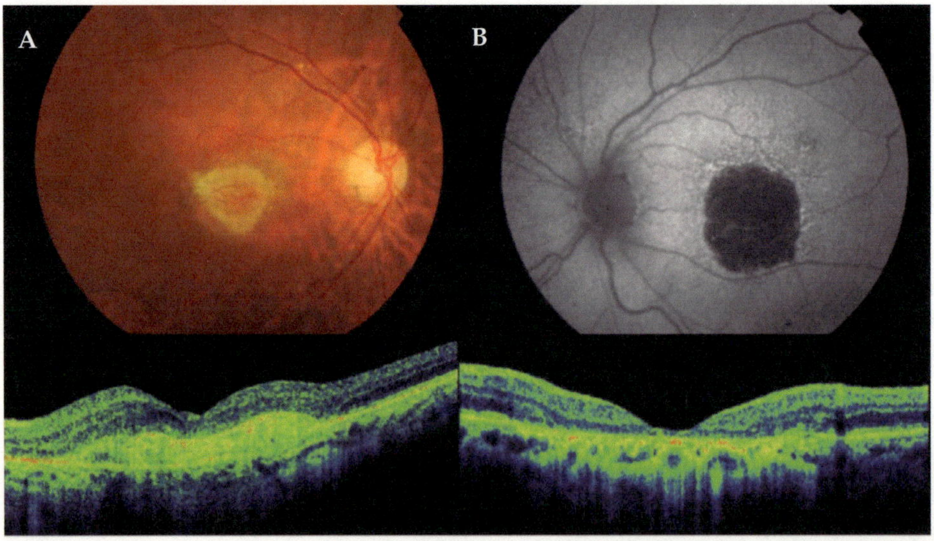

Fig. 5. (A) Retinograph and OCT of subretinal fibrosis of an AMD patient treated with anti-VEGF. (B) Autofluorescence of macular atrophy in the context of wet AMD that had already been treated. In both cases, the evolution of visual acuity was poor despite inactivating the lesion with repeated doses of anti-VEGF.

In a study in which 82 patients, treated with Ranibizumab monotherapy, were monitored in a follow-up of two to six years, reported that the rate of fibrosis was 50% and the rate of atrophy of the retinal pigment epithelium was 40%; 8% percent had both. The fibrosis may have been caused by ongoing inflammation and by maturation of vascular tissue. Hemorrhage above or below the subretinal pigment epithelium may have played a contributing role. Fibrosis was often observed after several years of antiangiogenesis therapy even among responders (Kaiser PK, 2009c).

These findings reinforce other evidence that fibrosis may be an important additional target to expand or preserve the benefits of Ranibizumab and other VEGF inhibitors in the treatment of AMD. Several strategies are being pursued. These include antagonists of integrin, inhibitors of the mammalian target of rapamycin, vascular disrupting agents, and radiation. Control of atrophy, which is generally observed at an earlier stage of AMD progression than fibrosis, is another potential target for improving outcome. The candidate targets for preventing atrophy include neurotrophic factors, free radical scavengers, and retinol binding competitors. Complement inhibition may be another viable strategy (Heier JS, 2009).

3.5 Several pathogenic pathways involved

Even the maximum inhibition of VEGF does not stop vascular growth due to the presence of redundant signaling pathways. Controlling one pathway, the inhibition of neovascularization is relatively modest due to the presence of redundant signaling pathways. The combination of molecules inhibit different parts of the angiogenic process and provide more profound inhibition of neovascularization relative to blocking a single proangiogenic signal (Frielander, 2009).

When one of two inhibitors of angiogenesis was used in experimental studies (Dorrell et al., 2007) complete inhibition of new vessel formation was achieved in a small proportion of animals. In contrast, complete inhibition of neovascularization was observed in more than half of the animals treated with triple combination therapy.

3.6 Route of administration, number and frequency of doses

Transscleral and intravitreal injections are alternative methods of local delivery. These methods may reduce the risk of systemic absorption, because topical therapy results in a significant amount of the drug draining away from the eye through the nasal lacrimal duct into the gut. Transscleral and intravitreal injections may also increase the percentage of the dose that reaches a posterior target. The efficacy of this approach is well documented with antiangiogenic therapies for AMD, but it is not risk-free for the patient, and moreover, it requires surgical administration, which in many cases can cause saturation of operating rooms and delays to the detriment of the patient. Moreover, as it is a chronic disease, retreatment is often necessary which increases these problems. Association of anti-VEGF with other therapies can be useful in reducing the number of anti-VEGF doses without reducing its effectiveness.

Not least important is the potential for unwanted effects on the biologic function controlled by drug targets, such as prolonged suppression of a complex molecule like VEGF, which while being a key factor in causing CNV associated with AMD, also plays an important role as a neuroprotectant in the mature retina.

Exudative AMD is a sub-acute process. Its natural progress from the first symptoms of CNV to scar formation takes over a year in most cases, but can even be active for years (Holz et al., 2004). In fact, the disease evolves to final subfoveal scarring, including the cases where the disease was extrafoveal initially. A well-known fact is that unfortunately, sometimes after years of thermal laser treatment of an extrafoveal lesion, there is foveal recurrence. Antiangiogenic drugs can prevent the growth of new blood vessels but it is not known how long antiangiogenic activity must be kept up to prevent CNV reactivation; it may be needed for years.

There is good justification for considering combination strategies in AMD to build on the initial success achieved with VEGF inhibitors, but combination strategies impose considerable challenges. The frequency of intravitreal injections causes significant difficulties in terms of clinical management and patient convenience and available devices for implantation do not seem to be viable for chronic treatment in their current form.

4. Combined therapies with anti-VEGF

Mediation synergies are used in medicine to potentiate the effect that two or more drugs provide separately, acting on the disease from a different etiopathogenic approach. As AMD is a complex process, it seems logical to focus its treatment from different physiopathological strategies. The combination of agents with different action mechanisms can give rise to a synergic effect, a lower number of overall treatments, and a greater duration of the response when compared with Ranibizumab monotherapy, while the outcome on visual acuity persists.

4.1 Action mechanisms: PDT and anti-VEGF

Photodynamic therapy with verteporfin has been used for years in the treatment of CNV in AMD and its action mechanism has been described repeatedly. Briefly, the action of verteporfin with non-thermal laser in the macular area where the CNV is present triggers processes that lead to apoptosis (Granville et al., 2001), alters the lipids of the cellular membranes of the endothelium, triggers plaquetary aggregation and thrombosis, and increases vascular permeability, blood stasis, and tissue hypoxia (Fingar, 1996). There is an increase in VEGF expression in this process which is the cause of the growth and reactivation of the common membrane before the third month; association of an anti-VEGF inhibits this effect.

Pharmacologic inhibition of VEGF-A decreases the proliferation of endothelial cells and recruitment of others, such as leukocytes, which can express the cytokines and proteases necessary to develop and maintain neovessels (Witmer, 2003; Ferrara, 2003). However, once neovascularization is stabilized, it will not respond to anti-VEGF treatment (Benjamin, 1999). This would explain the added benefit of associating PDT to destroy the architecture of the different components of the neovascular membrane that do not respond to anti-VEGF.

In 2003, Schmidt-Erfurth evaluated the impact PDT has on the expression and distribution of VEGF, VEGF receptor (VEGFR)-3, and pigment epithelium-derived factor (PEDF) after applying it to the retina. Said author reported that PDT using verteporfin induces a reproducible angiogenic response in elderly human eyes. Vascular endothelial growth factor, VEGFR-3, and PEDF expression is enhanced after PDT. Choroidal endothelial cells appear to be the primary site of angiogenic stimulation (Schmidt-Erfurth et al., 2003). This suggests that combining PDT with anti-VEGF for decreasing the PDT response is advisable. The increase in the formation of VEGF, VEGF-3, and PEDF can favor the growth of CNV after initial PDT treatment. This has been observed constantly in our series of 262 cases treated with PDT with a 48-month follow-up. We noted an increase in the CNV size throughout the observation period. This growth was nearly 60% of the total size increase at month three after the first PDT treatment (Mataix et al. 2009).

Photodynamic therapy is very effective in the initial control of CNV because it achieves almost 100% closure of the neovessels in all patients in a period of seven days to one month (Miller et al., 1999). Its side effects include hypoxia, stimulation of inflammatory factors, and upregulation of VEGF expression (Schmith-Erfurth et al., 2001), which can be prevented by associating an anti-VEGF. Although monotherapy with PDT achieves inactivation of the lesion, it does not inhibit subsequent growth, bringing about a loss of vision that in many cases is difficult to recover (Awan, et al., 2009).

The benefits of PDT are documented in a great variety of cases with CNV due to AMD and there is encouraging evidence of improved outcomes when this angioocclusive modality is combined with antiangiogenic agents (Schmidt-Erfurth et al., 2009). It is known that treatment with verteporfin produces hypoperfusion in the treated area and that concomitant use of anti-VEGF can prolong this effect. Moreover, numerous analyses show minimal evidence that there is association with visual deterioration or other adverse effects. Furthermore, hypoperfusion helps to reduce recanalization of CNV and permits neuronal recovery by decreasing exposure to oxygen and oxidative radicals. The reduced need for frequent retreatments clearly has a major appeal due to the lower costs associated with fewer interventions and reduced burden of clinical monitoring and diagnostic reevaluations (Schmidt-Erfurth et al., 2009).

4.2 Clinical trials combining PDT + Ranibizumab

Various clinical assays have been performed with different designs in which combined treatment has been compared with monotherapy. A previous study - PROTECT (Schmidt-Erfurth, 2008) – evaluated the safety and efficacy of administering PDT and Ranibizumab on the same day. Photodynamic therapy was applied and an hour later the intravitreal injection was given. Photodynamic therapy was repeated every three months in accordance with the investigator's opinion and Ranibizumab was administered the first three months, then as required. The study served to show that combined treatment performed on the same day is safe and effective.

The FOCUS study (Heier, 2006) was designed to evaluate, in wet AMD with predominantly classic CNV the safety and efficacy of the combination of Ranibizumab and PDT as the first treatment, followed by monthly Ranibizumab for the first twelve months and PDT every three months according to the investigator's opinion. The control group only received PDT and a simulation injection. After twelve months, the study group showed 90.5% of eyes had lost less than 15 letters as opposed to 67.9% in the control group. The combined treatment group received a mean of 1.32 PDT and the control group 4 PDT per year the first year. After 24 months there was a difference of 12.4 letters in favor of the combined treatment group.

The most interesting assays are the SUMMIT with its two groups, the DENALI which was carried out in the United States and Canada, and the MONTBLANC which was performed in Europe. They were designed to determine whether PDT combined with Ranibizumab was better than monotherapy with Ranibizumab and they included patients with all types of lesions. They were divided randomly into two groups in the MONTBLANC study: in one, PDT was performed and basal intravitreal Ranibizumab and two more injections of Ranibizumab were administered; subsequent treatments were as required and PDT was associated in accordance with the investigator's opinion every three months. Monotherapy and simulating PDT were used in the control group. In the American group, a third group with combined treatment of low fluence PDT was added.

According to the results after twelve months of the MONTBLANC study presented at the European Retina Society in Amsterdam in 2010, the differences between combined and monotherapy treatment were slight in overall terms. The visual behavior was similar between the study and control groups. Neither was there a very significant difference regarding the need for retreatments in the two groups, although with combination therapy a tendency towards a decrease in repeated treatments with Ranibizumab was observed. After twelve months, the mean change in best-corrected visual acuity (BCVA) was +2.5 in the combined treatment group and +4.4 in the monotherapy group. Over 50% of the patients in the two groups gained at least one line of vision compared with their basal value. There was a mean improvement in VA of +2 letters in the combined group and +1.6 letters in the monotherapy group after twelve months in the predominantly classic lesions. Patients with ≤2 area of disc (AD) lesions experienced a mean improvement in VA of +9.7 letters in the combination group and +7.1 letters in the monotherapy group after twelve months.

The patients in the combination group received, on average, 0.3 times fewer Ranibizumab injections. The mean number of treatment repetitions with Ranibizumab after the loading phase in the combination group was 1.8 compared with 2.2 in the Ranibizumab monotherapy group. A tendency towards a decrease in repeated treatments with Lucentis was observed in the combination group. Patients with predominantly classic lesions and smaller lesions who received combined treatment seemed to present better visual results with combined treatment than with monotherapy. It was also observed that the monotherapy group conserved the vision obtained after the initial three loading injections when these were followed by individualized therapy and, on average, fewer injections were necessary.

In the RADICAL (*Reduced Fluence Visudyne-Anti-VEGF-Dexamethasone In Combination for AMD Lesions)* study, other combinations, as opposed to monotherapy, were analyzed which included PDT with reduced fluence + Ranibizumab, PDT with reduced fluence + Ranibizumab + dexamethasone, and PDT with very reduced fluence + Ranibizumab + dexamethasone. In general, there was a tendency to fewer repetitions in the combined groups, with similar outcomes and adverse effects in all the groups (Hughes et al., 2009).

4.3 Other studies

Several studies have been published in which combination treatments were used. Most of them were made up of small groups or with short follow-ups. An interesting study by Augustin's group (2007) included 104 eyes; a triple treatment of PDT, dexamethasone, and

Bevacizumab intravitreal injections was used. The mean improvement obtained was 1.8 lines in almost ten months with a low number of retreatments. A vitrectomy was associated to inject a greater volume of liquid. In a record of cases published recently, 1,073 patients were treated with PDT and Bevacizumab as required, with 1.6 PDT and three injections in twelve months, achieving 82% of patients with a loss of fewer than three lines (Kaiser, 2009a).

An increase in the treatment-free interval was observed in the PDT + anti-VEGF combination. Wan (Wan et al., 2010) in their study on 174 patients with AMD treated with PDT followed by intravitreal injection of Bevacizumab, obtained a mean of 193 days of treatment-free interval, and 52% of the patients did not require postinduction retreatment in the ten months of follow-up. Moreover, other studies report stabilizing the lesion with one single dose of PDT induction + anti-VEGF after twelve months follow-up. The percentage of cases varies in different studies ranging from 39.6% to 46% to 48% (Mataix, 2010; Navea 2009; Smith, 2008).

A systematic review published recently (Das et al., 2011) establishes that intravitreal treatment with anti-VEGF obtains an increase in vision in AMD patients. Combination with PDT brings about a reduction in the number and frequency of retreatments and maintains the improvement in the long term. It seems fairly conclusive that combined treatment for neovascular AMD is a therapeutic option for diseases which do not respond to monotherapy. Moreover, it has the advantage of minimizing the risk monotherapy does have, that of potentiating other chronification pathways of the neovascular disease as it could allow compensatory stimulation of other pathogenic mechanisms of the disease. Tao and Jonas used a combination of Bevacizumab and high-dose-triamcinolone-acetonide in a group of 29 patients who were being treated with Bevacizumab in monotherapy and obtaining no visual or anatomic response. They achieved a visual improvement and reduction in macular thickness (Tao & Jonas, 2010). However, Rudinsky reported finding no benefit in combination therapy in a retrospective study which compared 139 eyes treated with Bevacizumab with 236 treated with PDT + Bevacizumab. The monotherapy eyes showed an improvement of 5.05 letters versus 4.8 letters with combination therapy; there was no difference between the groups. The monotherapy eyes received 3.32 injections versus 3.14 injections in the combination therapy group (Rudinsky et al., 2010).

A recent study (Forte et al., 2011) compared PDT + dexamethasone + anti-VEGF (Ranibizumab or Bevacizumab) triple therapy with Ranibizumab or Bevacizumab monotherapy. Sixty-one eyes were included in the first group and 40 in the second. The mean follow-up was between 14 and 16 months. The triple-therapy group required fewer treatments (1.92 vs 3.12); furthermore, on average, this group took longer to require the first retreatment (5.4 vs 3.6 months). There was a significant improvement in vision and foveal thickness in both groups, therefore it can be concluded that triple therapy reduces the number of retreatments when compared with anti-VEGF monotherapy.

Use of reduced-fluence PDT in combination with anti-VEGF is another method that is obtaining good outcomes. Spielberg treated 27 cases with reduced-fluence PDT followed by intravitreal Ranibizumab on the same day. Retreatments administered with Ranibizumab during the 24-month follow-up stabilized 84% of the patients' vision or improved it at month 24 (Spielberg & Leys, 2010). A prospective comparative study was performed on 85 AMD patients divided into two groups, one treated with intravitreal Bevacizumab (IVB) monotherapy and the other with IVB combined with low-fluence PDT (300 mW/cm2 for 83 s, 25 J/cm2) with a twelve-month follow-up. The combination of IVB with low fluence PDT for the treatment of classic or predominantly classic neovascular AMD worked in a synergistic fashion with a significant reduction in IVB reinjection rate (Costagliola et al., 2009).

Kovacs recently published a retrospective analysis of triple combination therapy with IVB, posterior sub-tenon's triamcinolon acetonide and low fluence verteporfin PDT with good visual results and a reduction in macular thickness with a twelve-month follow-up (Kovacs et al., 2011).

4.4 Our experience

Our group has considerable experience in treatment combining PDT with anti-VEGF. In 2006 we began to treat patients with wet AMD using this method. A sample of this work appears in two publications showing the results of two groups using different treatments, one PDT + Bevacizumab and the other PDT + Ranibizumab.

The study groups included patients with active subfoveal and juxtafoveal CNV secondary to AMD, naïve cases, initial BCVA ≥ 20/400, and maximum lesion size under 5.400 μm defined on fluorescein angiography (FA).

The treatment included a single, initial dose of PDT + Bevacizumab/Ranibizumab. Criteria for retreatment were based on OCT, BCVA, and FA; an increase in central retinal thickness of over 100 μm or the presence of subretinal fluid was a criterion for retreatment. Loss of more than five letters of vision since the previous visit or the presence of new macular bleeding was also a criterion for retreatment if any kind of fluid was present on the OCT. In both situations an FA was performed and treatment with PDT + Bevacizumab/Ranibizumab was provided if a CNV increase or fluorescein leakage was observed. If the FA did not show a CNV increase or fluorescein leakage, treatment was provided with Ranibizumab alone. Photodynamic treatment was only provided when over three months had elapsed since the previous PDT. If development of macular atrophic changes seemed to be the cause of vision loss, it was not treated.

We studied 53 eyes of 53 patients treated with PDT + Ranibizumab and 63 eyes of 63 patients treated with PDT + Bevacizumab, with a twelve-month follow-up. The demographic characteristics and the characteristics of the CNV were similar in both groups. The CNV localization was mainly subfoveal in both groups, with a mean size of 2386 and 2064 μm in the Ranibizumab and Bevacizumab groups, respectively.

Evolution of retinal thickness: The OCT baseline central retinal thickness was 372 μm. It decreased to 251 μm in the first month of treatment and remained the same throughout the follow-up, reaching a mean thickness of 254 μm twelve months later in the group with the Ranibizumab combination, with a mean reduction of -118 μm. The OCT baseline central retinal thickness was 357 μm, decreasing to 246 μm in the first month of treatment and reaching a mean thickness of 227 μm twelve months later in the group with the Bevacizumab combination, with a mean reduction of -129 μm. Separate analysis of the two groups with Student's t-test showed the reduction in retinal thickness was statistically significant ($p<0.05$) from the first month, remaining the same throughout the year.

	N	Follow-up (months)	Treatment	Loss < 15 letters	Gain ≥ 25 letters	VA change from baseline	Number of treatments (average)
MARINA	240	12	Ranibizumab 0,5 mg. (monthly)	94,6 %	33,8 %	+7,2	13 Ranibizumab
ANCHOR	146	12	Ranibizumab 0,5 mg. (monthly)	96,4%	40,3%	+11,3	13 Ranibizumab
PROTECT	32	4	PDT + Ranibizumab 0,5mg monthly	96,9%			1 PDT 4 Ranibizumab
FOCUS	106	12	PDT + Ranibizumab 0,5mg monthly	90,5%	23,8%	+4,9	1,4 PDT 13 Ranibizumab
MONT BLANC	122	12	PDT + Ranibizumab (3 initial doses) retreatments as required	87%	18%	+2,5	1,7 PDT 4,8 Ranibizumab
RADICAL	43	12	PDT (1/2 fluence) + Ranibizumab 0,5mg (3 initial doses) retreatments as required	88%	26%	+5	
Navea et. al.	63	12	PDT + Bevacizumab 1,25mg (single initial doses) retreatments as required	95,2%	19%	+5,7	1,46 PDT 2 Bevacizumab
Mataix et. al.	53	12	PDT + Ranibizumab (single initial doses) retreatments as required	92,3%	32,7%	+7,2	1,22 PDT 2,37 Ranibizumab
Kaiser et. al.	701	12	PDT + Ranibizumab (single initial doses) retreatments as required	82%	36%	+6	1,6 PDT 3,2 Bevacizumab
Rudinsky et. al.	236	12	PDT + Bevacizumab			+4,8	3,14 Bevacizumab
Spielberg et. al.	27	12 / 24	PDT (1/2 fluence) + Ranibizumab 0,5mg (3 initial doses) retreatments as required	84% (24 months)	16% (24 months)	+7,2 (24 months)	5,1 Bevacizumab (12 months) 7,1 Bevacizumab (24 months)

Table 1. Summary of studies with PDT + Anti-VEGF

Visual Acuity Evolution: In the Ranibizumab group, the mean initial BCVA was 8.26 lines which increased to 10.3 lines in the first month of treatment. This gain was maintained until the sixth month, after which it decreased slightly to 9.72 lines twelve month later, thus obtaining a mean increase of 1.21 lines, which is equivalent to a gain of 6.05 letters after twelve months. This slight decrease is due to the severe and occasional loss of vision in a few cases after the sixth month which affected the total mean. The mean initial BCVA was 8.41 lines in the Bevacizumab group and increased from the first month of treatment to 9.38 lines. This gain was maintained throughout the twelve months, undergoing small variations and reaching 9.54 lines, obtaining a mean increase of 1.12 lines after twelve months, which is a gain of 5.6 letters. The percentage of cases that lost 15 letters was 95.2% in the PDT + Bevacizumab group and 92.3% in the PDT + Ranibizumab group. Visual gain was 58.7% and 57.7%, respectively (Figures 6, 7).

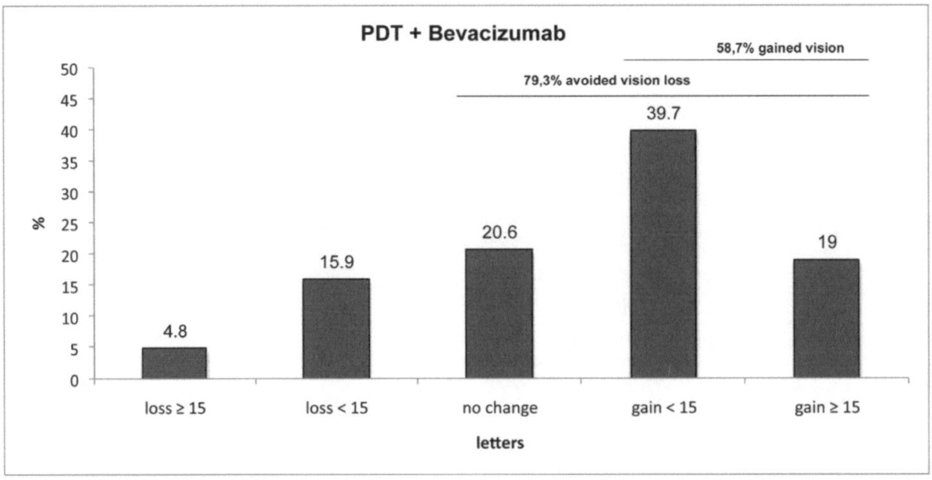

Fig. 6. Percentage of visual acuity variations throughout the follow-up in patients treated with PDT + Bevacizumab: 95.2% of cases lost fewer than 15 letters after twelve months. Visual loss was avoided in 79.3% of cases and 58.7% gained vision.

The distribution of the lines of vision between the beginning and end of the follow-up is statistically significant (p-value <0.001) in both groups. The Mann-Whitney test concludes that the visual gain is significantly better (p-value <0.05) in the first six months in the Ranibizumab group, but there were no differences between the two groups after one year.

Retreatments: A record of the number of treatments was kept throughout the study for both groups. The patients in the group treated with Bevacizumab received a mean of 1.46 therapies and 1.92 intravitreal injections, and those treated with Ranibizumab received a mean of 1.23 therapies and 2.38 intravitreal injections. The Mann-Whitney test showed that the Bevacizumab group received significantly more therapies (p-value <0.05), but there was no difference in the number of intravitreal injections. In 21 cases (39.6%) only a single initial combination therapy was required in the Ranibizumab group versus 29 cases (46%) in the Bevacizumab group to keep the lesion stable until the end of the follow-up. In the Ranibizumab group, 77.4% of the patients were treated with a maximum of three injections and 79.2% of the patients needed a single PDT treatment at the initiation of the treatment. In the Bevacizumab group, 87.3% and 61.9% of the patients were treated, respectively.

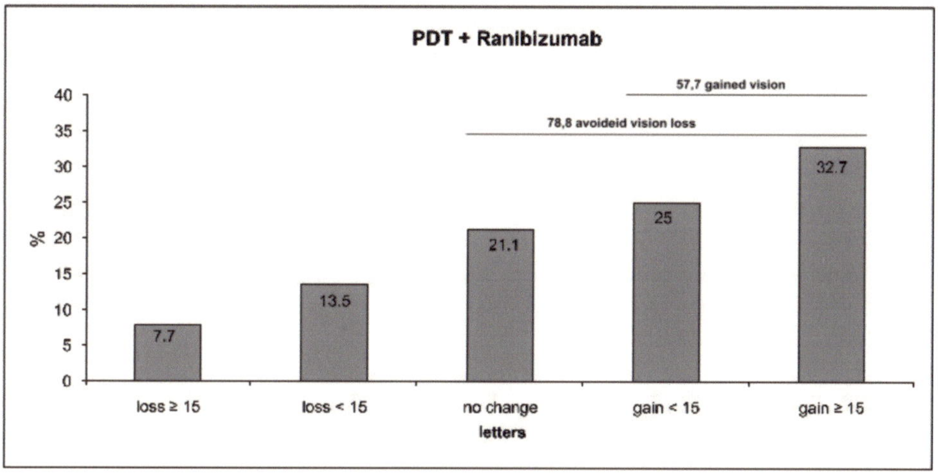

Fig. 7. Percentage of visual acuity variations throughout the follow-up in patients treated with PDT + Ranibizumab: 92.3% of cases lost fewer than 15 letters after twelve months. Visual loss was avoided in 78.8% of cases and 57.7% gained vision.

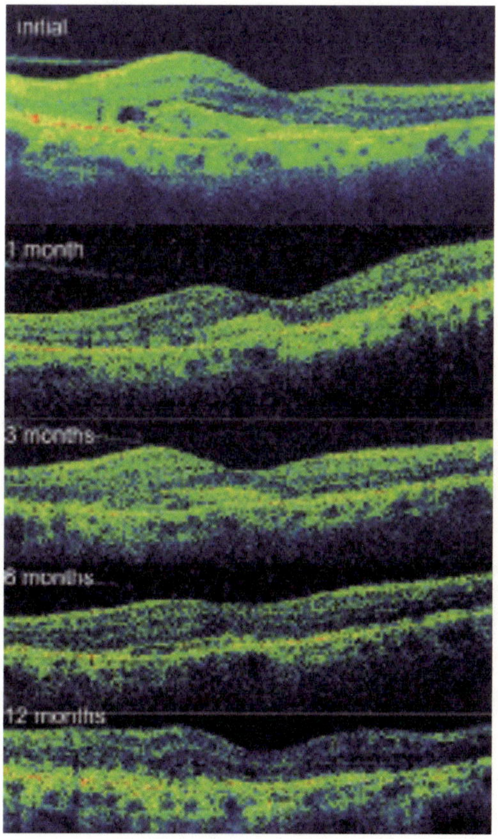

Fig. 8. Evolution of OCT from the beginning of the treatment until the end of the follow-up twelve months later.

Our results suggest that a combination of PDT and anti-VEGF is a good option for treating CNV in AMD more effectively by maintaining good visual results and decreasing the need for retreatments.

5. Other therapies

The etiology of AMD is multifactorial and there are several mechanisms that can lead to irreversible loss of vision. To achieve a complete therapy for CNV, we should not simply focus on neovessels, but rather act on both the vascular component (mature and immature vessels) and the non-vascular component (inflammatory cells, cytokines, glial cells, myofibroblasts, fibrocytes, etc.).

5.1 The vascular component (immature and mature vessels)

The antiangiogenesis agents currently used in the treatment of AMD inhibit VEGF by blocking the growth factor in the extra-cellular space, thereby preventing access to its receptor. Several VEGF inhibitors, including **Bevacizumab and Ranibizumab**, have demonstrated excellent safety and efficacy in exudative AMD (Rosenfeld PJ et al., 2006; Spaide RF et al., 2006b). The current strategy of blocking VEGF in the extracellular space may be an inadequate approach for long-term control of AMD. Combining drugs that act at different points of the angiogenesis pathway has the potential to build on the benefits of extracellular VEGF inhibitors, but a more profound inhibition of the disease process may require activity in additional pathways of the disease.

VEGF Trap-Eye is a fully human soluble VEGF receptor fusion protein that binds all forms of VEGF-A along with the related placental growth factor (PlGF). VEGF Trap-Eye is made by fusing two different domains from VEGF receptors 1 and 2 onto a human Fc fragment. VEGF Trap-Eye has tighter VEGF binding than the natural receptor and has greater affinity than the current VEGF inhibitors (Steward & Rosenfeld, 2007). Two parallel Phase 3 trials have been developed in patients with wet AMD (VIEW 1 and VIEW 2). VEGF Trap-Eye is being dosed at 0.5 mg every four weeks, 2 mg every four weeks, and 2 mg every eight weeks in direct comparison with Ranibizumab administered at 0.5 mg every four weeks during the first year of the studies. The primary endpoint was statistical non-inferiority in the proportion of patients who maintained (or improved) vision over 52 weeks compared to Ranibizumab. A generally favorable safety profile was observed for both VEGF Trap-Eye and Ranibizumab.

Small interfering RNA agents, such as **RTP-801i and Bevasiranib**, which turn off target genes, are extremely promising in a variety of therapeutic areas. **Bevasiranib** is designed to block the production of VEGF directly by inhibiting the messenger RNA from the VEGF gene. Studies in mice have demonstrated that Bevasiranib can inhibit and regress ocular neovascularization (Reich et al., 2003). Studies in rabbits have shown that an intravitreal injection of Bevasiranib achieved good distribution in the retina and in RPE (Dejneka NS et al., 2008). The agent is well distributed after intravitreal injection and well tolerated by human subjects (Karagiannis & El-Osta, 2005). A Phase 3 Clinical Trial tests this agent in combination with Ranibizumab because potentially the drug may prevent further production of VEGF while Ranibizumab blocks the VEGF that is present.

Experimental models show that monotherapy with anti-VEGF agents inhibits new vascular formation but has little effect on existing capillaries. Pericyte coverage provides survival signals to neovascular endothelial cells and hence makes them resistant to VEGF (Bergers et al., 2003). Pericytes are essential in vascular maturation so their inhibition is important in inhibiting neovascularization and the regression of new mature vessels. **Anti-PDGF (Platelet-derived growth factor)** treatment strips away pericytes to leave the endothelial cells unprotected and vulnerable to anti-VEGF treatment (Erber R. et al., 2004). The combination of anti-VEGF and anti–PDGF produces inhibition and regression of corneal and choroidal neovascularization compared with anti-VEGF treatment alone. In models of pathologic tumor angiogenesis, strategies involving both anti-VEGF and anti-PDGF have also produced regression when an anti-VEGF therapy alone failed (Jo N et al., 2006).

Platelet-derived growth factor, which has an important role in recruiting the pericytes critical to maturation of vessel walls, may also be a viable target to augment the effects of a VEGF inhibitor. A recent phase 1 clinical trial with anti-PDGF (E10030) included patients with subfoveal CNV who received three monthly doses of E10030 in combination with a standard dose of Ranibizumab. The preliminary findings reveal a reduction in neovascular size (neovascular regression) in all patients. This regression is associated with a marked improvement in visual acuity, gain ≥ 15 ETDRS letters: 4 weeks (32%) 12 weeks (59%) and gain in numbers of letters: 4 weeks (10.9%) 12 weeks (14%). However, it is not yet clear whether the improvement was due to the E10030/Ranibizumab combination or simply a Ranibizumab effect (Boyer DS et al., 2009).

The inhibition of **Insulin-like growth factor** could be another option in the treatment of neovessels. It leads to endothelial cell proliferation and inhibits apoptosis of endothelial cells, the nicotinic acetylcholine receptor, which also induces endothelial cell migration, and tubular binding proteins, which govern endothelial cell shape formation.

5.2 The nonvascular component (inflammatory cells, cytokines, glial cells, myofibroblasts, and fibrocytes)

Antiangiogenesis agents are effective for preventing progression of CNV in a substantial proportion of patients, although regression is not typically observed. Experimental studies indicate that newly formed capillaries are no longer susceptible to regression with anti-VEGF agents within about two weeks after formation. Antiangiogenesis agents may still be effective for preventing the development of additional capillaries or reducing leakage in vessels invading the retina, but the persistence of CNV may stimulate inflammation or other pathologic processes that eventually result in vision loss due to the formation of fibrosis. Prevention of fibrosis is essential to the preservation of VA.

Radiation therapy has long been used to control fibrosis in a variety of tissues. In AMD, radiation may be particularly attractive because there is evidence of synergistic inhibition of neovascularization when radiation is combined with antiangiogenesis drugs (Nieder C. et al., 2007). Historically, radiation monotherapy sufficient to eradicate CNV effectively has been associated with a modest benefit for AMD. The growing evidence that antiangiogenic agents can increase the antitumor efficacy of radiotherapy includes studies in animal models: the combination of radiation and antiangiogenesis agents had a greater effect in reducing tumor regrowth than either alone (Gorski DH et al., 1999). In another animal study, the use of anti-VEGF and anti-PDGF agents in combination with radiation showed a significantly greater antitumor effect relative to radiation alone (Timke C et al., 2008). Mammalian target of rapamycin (mTOR) inhibitors (Sirolimus) radiosensitize cancer cells *in* *vitro* and several studies have demonstrated their ability to radiosensitize *in vivo* (Shinohara ET et al., 2005). In a Phase I recent report, CNV was irradiated in a few patients with strontium 90 delivered by a specialized, 20-gauge, intravitreal probe that is placed over the lesion intraoperatively. All patients underwent a vitrectomy before radiotherapy and were treated with Bevacizumab before and after radiation. In a 4-minute exposure, the estimated dose at the lesion was 24 Gy. Results were excellent, with 76% of patients gaining at least 10 letters of visual acuity. Most of the responders required no more than one additional injection of Bevacizumab over the first year of follow-up.

Integrins as a mediator of adhesion both between cells and between cells and extracellular matrix, have a role in a variety of proliferative processes, including fibrosis. Integrin also seems to have a direct influence on proliferative kinase signalingare, a mediator of adhesion between cells and extracellular matrix. It is a transmembrane protein that binds to extracellular matrix proteins (fibronectin) allowing cell adhesion and cytoskeletal organization. The $\alpha5\beta1$ is especially important in pathologic angiogenesis (not in normal vasculature) (Kim S et al., 2000). Many of the cellular effects of VEGF are duplicated downstream in the angiogenic cascade by the interaction between the transmembrane integrin $\alpha5\beta1$receptor and its natural ligand, fibronectin. In addition to VEGF, the interaction of integrin $\alpha5\beta1$ with fibronectin is critical to endothelial cell survival. Integrin $\alpha5\beta1$ has been shown to be upregulated in all the cells associated with AMD pathogenesis, including endothelial cells, retinal pigment epithelium cells, macrophages, and fibroblasts. This implicates this molecule in multiple pathogenic processes involved in AMD, including neovascularization, vascular leakage, and inflammation (Klatt K et al., 2007). Two studies have demonstrated that once neovascular tissue begins to grow, the extracellular matrix needs to adhere to the neovascular endothelial cells for them to survive (Hynes RO, 2002; Hodivala-Dilke et al., 2003). Inhibiting the ligation of integrin $\alpha5\beta1$ and fibronectin may disrupt the process of neovascularization, regardless of the upstream growth factor pathway. **Volociximab** (M200), a chimeric monoclonal antibody targeting integrin $\alpha5\beta1$ to block its ligation of fibronectin, has robustly inhibited human umbilical vein endothelial cell tube formation in laboratory tests. It does so regardless of an initial growth factor stimulant. It has also inhibited neovascularization in primate choroid tissue and tumor angiogenesis in rabbits (Ramakrishnan V et al., 2006; Bhaskar V et al., 2008).

Vascular disrupting agents also have potential for the inhibition of fibrosis as well as formation of new blood vessels. Unlike antiangiogenesis agents that block formation of new blood vessels, vascular-disrupting agents attack newly formed endothelium by disrupting connectivity between cells. This activity is expected to be complementary to anti-VEGF agents because it takes place at a later stage of neovascularization. It may also exert an important antifibrotic effect. A vascular-disrupting agent called **combretastatin** A4P (CA4P) has been evaluated in a Phase 1 study in humans with myopic macular degeneration, where it demonstrated relatively modest effects, but the characteristics of AMD may be more suitable for its activity.

Compared with age-matched controls, individuals with AMD demonstrate elevations in a variety of systemic biomarkers of inflammation, including activated monocytes and interleukin-6 (Vine AK et al., 2005 & Seddon et al., 2005). An increased risk of AMD in individuals with polymorphisms in their genes coding for the complement regulatory proteins is another signal that complement driven inflammation is perhaps an important mediator of this disease (Klein RJ et al., 2005). Although terminal elements of the complement pathway are implicated in the formation of drusen in primate models and human postmortem specimens (Anderson DH et al., 2002), patients with membranoproliferative glomerulonephritis type II, a disorder characterized by uncontrolled complement cascade activation, develop drusen histologically identical to drusen associated with AMD (Mullins RF et al., 2001). These findings support the potential for adding therapies directed at complement activation to those that already demonstrate activity in AMD, but it is not yet clear what incites the complement cascade or how to inhibit it at its source. Therefore, to attack the complement pathway, it may be necessary to address both membrane attack complex and C5a, while preserving the beneficial antimicrobial function of C3 (Giese MJ et al., 1994). There are numerous questions about where and when to block complement to inhibit best progression of AMD. An experimental treatment, known as ARC 1905, has been associated with the inhibition of C5a and C5b-9. In experimental models, this **inhibitor of C5aR** has demonstrated measurable activity in reducing the influx of neutrophils and macrophages and has also been associated with suppression of CNV (Adamis AP, 2009).

Mammalian target of rapamycin, a protein kinase linked to a variety of gene transcriptions and protein production, including VEGF, is strongly implicated in a number of proliferative processes and is a targetable mediator of fibrosis. Palomid 529 (mTOR inhibitor) has demonstrated a strong antifibrotic effect in retinal fibrosis models, including laser-induced retinopathy. The antifibrotic activity of this inhibitor has been measured, across a variety of endpoints, including inhibition of the inflammatory response as well as the extent of the fibrotic scar. Other mammalian targets of rapamycin inhibitors, such as sirolimus, have demonstrated good antiangiogenic, antiinflammatory, and antifibrotic effects (Chiang GC et al., 2007) and inhibit the response to interleukin-2 (IL-2) and thereby block activation of T- and B-cells.

6. Conclusion

The potential for a single therapy to control the complex process of AMD seems to be relatively remote. It is not clear that a combination of different agents, working on the same pathway of extracellular VEGF inhibition, will reduce AMD progression, but there may be a strong potential for additive or synergistic effects from combining drugs with independent mechanisms. The current strategy of blocking VEGF in the extracellular space may be an inadequate approach for long-term control of AMD. Combining drugs that act at different points of the angiogenesis pathway has the potential to build on the benefits of extracellular VEGF inhibitors, but a more profound inhibition of the disease process may require activity in additional pathways of the disease.

7. References

Adamis AP. (2009). The Rationale for drug combinations in Age related macular degeneration. *Retina*, Vol. 29, No. Supplement 6, (June 2009), pp. 42-44, ISSN 0275-004X

Anderson DH.; Mullins RF.; Hageman GS. &J ohnson LV. (2002). A role for local inflammation in the formation of drusen in the aging eye. *American Journal Ophthalmology*, Vol. 134, No. 3, (September 2002), pp.411–431, ISSN 0002-9394

Augustin AJ.; Puls S. & Offermann I. (2007). Triple therapy for choroidal neovascularization due to age-related macular degeneration: verteporfin PDT, bevacizumab, and dexamethasone. *Retina*, Vol. 27, No. 2, (February 2007), pp. 133-140, ISSN 0275-004X

Awan MA.; Chavan R.; Peh KK. & Yang YC. (2009). The effect of the first application of verteporfin photodynamic therapy on lesion growth in choroidal neovascularisation and its potential impact on combination therapy. *Clinical & Experimental Optometry*, Vol. 92, No. 5, (September 2009), pp. 440–443, ISSN 144-0938

Benjamin LE.; Golijanin D.; Itin A.; Pode D. & Keshet E. (1999). Selective ablation of immature blood vessels in established human tumors follows vascular endothelial growth factor withdrawal. *The Journal of Clinical Investigation*. Vol. 103, No. 2, (January 1999), pp.159-165, ISSN 0021-9738

Bergers G.; Song S.; Meyer-Morse N.; Bergsland E. & Hanahan D. (2003). Benefits of targeting both pericytes and endothelial cells in the tumor vasculature with kinase inhibitors. *The Journal of Clinical Investigation*. Vol 111, No. 9, (May 2003), pp. 1287–1295, ISSN 0021-9738

Bhaskar V.; Fox M.; Breinberg D.; Wong MH. & Wales PE. (2008). Volociximab, a chimeric integrin alpha5beta1 antibody, inhibits the growth of VX2 tumors in rabbits. *Investigational New Drugs*, Vol. 26, No. 1, (February 2008), pp. 7–12, ISSN 0167-6997

Boyer DS. & Ophthotec Anti-PDGF in AMD Study Group. (2009). Combined Inhibition of Platelet Derived (PDGF) and Vascular endothelial Growth Factor (VEGF) for the Treatment of Nevascular Age-Related Macular Degeneration : Results of a Phase 1 study. *Proceedings of ARVO 2009 Annual Meeting*, IOVS E-abstract 1260, ISSN 1552-5783 Fort Lauderdale, Florida, USA, may 3-7, 2009

Brown DM.; Kaiser PK.; Michels M.; Soubrane G. & Heier JS. (2006). ANCHOR Study Group. Ranibizumab versus verteporfin for neovascular age- related macular degeneration. *The New England Journal of Medicine*, Vol. 355, No. 14, (Octuber 2006), pp. 1432– 1444, ISSN 0028-4793

Costagliola C.; Romano MR.; Rinaldi M.; dell'Omo R. & Chiosi F. (2010). Low fluence rate photodynamic therapy combined with intravitreal bevacizumab for neovascular age-related macular degeneration. *The British Journal of Ophthalmology*, Vol. 94, No. 94, (February 2010), pp. 180-184, ISSN 0007-1161

Chiang GG. & Abraham RT. (2007). Targeting the mTOR signaling net-work in cancer. *Trends in Molecular Medicine*, Vol. 13, No. 10, (Octuber 2007), pp. 433–442, ISSN 1471-4914

Das RA.; Romano A,; Chiosi F,; Menzione M, & Rinaldi M. (2011). Combined treatment modalities for age related macular degeneration. *Current Drug Targets*, Vol. 12, No. 2, (February 2011), pp. 182-189, ISSN 1389-4501

Dejneka NS.; Wan S.; Bond OS.; Kornbrust DJ. & Reich SJ. (2008). Ocular biodistribution of bevasiranib following a single intravitreal injection to rabbit eyes. *Molecular Vision*, Vol. 18, No. 14. (May 2008), pp. 997-1005, ISSN 1090-0535.

Dorrell MI.; Aguilar E,; Scheppke L.; Barnett FH. & Friedlander M. (2007). Combination angiostatic therapy completely inhibits ocular and tumor angiogenesis. *Proc Natl Acad Sci U S A*. Vol. 104, No. 3, (January 2007), pp. 967– 972, ISSN 0027-8424

Erber R.; Thurnher A.; Katsen AD.; Groth G. & Kerger H. (2004). Combined inhibition of VEGF and PDGF signaling enforces tumor vessel regression by interfering with pericyte-mediated endothelial cell survival mechanisms. *FASEB J*. Vol. 18, No. 2, (February 2004), pp. 338–340, ISSN 1530-6860

Ferrara N. & Gerber HP. (2001). The role of vascular endothelial growth factor in angiogenesis. *Acta Haematologica,* Vol. 106, No. 4, (2001), pp. 148-156, ISSN 0001-5792

Ferrara N.; Gerber HP. & Le Couter J. (2003). The Biology of VEGF and it's receptors. *Nature Medicine,* Vol. 9, No. 6, (June 2003), pp. 669-676, ISSN 1078-8956

Fingar VH. (1996). Vascular effects of photodynamic therapy. *Journal of clinical laser medicine & surgery,* Vol. 14, No. 5, (October 1996), pp. 323-328, ISSN 1044-5471

Forooghian F.; Cukras C.; Meyerle CB.; Chew EY. & Wong WT. (2009). Tachyphylaxis after intravitreal bevacizumab for exudative age-related macular degeneration. *Retina,* Vol. 29, No. 6, (June 2009), pp. 723-731, ISSN 0275-004X

Forte R.; Bonavolontà P.; Benayoun Y.; Adenis JP. & Robert PY. (2011). Intravitreal ranibizumab and bevacizumab in combination with full-fluence verteporfin therapy and dexamethasone for exudative age-related macular degeneration. *Ophthalmic Research,* Vol. 45, No. 3, (September 2011), pp. 129-134, ISSN 0030-3747

Gerber HP.; Dixit V. & Ferrara N. (1998). Vascular endothelial growth factor induces expression of the antiapoptotic proteins Bcl-2 and A1 in vascular endothelial cells. *Journal of biological chemistry,* Vol. 273, No 21, (May 1998), pp. 13313-13316, ISSN 0021-9258

Giese MJ.; Mondino BJ.; Glasgow BJ.; Sumner HL. & Adamu SA- (1994). Complement system and host defense against staphylococcal endophthalmitis. *Investigative ophthalmology & visual science,* Vol. 35, No 3, (March 1994), pp. 1026–1032, ISSN 0146-0404

Gorski DH.; Becket MA.; Jaskowiat NT.; Calvin DP. & Mauceri HJ. (1999). Blockage of the endothelial growth factor stress response increases the antitumor effects of ionizing radiation. *Cancer Research.* Vol. 59, No. 14, (July 1999), pp. 3374–3378, ISSN 0008- 5472

Granville DJ.; Jiang H.; McManus BM. & Hunt DW. (2001). Fas ligand and TRAIL augment the effect of photodynamic therapy on the i.nduction of apoptosis in JURKAT cells. *International Immunopharmacology,* Vol. 1, No 9-10, (September 2001), pp. 1832-1840. ISSN 1567-5769

Gragoudas ES.; Adamis AP.; Cunningham ET Jr.; Feinsod M. & Guyer DR. (2004). VEGF Inhibition Study in Ocular Neovascularization Clinical Trial Group. Pegaptanib for neovascular age-related macular degeneration. *New england journal of medicine,* Vol. 351, No 27, (December 2004), pp. 2805–281, ISSN 0028-4793

Heier JS.; Boyer DS.; Ciulla TA.; Ferrone PJ. & Jumper JM. (2006). FOCUS Study Group. Ranibizumab combined with verteporfin photodynamic therapy in neovascular age-related macular degeneration: year 1 results of the FOCUS Study. *Archives Ophthalmology,* Vol. 124, No. 11, (November 2006), pp. 1532-1542, ISSN 0003-9950

Heier JS. (2009). Pathology beyond neovascularization. New targets in Age-Related Macular Degeneration.. *Retina,* Vol. 29, No 6, (June 2009), pp. 39–41, ISSN 0275-004X

Hodivala-Dilke KM.; Reynolds AR. & Reynolds LE. (2003). Integrins in angiogenesis: multitalented molecules in a balancing act. *Cell and tissue research,* Vol. 314, No. 1, (Octuber 2003), pp. 131–144, ISSN 0302-766X

Holz FG., Pauleikhoff D.; Klein R. & Bird AC. (2004). Pathogenesis of lesions in late age-related macular disease. *American Journal Ophthalmology,* Vol. 137, No. 3, (March 2004), pp. 504-510, ISNN 002-9394

Hynes RO. (2002). Integrins: bidirectional, allosteric signaling machines. Cell, Vol. 110, No. 6, (September 2002), pp. 673–687, ISSN 0092-8674

Hughes M. & Sang DN. (2009). Triple plus therapy compared with monthly ranibizumab redices the retreatment rate in a randomized study in age-related macular degeneration. Proceeding of ARVO 2009 anuual meeting, IOVS 2009 E-abstract 1903, ISSN 1552-5783, Fort Lauderdale, florida, USA, May 3-7, 2009.

Jain RK. (2005). Normalization of tumor vasculature: an emerging concept in antiangiogenic therapy. *Science*, Vol. 307, No. 5706, (January 2005), pp. 58–62, ISSN 1095-9203

Jiménez Cuenca B. (2003). Mechanism of inhibition of tumoral angiogenesis by thrombospondin-1. *Nefrologia,* Vol. 23, No. suppl 3, (2003), pp. 49-53, ISSN 0211-6995

Jo N.; Mailhos C.; Ju M.; Cheung E. & Bradley J. (2006). Inhibition of platelet-derived growth factor B signaling enhances the efficacy of anti-vascular endothelial growth factor therapy in multiple models of ocular neovascularization. *American Journal of Pathology*, Vol. 168, No. 6, (June 2006), pp. 2036–2053, ISSN 0002-9440

Kaiser PK.; Boyer DS.; Garcia R.; Hao Y. & Hughes MS. (2009a) Verteporfin photodynamic therapy combined with intravitreal bevacizumab for neovascular age-related macular degeneration. *Ophthalmology*. Vol. 116, No. 4, (April 2009), pp. 747-755, ISSN 0161-6420

Kaiser PK. (2009b). Overview of radiation trials for age-related macular degeneration. *Retina*. Vol. 29, No. suppl 6, (June 2009), pp. 34-35, ISSN 0275-004X

Kaiser PK. (2009c). Strategies for inhibiting vascular endothelial growth factor. *Retina*. Vol 29, No. suppl 6, (June 2009), pp. 15-17, ISSN 0275-004X

Karagiannis TC. & El-Osta A. (2005). RNA interference and potential therapeutic applications of short interfering RNAs. *Cancer Gene Therapy*, Vol. 12, No. 10, (Octuber 2005), pp. 787–795, ISSN 0929-1903

Kim S.; Bell K.; Mousa SA. & Varner JA. (2000). Regulation of angiogenesis in vivo by ligation of integrin alpha5beta1 with the central cell-binding domain of fibronectin. *American Journal of Pathology*, Vol. 156, No 4, (April 2000), pp. 1345–1362, ISSN 0002-9440

Klatt K.; Zahn CG., Heier JS.; Daniel P.; Holz FG. & Loeffler KU. (2007). Integrin $\alpha 5\beta 1$ in preretinal membranes associated with proliferative vitreoretinopathy (PVR). Proceedings of ARVO 2007 Annual meeting, Invest ophthalmol Vis Sci 2007 E-abstract 1233, ISSN 1552-5783, Fort Lauderdale, Florida, USA, May -10, 2007

Klein RJ.; Zeiss C.; Chew EY.; Tsai JY. & Sackler RS. (2005). Complement factor H polymorphism in age-related macular degeneration. *Science*, Vol 308, No 5720, (April 2005), pp. 385–390, ISSN 1095-9203

Kovacs KD.; Quirk MT.; Kinoshita T.; Gautam S. & Ceron OM. (2011). A retrospective analysis of triple combination therapy with intravitreal bevacizumab, posterior sub-tenon's triamcinolone acetonide, and low-fluence verteporfin photodynamic therapy in patients with neovascular age-related macular degeneration. *Retina*, Vol 31, No 3, (March 2011), pp. 446-452, ISSN 0275-004X

Mataix J.; Desco MC.; Palacios E.; Garcia-Pous M. & Navea A. (2009). Photodynamic therapy for age-related macular degeneration treatment: epidemiological and clinical analysis of a long-term study. *Ophthalmic surgery lasers & imaging*. Vol. 40, No 3. (May-June 2009), pp. 277-284, ISSN 1542- 8877

Mataix J.; Palacios E.; Carmen DM.; Garcia-Pous M. & Navea A. (2010). Combined ranibizumab and photodynamic therapy to treat exudative age-related macular degeneration: an option for improving treatment efficiency. *Retina*. Vol. 30, No 8. (September 2010), pp. 1190-1196, ISSN 0275-004X

Miller JW.; Schmidt-Erfurth U.; Sickenberg M.; Pournaras CJ. & Laqua H. (1999). Photodynamic therapy with verteporfin for choroidal neovascularization caused by age-related macular degeneration: results of a single treatment in a phase 1 and 2 study. *Archives of Ophthalmology*, Vol. 117, No 9, (September 1999), pp. 1161–1173, ISSN 0003-9950

Mullins RF.; Aptsiauri N. & Hageman GS. (2001). Structure and composition of drusen associated with glomerulonephritis: implications for the role of complement activation in drusen biogenesis. *Eye*, Vol. 15, No 3, (June 2001), pp. 390–395, ISSN 0950-222X

Navea A.; Mataix J.; Desco MC.; Garcia-Pous M. & Palacios E. (2009). One-year follow-up of combined customized therapy. Photodynamic therapy and bevacizumab for exudative age-related macular degeneration. *Retina*; Vol. 29, No. 1, (January 2009), pp. 13-9, ISSN 0275-004X

Nieder C.; Wiedenmann N.; Andratschke NH.; Astner ST. & Molls M. (2007). Radiation therapy plus angiogenesis inhibition with bevacizumab: rationale and initial experience. *Reviews of recent clinical trials*, Vol. 2, No. 3, (September 2007), pp. 163–168, ISSN 1574-8871

Ramakrishnan V.; Bhaskar V.; Law DA.; Wong MH. & DuBridge RB. (2006). Preclinical evaluation of an anti-alpha5beta1 integrin antibody as a novel anti-angiogenic agent. *Journal of experimental therapeutics & oncology*, Vol. 5, No.4, (2006), pp. 273–286, ISSN 1533-869X

Regillo CD.; Brown DM.; Abraham P. Yue H. & Ianchulev T. (2008). Randomized, double-masked, sham-controlled trial of ranibizumab for neovascular age-related macular degeneration: PIER Study year 1. *American Journal of Ophthtalmology*, Vol 145, No 2, (February 2008), pp. 239 –248, ISSN 0002-9343

Rosenfeld PJ.; Brown DM.; Heier JS.; Boyer DS. & Kaiser PK. (2006) MARINA Study Group. Ranibizumab for neovascular age-related macular de- generation. *N Engl J Med*, Vol. 355, No 14. (Octuber 2006), pp. 1419–1431, ISSN 0028-4793

Rudnisky CJ.; Liu C.; Ng M.; Weis E. & Tennant MT. (2010). Intravitreal bevacizumab alone versus combined verteporfin photodynamic therapy and intravitreal bevacizumab for choroidal neovascularization in age-related macular degeneration: visual acuity after 1 year of follow-up. *Retina*; Vol. 30, No. 4, (April 2010), pp. 548-554, ISSN 0275-004X

Schaal S.; Kaplan HJ. & Tezel TH. (2008). Is there tachyphylaxis to intravitreal anti-vascular endothelial growth factor pharmacotherapy in age-related macular degeneration?. *Ophthalmology*. Vol. 115, No. 12, (December 2008), pp. 2199-2205, ISSN ISSN 0161-6420

Schmidt-Erfurth U.; Scholtzer-Schrehard U.; Cursiefen C.; Michels S. & Beckendorf A. (2003). Influence of photodynamic therapy on expression of vascular endotelial growth factor (VEGF), VEGF receptor 3, and pigmento epithelium-derived factor. *Invest Ophthalmol Vis Sci*, Vol. 44, No. 10, (Octuber 2003), pp. 4473–4480, ISSN 0146-0404

Schmidt-Erfurth U.; Wolf S.; PROTECT Study Group. (2008). Same-day administration of verteporfin and ranibizumab 0.5 mg in patients with choroidal neovascularisation due to age-related macular degeneration. *Br J Ophthalmol*, Vol. 92, No. 12, (December 2008), pp. 1628-35, ISSN 1468-2079

Schmidt-Erfurth U.; Kiss C. & Sacu S. (2009). The role of choroidal hypoperfusion associated with photodynamic therapy in neovascular age-related macular degeneration and the consequences for combination strategies. *Prog Retin Eye Res*, Vol. 28, No.2, (March 2009), pp. 145-54, ISSN 1350-9462

Seddon JM.; George S.; Rosner B. & Rifai N. (2005). Progression of age-related macular degeneration: prospective assessment of C-reactive protein, interleukin 6, and other cardiovascular biomarkers. *Arch Ophthalmol*. Vol. 123, No. 6, (June 2005), pp. 774–782. ISSN 0003-9950

Shinohara ET.; Cao C.; Niermann K.; Mu Y. & Zeng F. (2005). Enhanced radiation damage of tumor vasculator by mTOR inhibitors. *Oncogene*, Vol. 24, No. 35. (August 2005), pp. 5414 –5422, ISSN 1476-5594

Smith BT.; Dhalla MS.; Shah GK.; Blinder KJ. & Ryan EH. Jr. (2008). Intravitreal injection of bevacizumab combined with verteporfin photodynamic therapy for choroidal neovascularization in age-related macular degeneration. *Retina*, Vol. 28, No. 5, (may 2008), pp. 675-681, ISSN 0275-004X

Spaide RF. (2006a). Rationale for combination therapies for choroidal neovascularization. *Am J Ophthalmol*. Vol. 141, No. 1, (January 2006), pp. 149–156, ISSN 0002-9394

Spaide RF.; Laud K.; Fine HF.; klancnik JM. Jr. & Meyerle CB. (2006b). Intravitreal bevacizumab treatment of choroidal neovascularization secondary to age- related macular degeneration. *Retina*, Vol. 26, No. 4, (April 2006), pp. 383–390, ISSN 0275-004X

Spaide RF. (2009). Rationale for combination theray in age-related macular degeneration. *Retina*, Vol. 29, No. suppl 6, (June 2009), pp. 5-7, ISSN 0275-004X

Spielberg L. & Leys A. (2010). Treatment of neovascular age-related macular degeneration with a variable ranibizumab dosing regimen and one-time reduced-fluence photodynamic therapy: the TORPEDO trial at 2 years. *Graefes Arch Clin Exp Ophthalmol*. Vol. 248, No. 7, (July 2010), pp. 943-956, ISSN 1435-702X

Steward MW. & Rosenfeld PJ. (2008). Predicted biological activity of intravitreal VEGF Trap. *Br J Ophthalmol*, Vol. 92, No. 5, (May 2008), pp. 667–668. ISSN 1468-2079

Reich SJ.; Fosnot J.; Kuroki A.; tang W. & Yang X. (2003). Small interfering RNA (siRNA) targeting VEGF effectively inhibits ocular neovascularization in a mouse model. *Molecular Vision*, Vol. 30, No. 9, (May 2003), pp. 210–216, ISSN 1090-0535

Tao Y. & Jonas JB. (2010). Intravitreal bevacizumab combined with intravitreal triamcinolone for therapy-resistant exudative age-related macular degeneration. *J Ocul Pharmacol Ther*. Vol. 26, No. 2, (April 2010), pp. 207-212, ISSN 1557-7732

Timke C.; Zieher H.; Roth A.; Hauser K. & Lipson KE. (2008). Combination of vascular endothelial growth factor receptor/platelet derived growth factor receptor inhibition markedly improves radiation tumor therapy. *Clin Cancer Res*. Vol. 14, No. 7, (April 2008), pp. 2210–2219, ISSN 1557-3265

Tatar O.; Shinoda K.; Kaiserling E.; Claes C. & Eckardt C. (2009). Implications of bevacizumab on vascular endothelial growth factor and endostatin in human choroidal neovascularisation. *Br J Ophthalmol*, Vol. 93, No. 2, (February 2009), pp. 159-165, ISSN 1468-2079

Vine AK.; Stader J.; Branham K.; Musch DC. &, Swaroop A. (2005). Biomarkers of cardiovascular disease as risk factors for age-related macular degeneration. *Ophthalmology*, Vol. 112, No. 12, (December 2005), pp. 2076–2080, ISSN 0161-6420

Wan MJ.; Hooper PL. & Sheidow TG. (2010). Combination therapy in exudative age-related macular degeneration: visual outcomes following combined treatment with photodynamic therapy and intravitreal bevacizumab. *Can J Ophthalmol*. Vol. 45, No. 4, (August 2010), pp. 375-380, ISSN 0008-4182

Witmer AN.; Vrensen GF.; Van Noorden CJF. & Schlingemann RO. (2003). Vascular endothelial growth factors and angiogenesis in eye disease. *Prog Retin Eye Res*. Vol. 22, No. 1, (January 2003), pp. 1-29, ISSN 1350-9462

10

Nutritional Supplement Use and Age-Related Macular Degeneration

Amy C. Y. Lo and Ian Y. Wong
Eye Institute, The University of Hong Kong
Hong Kong

1. Introduction

Age-related macular degeneration (AMD) is a leading cause of irreversible visual impairment and blindness in the aging population [1]. Yet, individuals with AMD have limited treatment options. Given the high prevalence and considerable public health burden, it is essential to understand the etiology and pathogenesis of AMD.

AMD is a multifactorial disease, with complex genetics and confounding environmental risk factors. The etiology of AMD still remains unknown, but oxidative stress to the retina and the retinal pigment epithelium (RPE) is one of the leading hypotheses in AMD pathogenesis.

2. Oxidative stress and AMD

Oxidative stress and the cellular damages caused by reactive oxygen species (ROS) has been implicated in aging and age-related eye diseases [2]. Most intracellular ROS are derived from the mitochondria in the electron transport chain. During fuel metabolism, oxygen consumption and ATP synthesis in the mitochondria, electrons are shuffled in sequential reduction and oxidation reactions in the electron transport chain. Yet, these reactions are not 100% efficient; electrons may "leak" out and result in the formation of ROS. ROS are highly reactive and unstable oxygen-containing atoms, ions, or molecules such as hydroxyl radical (OH·), superoxide anion ($O_2^{-\cdot}$) and hydrogen peroxide (H_2O_2). Due to the presence of the "unpaired" electron in the outer shell, ROS are very unstable. In trying to achieve stability, ROS will then participate in further reduction and oxidation reactions, oxidizing target molecules and resulting in generation of other free radicals by chain reaction.

Oxidative damages by ROS affect DNA and lipids inside the cell. Earlier senescence, which may be related to shortening of telomeric DNA, occurs after oxidative damage [3-6]. Oxidative damage also results in point mutations and deletions in mitochondrial DNA [7]. In fact, mitochondrial DNA is more susceptible to ROS-induced damage than nuclear DNA [8]. As for lipids, ROS causes oxidation of lipid in a process called lipid peroxidation. The polyunsaturated fatty acids, a common and significant component of cell membrane, are particularly vulnerable to oxidation by ROS as a result of their many conjugated double bonds. Oxidation of polyunsaturated fatty acids results in the formation of reactive aldehyde intermediates which are toxic to the cell [9].

The retina is a structure that is particularly susceptible to oxidative damage by ROS. Firstly, the retina has the highest oxygen consumption in the body [10]. In addition, constant exposure to incoming light in the retina can lead to photo-oxidation. The high oxygen consumption and high light exposure in the retina may in turn generate ROS. Moreover, the retina has a high lipid content, with abundant polyunsaturated fatty acids in the photoreceptor outer segments which are most prone to lipid peroxidation. In the neighborhood of photoreceptors are the RPE cells. Besides providing metabolic support to the photoreceptors, they also phagocytose the constantly shed parts of the photoreceptor outer segments. All these factors contribute to the susceptibility of the retina and RPE to oxidative stress.

With age, the susceptibility to oxidative damage in the retina increases. Aged rat retina showed decreased GSH-Px and catalase activities, which are related to increased lipid peroxidation with age [11]. In particular, RPE cells accumulate lipofuscin granules during life. Lipofuscin granules are lysosomal residual bodies containing undigested end products from phagocytosis of photoreceptor outer segments [12]. It was estimated that lipofuscin can occupy up to 19% of RPE cytoplasmic volume by the age of 80 when compared with only 1 % during the first decade of life [13]. Lipofuscin has been shown to contain toxic substances, such as retinoids (products of the visual cycle) and oxidized proteins [14]. Lipofuscin was also able to reduce RPE lysosomal and antioxidant activity [15]. *In vitro* studies using porcine RPE cells showed that visible light irradiation can degrade RPE melanosomes, reduce melanin amount and increase ROS production, changes that also occur in human RPE melanosomes with aging [16].

3. Nutritional supplements and AMD

Oxidative stress has a recognized role in aging and AMD; treatments for AMD are therefore aimed at reducing oxidative stress-induced damage within the retina and RPE cells. This can be approached in two ways, either by decreasing the source of oxidative stress or by increasing the defense against oxidative stress. Among them, a tempting measure in lowering oxidative damage would be by dietary antioxidant supplementation. Data from observational studies have supported a link between nutritional factors with antioxidant properties and risks of AMD [17,18]. Carotenoids, vitamin C and vitamin E with their antioxidant properties have been identified as having a potentially protective role. Other nutrients such as zinc and omega-3 fatty acids have been shown to be associated with reduced risk of AMD. Recently, B vitamins (folic acid, B_6 and B_{12}) have also been proposed to provide protection by a non-oxidative mechanism. Another nutritional supplement that has gained interest recently is the extracts from a group of fruit, berries.

Common nutrition supplements include:

1. AREDS and AREDS-type formulation
2. Carotenoids (β-carotene, lutein and zeaxanthin)
3. Vitamin C (L-ascorbic acid)
4. Vitamin E (α-tocopherol))
5. Zinc
6. Omega-3 Long chain polyunsaturated fatty acids
7. B vitamins
8. Berry extracts

A summary of studies investigating the effect of nutritional supplements on the prevention and progression of AMD is shown in Tables 1 and 2.

	Study	**Nutrients investigated**	**participants (number; age)**	**Follow-up**
Randomized trials				
Teikari 1998 [43]	Alpha-tocopherol and beta-carotene study (ATBC)	beta-carotene; vitamin E	Finland (941; ≥65 years old)	6-year prevalence
Taylor 2002 [74]	Vitamin E, cataract, and age related maculopathy trial (VECAT)	vitamin E	Australia (1,193; 55-80 years old)	4-year incidence
Christen 2009 [132]	Women's Antioxidant and Folic Acid Cardiovascular Study (WAFACS)	folic acid/B_6/B_{12}	Female health care professionals in USA (5,442; ≥40 years)	Av 7.3 years
Christen 2010 [75]	Women's Health Study (WHS)	vitamin E	Female health professionals in USA (39,876; ≥45 years)	Av 10 years follow up
Weigert 2011 [61]	Lutein Intervention Study Austria (LISA)	lutein	126 AMD patients	6-month follow up
Population-based studies				
VandenLangenberg et al [23]	Beaver Dam study	alpha-carotene; beta-carotene; beta cryptoxanthin; lutein + zeaxanthin; lycopene; vitamin E; zinc; fruit and vegetables; supplements	USA (1,709; 43-84 years old)	5-year incidence
Smith 2000 [107]	The Blue Mountains Eye Study (BMES)	dietary fat, fish	Australia (3654; ≥49 years old)	
Cho 2001 [88]	Nurses' Health Study (NHS) and Health Professional Follow-up Study (HPFS)	zinc	Health professionals in USA (104,208: 66,572 women, 37,636 men; ≥50 years old)	8-10 year incidence
Cho 2001 [108]	Nurses' Health Study (NHS) and Health Professional Follow-up Study (HPFS)	Dietary fat	Health professionals in USA (72,489: 42,743 women, 29,746 men; ≥50 years old)	
Heuberger 2001 [145]	Third National Health and Nutrition Examination Study (NHANES III)	Dietary fat	USA (11,448; 40-79 years old)	

	Study	Nutrients investigated	participants (number; age)	Follow-up
Flood 2002 [44]	The Blue Mountains Eye Study (BMES)	alpha-carotene; beta-carotene; beta cryptoxanthin; lutein + zeaxanthin; lycopene; vitamin A; vitamin C; zinc; supplements	Australia (1,989; ≥49 years old)	5-year incidence
Cho, 2004 [52]	Nurses' Health Study and men in the Health Professionals Follow-up Study	alpha-carotene; beta-carotene; beta cryptoxanthin; lutein + zeaxanthin; lycopene; vitamin A; vitamin C; vitamin E; fruits and vegetables; supplements	Health professionals in USA (118,428; ≥50 years old)	12-18 year incidence
van Leeuwen 2005 [42]	Rotterdam Eye Study	alpha-carotene; beta-carotene; beta cryptoxanthin; lutein + zeaxanthin; lycopene; vitamin A; vitamin C; vitamin E; zinc	Netherlands (4,170; ≥55 years old)	Mean 8-year follow-up
Chua 2006 [110]	The Blue Mountains Eye Study (BMES)	omega-3 fatty acid; fish	Australia (3654; ≥49 years old)	5-year incidence
Moeller 2006 [53]	Carotenoids in Age-related Eye Disease Study (CAREDS)	lutein + zeaxanthin; fruit and vegetable	Women's Health Initiative (1,787; 50 to 79 years old), women only	6 year prevalence
Delcourt 2007 [112]	Pathologies Oculaires Liees a IAge (POLANUT)	total fish; white fish; fatty fish	France (832; ≥70 years old)	
Augood 2008 [114]	EUREYE	DHA; EPA; oily fish	Europe (4,753)	
Cho 2008 [54]	Nurses' health Study and Health Professionals Follow-up Study	lutein + zeaxanthin	(113,058: 71,494 women and 41,564 men; ≥50 years old)	Up to 16 years in men, Up to 18 years in women
Wang 2008 [117]	The Blue Mountains Eye Study (BMES)	fish	Australia (1,881; ≥49 years old; *CFH* genotype)	10 year
Tan 2008 [45]	The Blue Mountains Eye Study (BMES)	alpha-carotene; beta-carotene; beta cryptoxanthin; lutein + zeaxanthin; lycopene; vitamins A; vitamin C ; vitamin E; iron; zinc	Australia (2,454; ≥49 years old)	Mean 5.1 years and 10.5 years
Tan 2009 [116]	The Blue Mountains Eye Study (BMES)	omega-3 fatty acid; fish	Australia (3654; ≥49 years old)	10-year incidence
Ho 2011 [91]	The Rotterdam Study	beta-carotene; lutein/zeaxanthin; DHA; EPA; zinc;	Netherlands (2,167; ≥55 years old; *CFH* and *LOC387715/ARMS2* genotype)	Mean 8.6 years

	Study	Nutrients investigated	participants (number; age)	Follow-up
Retrospective study				
Mares-Perlman 1995	Beaver Dam Study and Nutritional Factors in Eye Disease Study	total fat; saturated fat; oleate; linoleate; cholesterol; seafood	USA (2,152; 45-84 years old)	
Klein 2008 [90]	AREDS	AREDS, zinc	USA (876; *CFH* and *LOC387715/ARMS2* genotype)	
Case controlled study				
Seddon 2006 [111]	US Twin Study of Age-Related Macular Degeneration	omega-3 fatty acids; fish	USA (681 twins; male only)	
SanGiovanni 2007 [113]	AREDS	DHA; omega-3 fatty acids; fish	USA (4,519; 60-80 years old)	
Cross-sectional study				
Chiu 2009 [146]	AREDS	DHA; EPA; lutein/zeaxanthin; vitamin C; vitamin E; zinc	USA (4,003)	

Table 1. Studies investigating nutritional supplements in the prevention of AMD

	Study	Nutrients investigated	participants (number; age)	Treatment duration
Newsome 1988 [24]		zinc	USA (151: 56 men, 95 women; 42-89 years old)	12-24 months
Stur 1996 [87]		Zinc	Austria (112: 48 men, 64 women; ≥50 years old)	24 months
AREDS [19]		beta-carotene;vitamin C; vitamin E; copper; zinc	USA (3640, 56% women; average 69 years old)	6 years
Seddon 2001 [109]		Dietary fat, fish	USA (349; 55-80 years old)	
Richer 2004 [55]	Veterans LAST study (Lutein Antioxidant Supplementation Trial)LAST	lutein /antioxidants/vitamins and minerals broad spectrum supplementation formula	USA (90: 86 men, 4 women)	12 months
SanGiovanni 2008 [115]	AREDS	omega-3 fatty acid; fish	USA (2,132)	
Weigert 2011 [61]	Lutein Intervention Study Austria (LISA)	lutein	Austria (126 AMD patients)	6 months

Table 2. Studies investigating nutritional supplements in the progression of AMD

3.1 AREDS and AREDS-type formulation

The Age-Related Eye Disease Study (AREDS) was a clinical trial sponsored by the National Eye Institute [19]. This was to date the largest prospective randomized controlled trial to investigate the effect of an active supplement formula on the risk of development of AMD. The dosages of the supplements were at a high-than-normal level, because it was considered a form of active treatment, instead of a simple supplement pill. There were a total of 3,640 subjects, being monitored for an average of 6.3 years. Each subject was given either the AREDS formula, or placebo, to be taken on a twice-daily basis. Main components of the AREDS formula are vitamin A, vitamin C, vitamin E, and zinc. These were chosen because of their anti-oxidative abilities [20-25]. When compared with the Dietary Reference Intake (DRI) issued by the Institute of Medicine, US National Academy, the dosage of ingredients in the AREDS formula was at a much higher level [26]. For instance, the dosage of vitamin C in the AREDS formula was 500 mg/day, while that of the DRI was only 90mg per day. As far as vitamin C was concerned, one has to take at least 7 to 8 oranges per day, just to match up with what is provided by the AREDS pill [27]. A comparison of the dosage in AREDS formulation with common fruits is given in Table 3.

Nutrients	Unit	AREDS	DRI*	Apple#	Orange#	Banana#	Blueberry#
Vitamin A@	International Unit (IU)	5000	3000	54	225	64	22
Vitamin C	milligram (mg)	500	90	4.6	53.2	8.7	0.7
Vitamin E	mg	400	15	0.18	0.1	0.1	0.23
Zinc	mg	80	11	0.04	0.07	0.15	0.1
Copper	mg	2	0.9	0.027	0.045	0.078	0.12
Lutein + Zeaxanthin	microgram (μg)	None	No data **	29	129	22	33

@ Vitamin A as beta-carotene
* Dietary Reference Intakes from the Institute of Medicine
** 2.0-2.3 mg/day for men and 1.7-2.0 mg/day for women in United States
(Food and Nutrition Board, 2001)
Nutrient contents of common fruits are expressed per 100 grams

Table 3. Dosages of the Age-Related Eye Disease Study (AREDS) type formulas in comparison to common fruit items

After categorizing the subjects according to their macular status (Table 4), they were then monitored serially with fundus photographs. Results of the AREDS were first released in 2001. It showed a 25% risk reduction in progression to advanced AMD, for category 3 and 4 subjects only. For other subjects, i.e. those under category 1 and 2, results were not statistically significant. In the US, 80% of those over 70 years of age fall under either category 1 or 2 [28]. Hence, the protection offered by the AREDS formula may not be applicable to all. Therefore, it was only recommended to high-risk individuals (those under category 3 or 4).

Risk associated with regular intake of the AREDS formula was of particular concern, mainly because it was meant for long-term use. In particular, the risk of regular intake of such a high level of vitamins and minerals was unknown. Potentially, vitamin A (in the form of beta-carotene) may be associated with an increased risk of lung cancer in smokers; vitamin C may cause renal stones; vitamin E may be associated with increased risk of hemorrhagic stroke; zinc can cause anemia, stomach upset, and may reduce serum high-density lipoprotein level.

	Brief description	Clinical features	Visual acuity
Category 1	No AMD in both eyes	<5 small drusen in one or both eyes	20/32 or better in both eyes
Category 2	Mild to borderline AMD in one or both eyes	Multiple small or intermediate drusen in one or both eyes Pigment abnormalities in one or both eyes	20/32 or better in both eyes
Category 3	Absence of advanced AMD in both eyes	Intermediate or large drusen Geographic atrophy Features not involving central macula	20/32 or better in better eye
Category 4	Advanced AMD in one eye	Advanced AMD or geographic atrophy in worse eye No such features in better eye	20/32 or better in better eye

Key: small drusen, <63 um in diameter (disc diameter around 1500 um); intermediate drusen, 63-124 um in diameter; large drusen, >125 um in diameter; pigment abnormalities refer to either hyperpigmentation or depigmentation [27]

Table 4. Categorization of AMD according to AREDS guidelines

However, observations from the AREDS cohort failed to show any statistically significant serious side effects as mentioned above. Documented minor side effects included 1) increased genitourinary symptoms; 2) increased self-reported anemia; and 3) yellow discoloration of skin due to high level of vitamin A. Self-reported anemia was not correlated with any genuine reduction in blood hematocrit level. Smokers in the AREDS were discouraged from smoking, therefore whether the risk of lung cancer was increased was not being addressed. However, this has already been confirmed in two other trials [29,30]. Hence, all smokers should be discouraged from smoking before the commencement of the AREDS formula. If he or she is not willing to quit smoking, the risk of having lung cancer may outweigh the potential benefit in AMD protection.

In general, the AREDS formula was deemed safe and effective, in selected high-risk individuals [31]. Inadequacy of the AREDS formula was that it did not include other potential ingredients such as lutein, zeaxanthin, and omega-3 fatty acid, which are also of particular interest due to their antioxidant abilities. In view of this, the National Eye Institute has launched the Age-Related Eye Disease Study 2 (AREDS2) in 2006, in hope to fill up the knowledge in this gap [32,33]. In the AREDS2 formula, lutein, zeaxanthin, and omega-3 fatty acid have been added to the existing AREDS formula, and vitamin A was removed, mainly due to the potential risk associated with lung cancer. Results of the AREDS2 are expected to be available in 2012. Until then, the AREDS formula remains the only evidenced-based formula to reducing the risk of development of advanced AMD.

3.2 Carotenoids (β-carotene, lutein and zeaxanthin)

Carotenoids are organic pigments naturally occurring in plants as well as in some algae, fungus and bacteria. Animals generally cannot synthesize carotenoids; they have to obtain carotenoids in their diet. There are two classes of carotenoids, xanthophylls (which contain oxygen) and carotenes (which are purely hydrocarbons, and contain no oxygen) accounting for over 600 known carotenoids. A well known carotene is beta-carotene, the pigment that makes carrots orange. Interestingly, there are only two carotenoids that are present in the human retina [34,35], namely lutein [(3R,3'R,6'R)-beta,epsilon-Carotene-3,3'-diol] and its stereoisomer, zeaxanthin [(3R,3'R)-beta,beta-Carotene-3,3'-diol]. These carotenoids are enriched in the macula in high concentrations, thus giving the macula its yellowish color.

In human, four carotenoids including beta-carotene, alpha-carotene, gamma-carotene, and beta-cryptoxanthin can be converted into retinal, which is an important molecule in the photo-transduction pathway and therefore vision. Carotenoids can also absorb light and act as antioxidants by scavenging ROS such as ·O2 and peroxyl radicals [36]. In particular, two xanthophylls, lutein and zeaxanthin, have been shown to absorb the damaging blue light [36] as well as protect the retina [37] and retinal ganglion cells [38] from oxidative damage *in vitro*. In animal studies, lutein protected the inner retina against acute retinal ischemia/reperfusion injury due to its antioxidant properties [39].

Due to their antioxidant properties and blue light-filtering effects, the association of carotenoids with risk of AMD was explored. There have been conflicting results. Decreased risk of neovascular AMD has been found to be associated with higher levels of carotenoids in the serum samples [40]. In monkeys, feeding a xanphophyll-free diet has been shown to promote drusen formation [41]. In an early study based on National Health and Nutrition Examination Survey I data, an inverse association between the consumption of fruits and vegetables rich in pro-vitamin A carotenoids and the prevalence of AMD was demonstrated [22]. In the Beaver Dam Eye Study, VandenLangenberg *et al* also found a significant but modest inverse association between intake of pro-vitamin A carotenoids and the incidence of large drusen [23]. Later studies using the AREDS formulation suggested a beneficial effect of beta-carotene [19]. The Rotterdam population-based study also reported a high dietary intake of beta-carotene together with vitamins C and E and zinc reduced the risk of AMD in elderly individuals [42]. A 35% reduced risk of AMD was observed when an above-median intake of these 4 nutrients was given.

On the other hand, opposing results were obtained from other clinical trials and population-based studies. The Alpha-Tocopherol and Beta-Carotene (ATBC) Study in Finland assessed the involvement of beta-carotene in occurrence of AMD among smoking males [43]. Over 29,000 smoking males aged 50 to 69 years were given alpha-tocopherol (50 mg/day), beta-carotene (20 mg/day), both of these, or placebo randomly. After 5 to 8 years of supplementation, Teikari *et al* found no beneficial effect of long-term beta-carotene supplementation on the incidence of AMD. The Blue Mountains Eye Study also reported no associations between beta-carotene intake and 5-year incidence of AMD [44]. This is a population-based study including 1,989 individuals who finished a food frequency questionnaire. This questionnaire assessed the baseline intake of nutrients including alpha-carotene, beta-carotene, beta-cryptoxanthin, lutein and zeaxanthin, lycopene, retinol, vitamin A, vitamin C, and zinc. For beta-carotene, Teikari *et al* suggested no evidence of protection by beta-carotene on the 5-year incidence of AMD. Further studies in the same population after 10-year of follow-up showed some interesting results. Instead of showing no effect of beta-carotene in AMD, Tan *et al* actually reported an increased risk of neovascular AMD with increasing beta-carotene intake [45]. The authors found that increasing beta-carotene intake, either from diet alone or diet plus supplementation, was associated with higher risk neovascular AMD. This association also existed when the smoking status of the individuals was adjusted.

In fact, one has to bear in mind about the possible harmful effect of beta-carotene supplementation. Apart from the skin coloration, changes in scotopic b-wave during electroretinography and crystal formation have also been shown with long-term beta-carotene use [46]. More importantly, daily supplementation of beta-carotene in smokers was associated with a higher mortality rate due to ischemic heart disease and lung cancer [29,30]. Since smoking also increases the risk of AMD, beta-carotene supplementation should be avoided in smokers. Currently, no biological explanation has been offered to clarify the harmful effect of beta-carotene in human.

Lutein and zeaxanthin are the only two carotenoids that exist in the human retina [34,35]. They are particularly dense in the macula in humans, where they are referred to as macular pigment [34]. Macular pigment is thought to be protective against retinal damage. Three case-controlled studies showed that there was an inverse association between the macular pigment density in the human retina and the risk of AMD [47-49]. In an early study investigating the effects of high dietary carotenoid intake, lutein and zeaxanthin were found to be the specific carotenoids that are most strongly associated with reduced risk of AMD [20]. This result was also supported by two other studies. The population-based Pathologies Oculaires Liees a l'Age (POLA) Study measured the plasma carotenoid levels by high-performance liquid chromatography (HPLC) in 899 subjects and correlated them with the risk of AMD [50]. It was shown that high plasma levels of lutein and zeaxanthin were associated with a significant reduced risk of AMD. Similarly, a study in U.K. involving men and women aged 66 to 75 found that subjects with the lowest plasma level of zeaxanthin has a two-fold increased risk when compared with those with the highest plasma zeaxanthin, supporting the view that zeaxanthin may protect against AMD [51].

Other studies also provide evidence in the association of lutein and zeaxanthin with AMD risk. In the Blue Mountains Eye Study, Flood *et al* reported a possible association between baseline intake of lutein and zeaxanthin and the 5-year incidence of early AMD [44]. A longer, 10-year follow-up study reported that high dietary lutein and zeaxanthin intake (top tertile) was associated reduced risk of incident neovascular AMD [45]. Participants with above median intakes had a reduced risk of indistinct soft or reticular drusen.

Conversely, several studies showed different results on the association of lutein and zeaxanthin. An early study in Beaver Dam (Beaver Dam Eye Study) reported no significant association between lutein and zeaxanthin and the risk of large drusen when 1,709 participants were followed up for 5 years [23]. In a prospective follow-up study of women in the Nurses' Health Study and men in the Health Professionals Follow-up Study, Cho *et al* followed 77,562 women and 40,866 men ≥50 years old for up to 18 years for women and up to 12 years for men. It was reported that lutein and zeaxanthin were not strongly related to either early or neovascular AMD risk [52]. The Carotenoids in Age-related Eye Disease Study (CAREDS), an ancillary study of the Women's Health Initiative, followed 1,787 female participants aged 50 to 79 for 4 to 7 years [53] and assessed their diet by a food frequency questionnaire. Subjects were divided according to their lutein and zeaxanthin intake, but there was no statistical difference between the amount of lutein and zeaxanthin intake and the prevalence of intermediate AMD. A later large prospective follow-up study also reported similar results [54]. Two cohorts, the Nurses' Health Study and the Health Professionals Follow-up Study which included 51,564 men and 71,494 women aged ≥50 years were followed up for up to 18 years. Cho *et al* reported that there was no association between lutein/zeaxanthin intake and the risk of self-reported early AMD. Yet, a non-significant and nonlinear inverse association between lutein/zeaxanthin intake and neovascular AMD risk was observed.

More recently, lutein itself has gained special interests. Two prospective randomized controlled trials have investigated the association of lutein supplementation and the incidence of AMD. The larger Veterans LAST study (Lutein Antioxidant Supplementation Trial) involved 90 subjects with atrophic AMD who were randomly divided into three groups: lutein (10mg) group, lutein (10mg) plus additional antioxidants and nutrients group, and maltodextrin placebo group [55]. Subjects were followed for 12 months and those who received lutein alone or lutein plus antioxidants and nutrients had improved visual acuity. Richer *et al* concluded that lutein alone or in combination with other nutritional supplements (including zinc, beta-carotene and vitamins C and E) is protective and slow down the progression of AMD. On the other hand, a smaller prospective trial measured the contrast sensitivity in 25 subjects after lutein supplementation (6mg) with vitamins and minerals or placebo over a 6-month period [56]. No statistical difference was observed between the lutein and placebo group, suggesting no significant association between lutein supplementation and AMD. However, one has to be careful about these findings. The sample sizes in both studies were fairly small and the follow-up periods were limited to 12 months or less.

More supportive evidence came from a recent study in which participants in AREDS were genotyped for the hepatic lipase (*LIPC*) gene [57]. Hepatic lipase is a protein in the high-density lipoprotein cholesterol pathway and has been shown in a large genome-wide association study to be a novel locus for advanced AMD risk [58]. It was observed in the AREDS participants that lower dietary lutein intake was significantly associated with increased risk of advance AMD, after controlling for the *LIPC* genotype. This suggests that high dietary lutein intake may reduce the risk of advanced AMD, after adjusting for genetic variants.

Lutein is also a macular pigment. Due to lutein's antioxidant properties and blue-light filtering capacity [36], it was hypothesized that macular pigment may provide protection against the development of AMD [59]. The first prospective follow-up study, Muenster Aging and Retina Study (MARS), recently investigated the determinants of macular pigment optical density and its relation to AMD [60]. Foveal macular pigment optical density was accessed in 369 participants including patients with different stages of AMD and healthy controls. In the 2.6-year follow-up study, it was observed that serum level of lutein, lutein supplementation in particular, was the strongest determinants of macular pigment optical density. However, the hypothetical protective effect of macular pigment in AMD could not be confirmed. On the other hand, a recent double-masked controlled study, Lutein Intervention Study Austria (LISA), investigated the association of 6-month lutein supplementation with macular pigment optical density and visual acuity in 126 AMD patients randomly assigned to lutein supplementation or placebo [61]. Weigert *et al* observed that lutein could significantly increase macular pigment optical density despite having no effect on mean differential light threshold or visual acuity. Interestingly, a significant correlation was found between the lutein-induced increase in macular pigment optical density and the change in mean differential light threshold and visual acuity. This finding suggests that patients who experience a pronounced increase in macular pigment optical density after lutein supplementation may benefit in terms of visual function.

As lutein and zeaxanthin were not ready for manufacturing as a research formula, neither of them was included in the AREDS formula [28]. The US Food and Drug Administration (FDA) has conducted an evidence-based review to evaluate the role of lutein and zeaxanthin in reducing the risk of AMD [62]. After reviewing a number of intervention and observational studies, the FDA denied a health claim about the intake of lutein or zeaxanthin (or both) and the risk of AMD in 2006. However, in view of the conflicting findings, the National Eye Institute (Bethesda, Maryland, USA) launched the Age-Related Eye Disease Study 2 (AREDS2) in 2006, hoping to resolve the link between carotenoids (lutein and zeaxanthin) intake and AMD protection [32,33]. The AREDS2, a large, multi-centered, randomized trial, is currently underway to address the effects of high dose lutein and zeaxanthin supplementation and/or omega-3 fatty acids on the progression of AMD. Beta-carotene, which increases the risk of lung cancer in smokers [29,30], is removed from the AREDS2 formula. Another on-going, similar randomized controlled trial is the Carotenoids in Age-Related Maculopathy (CARMA) Study [63]. In this study, 433 participants with either early AMD features or any level of AMD in one eye and advanced AMD in the fellow eye were recruited. Either lutein and zeaxanthin, in combination with antioxidants (including vitamin C, vitamin E, zinc, and copper) or placebo was given. Again, beta-carotene was excluded in the preparation due to the increased risk of lung cancer in smokers [29,30].

Although the beneficial effects have not been proven, lutein and zeaxanthin are included in daily supplements and food additives and can be obtained over the counter. Moreover, the addition of crystalline lutein into food and beverage products is considered GRAS (generally recognized as safe) and is approved by the FDA [64]. Lutein toxicity studies in animals using high doses of purified crystalline lutein revealed no unfavorable events [64] and no adverse events are reported for lutein and zeaxanthin at doses up to 40 mg/day in human for 2 months [65]. The risk profile of lutein was also recently reviewed in 2006 by the Council for Responsible Nutrition (CRN) in Washington, D.C. It was concluded that apart from the reversible skin discoloration, no other adverse effects were observed [66]. The CRN suggested an upper level of intake for lutein up to 20 mg/day. Currently, the average daily intake for lutein and zeaxanthin is 2.0-2.3 mg/day for men and 1.7-2.0 mg/day for women in United States (Food and Nutrition Board, 2001).

In view of their potential benefits as well as minimal side effects, lutein and zeaxanthin may be recommended for those who are keen and at risk of AMD [27].

3.3 Vitamin C (L-ascorbic acid)

Vitamin C is a water-soluble nutrient that is synthesized in almost all animals and plants. It is well known for its potent antioxidant activities [67,68]. It also acts as an important co-factor in mammals as in the synthesis of collagen; therefore vitamin C is used in the treatment and prevention of scurvy. In ophthalmology, there has not been any randomized controlled trial in assessing the efficacy of vitamin C as a single supplement in AMD. Yet, in other studies combining vitamin C with other supplements, data on the protective effects of vitamin C has been mixed. Vitamin C is shown to be beneficial in the AREDS study [19]. In two large prospective studies of 135 men and 329 women with up to 18 years of follow-up [52], it was found that higher fruit intake was related to a reduced risk of neovascular age-related maculopathy but none of the vitamins (including vitamin C) or carotenoids examined was clearly related to the disease. In a population-based cohort study involving 1,586 middle-aged and older adults, the researchers found no significant associations between the risk of large drusen and intake of vitamin C [23]. Another population-based cohort study even suggested that an increasing baseline vitamin C intake from diet and supplements was associated with an increased risk of incident early age-related maculopathy when compared with the lowest quintile [44]

3.4 Vitamin E (α-tocopherol)

Vitamin E is a collective term for a group of natural lipid-soluble compounds containing the tocopherols (α-, β-, γ- and δ-) and tocotrienols (α-, β-, γ- and δ-) with antioxidant properties. Among them, α-tocopherol is the only form to meet human requirements. In the eye, α-tocopherol can be found in the retina, RPE and choroid [69]. Its concentration in the retina increases after oral supplements [70].

As an antioxidant and a nutritional factor, vitamin E has been explored in its association with prevention of AMD. Again, data for vitamin E have been mixed. Some studies reported that higher intake are associated with lower risks of AMD or signs [23,42,71] whereas some concluded no associations [45,52,72,73].

In particular, three large randomized controlled trials have assessed vitamin E in the incidence of AMD. The Alpha-Tocopherol and Beta-Carotene (ATBC) Study involved over 29,000 smoking males aged 50 to 69 years who were randomly assigned to alpha-tocopherol (50 mg/day), beta-carotene (20 mg/day), both of these, or placebo [43]. Of these, an end-of-trial ophthalmological examination was performed in a random sample of 941 participants aged 65 years or more. No beneficial effect of long-term supplementation with alpha-tocopherol on the occurrence of AMD was detected among smoking males. In the Vitamin E Cataract and Age-related Maculopathy Trial (VECAT), 1,193 healthy volunteers aged between 55 and 80 years were randomly given either vitamin E (500IU = 335 mg) or placebo daily for 4 years [74]. In the study, the incidence of early AMD in those receiving vitamin E (8.6%) was similar to those on placebo (8.1%) whereas for late disease the incidence was 0.8% versus 0.6%. Again, daily vitamin E supplement does not prevent the development or progression of early or later stages of AMD. In the Women's Health Study (WHS) [75], a large scale randomized trial of women, 39,876 healthy female health professionals were randomly assigned to receive with natural source vitamin E (600IU) or placebo on alternate days. There were 117 AMD cases in the vitamin E group versus 128 cases in the placebo group after 10 years of treatment and follow-up. Similar to other studies, no large beneficial or harmful effect on risk of AMD was observed in long term vitamin E supplementation.

More importantly, a negative association between vitamin E and AMD was recently reported. In the Blue Mountains Eye Study involving an Australian population-based cohort, Tan *et al* reported that high vitamin E intake was associated with increased risk of late AMD, suggesting a harmful effect of dietary vitamin E on risk of AMD [45]. However, one has to be cautious about these results. There was a moderate loss of participants in this particular study, while the levels of vitamin E intake between participants followed up and not followed up were significantly different. The authors mentioned that this might affect the interpretation of the observed results.

3.5 Zinc

Zinc is an essential trace element for almost all organisms including plants, animals and microorganisms. It has a multitude of biological roles, playing a fundamental role in cellular metabolism. For example, it plays a structural role in a large number of transcription factors containing zinc fingers and similar structural motifs. Most importantly, it was first shown to be required for the catalytic activity of carbonic anhydrase [76]. Later studies showed that zinc has a catalytic or structural role in at least 300 zinc metalloenzymes [77-79], influencing many metabolic reactions. In fact, approximately 10% of the human genome encodes for proteins that can bind zinc [80].

In the human body, there are about 2-3 g of zinc, making it the second most abundant trace element [79,81]. In ocular tissues, the concentration of zinc is unusually high when compared with other tissues [82]. In the eye zinc is most abundant in the retina and choroid, followed by ciliary body, iris, optic nerve, sclera, cornea, and lens [83]. A number of functions of zinc in the retina have been suggested, including modulation of retinal synaptic transmission, modification of photoreceptor plasma membrane, involvement in retinal vitamin A metabolism, regulation of light-rhodopsin reaction within the photoreceptor, and antioxidant activity [84,85].

There are subtle ocular manifestations associated with zinc deficiency. In a prospective, randomized, double-masked, placebo-controlled investigation of the effects of oral zinc administration on the visual acuity outcome in 151 subjects with drusen or macular degeneration, the treatment group had significantly less visual loss than the placebo group [24]. As elderly patients are found to be at higher risk of zinc deficiency [86], this may suggest an increased risk of vision loss from AMD in elderly patients.

For the past three decades, there have been considerable interest and controversy related to zinc supplementation in AMD patients. To date, results on zinc supplementation and AMD have been mixed. As described above, Newsome *et al* reported significant reduction in visual loss in AMD patients when supplemented with oral zinc [24]. Moreover, Mares-Perlman *et al* reported a weak protective effect of dietary zinc on the development of some forms of early AMD [71]. In the large double-masked clinical trial, The Age-Related Eye Disease Study (AREDS), involving 11 centers, participants taking zinc alone demonstrated an odds reduction of 0.75 for the development of advanced AMD. Zinc significantly reduced the odds of developing advanced AMD in the higher-risk group. A population-based cohort study reported that high dietary zinc intake was associated with a lower risk of incident AMD [42]. In the Beaver Dam Eye Study, it was observed that there is a significant inverse association between zinc and the incidence of pigmentary abnormalities, but there was no relationship between zinc intake and incidence of early AMD [23]. In fact, an early study by the Eye Diseases Case-Control Study Group reported no association between serum zinc levels and risk of neovascular AMD [40]. In a 2-year, double-masked, randomized, placebo-controlled study, Stur *et al* reported that oral zinc substitution has no short-term effect in patients who have an exudative form of AMD in one eye [87]. Unfortunately, this study was prematurely terminated because of no beneficial effects found in first 40 patients at 24 months. In addition, two large prospective studies involving 66,572 women and 37,636 men do not support a lowered AMD risk associated with higher zinc intake [88]. The Blue Mountains Eye Study Group reported no significant association between baseline zinc intake from diet or supplements and the 5-year incidence of early Age-related maculopathy[44].

A systematic review and meta-analysis involving four prospective cohort studies [23,42,44,88]reported that a pooled odds ratio of zinc for early AMD was 0.91 (95% CI 0.74 to 1.11). Another meta-analysis reported that zinc supplementation can slow down AMD progression (adjusted odds ratio = 0.77, 95% CI 0.62 to 0.96) [89].

Although the evidence is conflicting, recent studies support a protective role of zinc in AMD progression. The AREDS study indicated that the beneficial effect of zinc supplementation was of a similar order to that of vitamin supplementation. Despite the 5-year findings by The Blue Mountains Eye Study Group [44], later studies by the same group published the 10-year data in which individuals with total zinc intake in the highest decile are less likely to develop early or any AMD [45].

Zinc intake and the genetic risk of AMD has also been assessed. In the AREDS population, the single nucleotide polymorphism in the *CFH* (Y402H, rs1061170) and *LOC387715/ARMS2* (A69S, rs10490924) genes of 876 participants who were considered at high risk was genotyped [90]. The findings suggest that there is an interaction between *CFH* genotype and treatment with antioxidant plus zinc when compared with placebo. Moreover, a recent study involving 2,167 individuals from the population-based Rotterdam Study at genetic risk of AMD assessed their dietary intake at baseline using a semi-quantitative food frequency questionnaire and determined the genetic variants using TaqMan assay [91]. In this nested case-control study, it was observed that there is a significant possibility of biological interaction between CFH Y402H and zinc as well as between LOC387715 A69S and zinc ($p < 0.05$). Moreover, individuals with homozygous CFH Y402H with dietary intake of zinc in the highest tertile reduced their hazard ratio of early AMD from 2.25 to 1.27.

Again, one has to be cautious about the risks of high dose supplementary intake of zinc. In the AREDS study, more people in the zinc group reported difficulty in swallowing the tablets (17.8% vs. 15.3%, $p < 0.04$) [19]. Circulatory adverse experiences were also more frequently reported in individuals receiving zinc. Hospitalizations due to genitourinary problems as well as mild or moderate symptoms are also more frequent in these participants. In fact, it was found that there is a significant increase in hospital admissions for urinary complications in patients with high zinc supplementation (11.1% vs 7.6%, $p = 0.0003$) [92]. The risk was greatest in male patients (RR 1.26, 95% CI 1.07-1.50, $p = 0.008$). Significant increase in urinary tract infections was also found ($p = 0.004$), especially in females. Another problem was gastrointestinal symptoms. Of 286 participants, 5/146 zinc-treated participants withdrew from the studies due to gastrointestinal symptoms when compared with 2/140 in the placebo group [24,87].

3.6 Omega-3 Long chain polyunsaturated fatty acids

The retina contains abundant fatty acids, about 30% of which are polyunsaturated fatty acids [93]. Polyunsaturated fatty acids are classified into 2 groups: ω-3 and ω-6 depending on the position of the first double bond from the methyl end of the molecule. Docosahexaenoic acid (DHA), an omega-3 fatty acid, is highly enriched in the retina, particularly in the disc membrane of photoreceptor outer segments [94]. DHA is the major polyunsaturated fatty acid in cerebral gray matter as well. Yet, the specific role of DHA in the eye is not clear. DHA has been shown to be important for photoreceptor survival [95-98]. DHA may have a role in modulating G protein-coupled signaling pathways that are involved in visual transduction [99]. DHA may also affect rhodopsin function during photoreception by influencing the membrane's biophysical properties [100,101]. In rhesus monkeys, dietary depletion of alpha-linolenic acid, a dietary precursor of DHA, resulted in undetectable plasma DHA level and more importantly, abnormal retinogram and visual impairment [102,103]. Nonetheless, DHA supplementation is effective in improving retinal function in a patient with autosomal dominant Stargardt-like retinal dystrophy [104]. The importance of DHA in retinal function may suggest a possible beneficial role of DHA in retinal disease such as AMD.

Another omega-3 fatty acid, eicosapentaenoic acid (EPA), is the precursor of eicosanoids in the body. It can act as a competitive inhibitor of arachidonic acid conversion to pro-inflammatory eicosanoids prostaglandin E(2) and leukotriene B(4) [105]. As inflammation plays a role in the pathogenesis of AMD, EPA may be one of the protective factors in AMD.

Supplementation of omega-3 fatty acids, DHA and EPA in particular, has received much interest in association with lowering the risk of AMD. Although DHA can be synthesized from alpha-linolenic acid in the body, the process is ineffective. DHA and EPA can readily be obtained from marine fish oils in the diet. Based on their roles in retinal function and inflammation, dietary modification and supplementation of omega-3 fatty acids have become attractive alternatives in lowering the risk of AMD.

Many studies have provided evidence for a protective role of omega-3 fatty acids supplementation in AMD risk [91,106-117]. The first study evaluating the relationship between dietary fat and AMD was published by Mares-Perlman et al [106]. They reported that high intake of saturated fat and cholesterol was associated with increased risk for early AMD. Later, a prospective follow-up study of participants in the Nurses' Health Study and the Health Professionals Follow-up Study showed that total fat intake was positively associated with increased risk of AMD [108]. Yet, a cross-sectional study involving participants in the Third National Health and Nutrition Examination Survey found no association between dietary fat and AMD risk. However, this study assessed only one eye per patient, thereby may have decreased the observed AMD prevalence.

There are further investigations into the association of omega-3 fatty acids with AMD risk. As dietary omega-3 fatty acids are obtained from marine fish oils, fish intake was also investigated. Earlier study on fish intake was performed in the Blue Mountain Eye Study population. In this cross-sectional, population based study, Smith et al showed that a higher fish consumption was associated with decreased odds of late AMD [107]. After 5 years of follow-up Chua *et al* reported that fish consumption at least once a week was protective against early AMD, whereas fish consumption at least 3 times per week could reduce the incidence of late AMD [110]. After 10 years of follow up in the same cohort, Tan *et al* suggested that a regular weekly serving of fish was associated with a reduced risk of early AMD [116]. Interestingly, it was also noted that fish consumption of more than one serving per week did not have a significant protective effect in reducing AMD risk in this cohort, suggesting a threshold effect. These findings are supported by other studies as well. Seddon *et al* in a multicenter eye disease case-control study reported that higher intake of omega-3 fatty acids and fish was associated with a lower risk for AMD among individuals with low linoleic acid intake [109]. More evidence on the protective role of omega-3 fatty acid came from a recent US Twin Study of Age-Related Macular Degeneration. This study investigated the association between dietary fat intake and fish consumption and risks of AMD in 681 twins [111] and found that both omega-3 and fish intake reduced the risk of AMD.

Oily fish rich in omega-3 fatty acids are also found to be beneficial in two European studies. The population-based POLANUT study from Southern France found that fatty fish intake was protective against AMD when comparing more than once a month and less than once a month and after multvariate adjustment [112]. Interestingly, total and white fish intake has no significant association with AMD risk. Another population-based study, EUREYE, showed that oily fish intake (at least once per week versus less than once per week) was associated with significant reduction of risk for neovascular AMD [114]. Similar findings were also observed for either DHA or EPA intake.

Among the AREDS participants, a prospective cohort of individuals with neovascular AMD and central geographic atrophy was also analyzed for the relationship of omega-3 fatty acids and AMD. It was observed that dietary total omega-3 fatty acids or DHA intake was inversely associated with neovascular AMD [113]. Similar findings were also observed with fish consumption. Further studies showed that dietary omega-3 fatty acids intake is associated with a decreased risk of progression from bilateral drusen to central geographic atrophy [115].

In addition, the association between omega-3 fatty acids and genetic risk of AMD is investigated. In the Blue Mountains Study group, 1881 participants were genotyped for complement factor H (CFH) genetic variants [117]. Wang *et al* reported that AMD risk increased with each additional C allele. Also, weekly compared with less than weekly consumption of fish was associated with reduced late AMD risk in participants with the CC genotype but not the CT or TT genotypes. This study provided evidence that weekly consumption of fish is protective on the development of late AMD, but not early AMD, among individuals with genetic susceptibility to AMD due to the Y402H variant. On the other hand, the dietary intake of 2167 individuals was assessed at baseline in a recent population-based Rotterdam study [91]. Ho *et al* reported a possible interaction between EPA/DHA and either *CFH* Y402H or *LOC387715* A69S. The authors also suggested that high dietary intake of omega-3 fatty acids may reduce the risk of early AMD in those who are at high genetic risk.

Taken together, much data suggests that dietary omega-3 fatty acids intake and fish consumption are protective against AMD. Results from a recent meta-analysis also supported the protective role of omega-3 fatty acids supplementation [118]. It was reported that dietary intake of omega-3 fatty acids was associated with reduced risk of late AMD while fish consumption (at least twice a week) was associated with reduced risk of both early and late AMD. However, the authors also cautioned that due to insufficient evidence, few prospective studies and no randomized clinical trials, recommendation for a routine omega-3 fatty acids supplementation and fish consumption for AMD prevention is not supported. A similar conclusion was also reached in another systematic review [119]. Hopefully, more definite answers on the protective role of omega-3 fatty acids will be provided by the ongoing AREDS2 randomized, multi-center trial.

3.7 B vitamins

B vitamins are a group of water-soluble compounds that are important in cell metabolism. The members of interest in AMD studies are folic acid, vitamin B_6 (pyridoxine) and vitamin B_{12} (cyanocobalamin) because of their ability to reduce homocysteine levels in intervention studies [120]. Homocysteine is an amino acid formed during the metabolism of methionine. It can either be recycled back into methionine or converted into cysteine with the help of B-vitamins.

Serum level of homocysteine has been implicated in increasing the risk of AMD. Recent cross-sectional [121-123]and case-control studies [124-128] showed that there may be a direct association between homocysteine level in the blood and AMD. Hyperhomocysteinemia (plasma homocysteine > 15μmol/L) can also induce vascular endothelial dysfunction [129-131]. It was therefore proposed that lowering blood homocysteine levels with folic acid, vitamin B_6 and vitamin B_{12} supplementation may help to reduce the risk of AMD.

In the Women's Antioxidant and Folic Acid Cardiovascular Study (WAFACS), 5,442 female health professionals participated in this randomized, double-masked, placebo controlled trial [132]. Christen *et al* reported that daily supplementation with folic acid/B_6/B_{12} reduce the risk of AMD in this large cohort of females after an average of 7.3 years of treatment and follow-up. Yet, disease report in this study was done by self-report questionnaires or medical records while no ophthalmic examinations were performed. More evidence and further research in other groups are needed despite the interesting association between folic acid/B_6/B_{12} supplementation and AMD prevention.

3.8 Berry extracts

Diets rich in fruits, nuts, and vegetables have long been considered to be an excellent source of antioxidants. There has been growing interest on berry extracts due to their high antioxidant properties. Among the berries, blueberries have been of specific interest because of their high antioxidant capacity (in some cases as high as 40−50 μmol Trolox equivalents/g) [133]. Indeed, of all the fresh fruits and vegetables tested to date, data indicate that blueberries have the highest antioxidant capacity, as estimated using the average oxygen radical absorbance capacity (ORAC) values [133-135]. Polyphenols in blueberries, specifically the anthocyanins that give the fruit its blue color, are the major contributors to antioxidant activity [133].

Anthocyanin is a water-soluble pigment present in all plants and is richly concentrated in berries. It is a powerful antioxidant *in vitro* [136]. It can absorb blue-green light and protects the cells from light stress in plant studies [137]. In laboratory studies, anthocyanin may protect the eyes from degenerative diseases such as AMD [138-140]. Yet, the evidence for the potential health effects of anthocyanin is mostly laboratory-based [141].

Another berry that recently received lots of interest is the fruit of *Lycium barbaurm*, also called wolfberry or Gouqizi, a commonly used herb in Chinese Traditional Medicine. It is also taken as food in Asian countries. It is well known for improving eye sight. Increasing lines of evidence showed that the polysaccharides in *Lycium barbaurm* can exhibit anti-aging [142] and anti-oxidative effects [143]. Other properties such as anti-tumor effects, cytoprotection, neuromodulation, and immune modulations have also been suggested [142,144]. Unfortunately, most evidence for its beneficial effects is limited to the laboratory level.

At this moment, there are no legal requirements for quality control in the preparation of these extracts. It is not obligatory to disclose the content and the production method. Moreover, the dosage and frequency are unclear while potential toxicity and long-term side effects remain to be investigated. A lot of investigation is needed before the potential of berry extracts in prevention of AMD can be hinted. Currently, berry extracts should not be recommended [27].

4. Future directions

Observational studies have shown beneficial effects from dietary supplementation of lutein and zeaxanthin as well as omega-3 fatty acids in the development of AMD. They are currently tested in AREDS2, the multi-centered randomized clinical trial launched by the National Eye Institute in 2006. The association of oral formulations containing lutein and zeaxanthin, and/or DHA and EPA, with the progression of AMD is being assessed. In AREDS2 participants will be followed for 5 years. Hopefully, data will be available by the end of 2012. Similarly, the ongoing CARMA study will also provide invaluable data on the protective effects of lutein and zeaxanthin in combination with antioxidants (vitamin C, vitamin E and zinc) with the exclusion of DHA and EPA.

5. Conclusions

To date a large body of evidence has supported a protective role of nutritional supplements in the development and progression of AMD. In particular, strongest evidence is present for the protective effect of lutein, zeaxanthin, DHA, and EPA. On the other hand, beta-carotene and vitamin E may have detrimental effects. While awaiting a further proof of the effects of lutein, zeaxanthin, DHA, and EPA, the AREDS formulation remains the best recommendation so far, although not without risk and maybe only for high-risk individuals. One concern for the AREDS formulation is the higher risk of lung cancer in smokers with daily beta-carotene supplementation. Therefore, in offering nutritional supplements to patients, physicians should consider on a case-by-case basis and fully explain the potential side effects from a long-term regular intake. It is also important to remind the patients that even with the AREDS formulation, AMD can still occur. It is equally important to teach the patients self-monitoring methods such as usage of the Amsler grid. Regular fundal examinations by ophthalmologists should also be strongly encouraged.

6. Reference

[1] Friedman DS, O'Colmain BJ, Munoz B, Tomany SC, McCarty C, de Jong PT, Nemesure B, Mitchell P, and Kempen J (2004) Prevalence of age-related macular degeneration in the United States. *Archives of ophthalmology* 122:564-72.

[2] Finkel T and Holbrook NJ (2000) Oxidants, oxidative stress and the biology of ageing. *Nature* 408:239-47.

[3] Hayflick L and Moorhead PS (1961) The serial cultivation of human diploid cell strains. *Experimental cell research* 25:585-621.

[4] Yuan H, Kaneko T, and Matsuo M (1995) Relevance of oxidative stress to the limited replicative capacity of cultured human diploid cells: the limit of cumulative population doublings increases under low concentrations of oxygen and decreases in response to aminotriazole. *Mechanisms of ageing and development* 81:159-68.

[5] Adelfalk C, Lorenz M, Serra V, von Zglinicki T, Hirsch-Kauffmann M, and Schweiger M (2001) Accelerated telomere shortening in Fanconi anemia fibroblasts--a longitudinal study. *FEBS letters* 506:22-6.

[6] Rubio MA, Davalos AR, and Campisi J (2004) Telomere length mediates the effects of telomerase on the cellular response to genotoxic stress. *Experimental cell research* 298:17-27.

[7] Golden TR and Melov S (2001) Mitochondrial DNA mutations, oxidative stress, and aging. *Mechanisms of ageing and development* 122:1577-89.

[8] Ballinger SW, Van Houten B, Jin GF, Conklin CA, and Godley BF (1999) Hydrogen peroxide causes significant mitochondrial DNA damage in human RPE cells. *Experimental eye research* 68:765-72.

[9] Catala A (2006) An overview of lipid peroxidation with emphasis in outer segments of photoreceptors and the chemiluminescence assay. *The international journal of biochemistry & cell biology* 38:1482-95.

[10] Sickel W (1972) Electrical and metabolic manifestations of receptor and higher-order neuron activity in vertebrate retina. *Advances in experimental medicine and biology* 24:101-18.

[11] Castorina C, Campisi A, Di Giacomo C, Sorrenti V, Russo A, and Vanella A (1992) Lipid peroxidation and antioxidant enzymatic systems in rat retina as a function of age. *Neurochem Res* 17:599-604.

[12] Kennedy CJ, Rakoczy PE, and Constable IJ (1995) Lipofuscin of the retinal pigment epithelium: a review. *Eye* 9 (Pt 6):763-71.

[13] Feeney-Burns L, Hilderbrand ES, and Eldridge S (1984) Aging human RPE: morphometric analysis of macular, equatorial, and peripheral cells. *Invest Ophthalmol Vis Sci* 25:195-200.

[14] Ng KP, Gugiu B, Renganathan K, Davies MW, Gu X, Crabb JS, Kim SR, Rozanowska MB, Bonilha VL, Rayborn ME, Salomon RG, Sparrow JR, Boulton ME, Hollyfield JG, and Crabb JW (2008) Retinal pigment epithelium lipofuscin proteomics. *Molecular & cellular proteomics : MCP* 7:1397-405.

[15] Shamsi FA and Boulton M (2001) Inhibition of RPE lysosomal and antioxidant activity by the age pigment lipofuscin. *Invest Ophthalmol Vis Sci* 42:3041-6.

[16] Zareba M, Szewczyk G, Sarna T, Hong L, Simon JD, Henry MM, and Burke JM (2006) Effects of photodegradation on the physical and antioxidant properties of

melanosomes isolated from retinal pigment epithelium. *Photochemistry and photobiology* 82:1024-9.

[17] Coleman H and Chew E (2007) Nutritional supplementation in age-related macular degeneration. *Curr Opin Ophthalmol* 18:220-3.

[18] Chiu CJ and Taylor A (2007) Nutritional antioxidants and age-related cataract and maculopathy. *Exp Eye Res* 84:229-45.

[19] Group A-REDSR (2001) A randomized, placebo-controlled, clinical trial of high-dose supplementation with vitamins C and E, beta carotene, and zinc for age-related macular degeneration and vision loss: AREDS report no. 8. *Arch Ophthalmol* 119:1417-36.

[20] Seddon JM, Ajani UA, Sperduto RD, Hiller R, Blair N, Burton TC, Farber MD, Gragoudas ES, Haller J, Miller DT, and et al. (1994) Dietary carotenoids, vitamins A, C, and E, and advanced age-related macular degeneration. Eye Disease Case-Control Study Group. *JAMA* 272:1413-20.

[21] Snellen EL, Verbeek AL, Van Den Hoogen GW, Cruysberg JR, and Hoyng CB (2002) Neovascular age-related macular degeneration and its relationship to antioxidant intake. *Acta Ophthalmol Scand* 80:368-71.

[22] Goldberg J, Flowerdew G, Smith E, Brody JA, and Tso MO (1988) Factors associated with age-related macular degeneration. An analysis of data from the first National Health and Nutrition Examination Survey. *Am J Epidemiol* 128:700-10.

[23] VandenLangenberg GM, Mares-Perlman JA, Klein R, Klein BE, Brady WE, and Palta M (1998) Associations between antioxidant and zinc intake and the 5-year incidence of early age-related maculopathy in the Beaver Dam Eye Study. *Am J Epidemiol* 148:204-14.

[24] Newsome DA, Swartz M, Leone NC, Elston RC, and Miller E (1988) Oral zinc in macular degeneration. *Arch Ophthalmol* 106:192-8.

[25] Moriarty-Craige SE, Ha KN, Sternberg P, Jr., Lynn M, Bressler S, Gensler G, and Jones DP (2007) Effects of long-term zinc supplementation on plasma thiol metabolites and redox status in patients with age-related macular degeneration. *Am J Ophthalmol* 143:206-211.

[26] website IoMotNA. *Dietary Reference Intakes*. [cited 2007 Dec 15]; Available from: http://www.iom.edu/CMS/3788/4574.aspx.

[27] Wong IY, Koo SC, and Chan CW (2011) Prevention of age-related macular degeneration. *International ophthalmology* 31:73-82.

[28] Klein R, Peto T, Bird A, and Vannewkirk MR (2004) The epidemiology of age-related macular degeneration. *Am J Ophthalmol* 137:486-95.

[29] The Alpha-Tocopherol BCCPSG (1994) The effect of vitamin E and beta carotene on the incidence of lung cancer and other cancers in male smokers. The Alpha-Tocopherol, Beta Carotene Cancer Prevention Study Group. *N Engl J Med* 330:1029-35.

[30] Omenn GS, Goodman GE, Thornquist MD, Balmes J, Cullen MR, Glass A, Keogh JP, Meyskens FL, Valanis B, Williams JH, Barnhart S, and Hammar S (1996) Effects of a combination of beta carotene and vitamin A on lung cancer and cardiovascular disease. *N Engl J Med* 334:1150-5.

[31] Evans JR (2006) Antioxidant vitamin and mineral supplements for slowing the progression of age-related macular degeneration. *Cochrane Database Syst Rev*:CD000254.
[32] website A. *Age-Related Eye Disease Study 2*. [cited 2011 Sep 7]; Available from: http://clinicaltrials.gov/ct2/show/NCT00345176?term=AREDS2&rank=1.
[33] AREDS2. *Age-Related Eye Disease Study 2. Manual of Procedures*. 2009 [cited 2011 Sep 7]; Available from: https://web.emmes.com/study/areds2/resources/areds2_mop.pdf.
[34] Bone RA, Landrum JT, and Tarsis SL (1985) Preliminary identification of the human macular pigment. *Vision Res* 25:1531-5.
[35] Parker RS (1989) Carotenoids in human blood and tissues. *J Nutr* 119:101-4.
[36] Diplock AT, Charleux JL, Crozier-Willi G, Kok FJ, Rice-Evans C, Roberfroid M, Stahl W, and Vina-Ribes J (1998) Functional food science and defence against reactive oxidative species. *Br J Nutr* 80 Suppl 1:S77-112.
[37] Gruszecki WI, Sujak A, Gabrielska J, Grudzinski W, Borc R, and Mazurek P (1999) Lutein and zeaxanthin as protectors of lipid membranes against oxidative damage: The structural aspects. *Arch Biochem Biophys* 371:301-307.
[38] Li SY and Lo AC (2010) Lutein Protects RGC-5 Cells Against Hypoxia and Oxidative Stress. *Int J Mol Sci* 11:2109-17.
[39] Li SY, Fu ZJ, Ma H, Jang WC, So KF, Wong D, and Lo AC (2009) Effect of lutein on retinal neurons and oxidative stress in a model of acute retinal ischemia/reperfusion. *Invest Ophthalmol Vis Sci* 50:836-43.
[40] Group TEDC-CS (1992) Risk factors for neovascular age-related macular degeneration. The Eye Disease Case-Control Study Group. *Arch Ophthalmol* 110:1701-8.
[41] Malinow MR, Feeney-Burns L, Peterson LH, Klein ML, and Neuringer M (1980) Diet-related macular anomalies in monkeys. *Invest Ophthalmol Vis Sci* 19:857-63.
[42] van Leeuwen R, Boekhoorn S, Vingerling JR, Witteman JC, Klaver CC, Hofman A, and de Jong PT (2005) Dietary intake of antioxidants and risk of age-related macular degeneration. *JAMA* 294:3101-7.
[43] Teikari JM, Laatikainen L, Virtamo J, Haukka J, Rautalahti M, Liesto K, Albanes D, Taylor P, and Heinonen OP (1998) Six-year supplementation with alpha-tocopherol and beta-carotene and age-related maculopathy. *Acta Ophthalmol Scand* 76:224-9.
[44] Flood V, Smith W, Wang JJ, Manzi F, Webb K, and Mitchell P (2002) Dietary antioxidant intake and incidence of early age-related maculopathy: the Blue Mountains Eye Study. *Ophthalmology* 109:2272-8.
[45] Tan JS, Wang JJ, Flood V, Rochtchina E, Smith W, and Mitchell P (2008) Dietary antioxidants and the long-term incidence of age-related macular degeneration: the Blue Mountains Eye Study. *Ophthalmology* 115:334-41.
[46] Yoser SL and Heckenlively JR (1989) The appearance of retinal crystals in retinitis pigmentosa patients using beta-carotene. *Invest Ophthalmol Vis Sci* 30 Suppl:305.
[47] Beatty S, Murray IJ, Henson DB, Carden D, Koh H, and Boulton ME (2001) Macular pigment and risk for age-related macular degeneration in subjects from a Northern European population. *Invest Ophthalmol Vis Sci* 42:439-46.
[48] Bone RA, Landrum JT, Mayne ST, Gomez CM, Tibor SE, and Twaroska EE (2001) Macular pigment in donor eyes with and without AMD: a case-control study. *Invest Ophthalmol Vis Sci* 42:235-40.

[49] Bernstein PS, Zhao DY, Wintch SW, Ermakov IV, McClane RW, and Gellermann W (2002) Resonance Raman measurement of macular carotenoids in normal subjects and in age-related macular degeneration patients. *Ophthalmology* 109:1780-7.

[50] Delcourt C, Carriere I, Delage M, Barberger-Gateau P, and Schalch W (2006) Plasma lutein and zeaxanthin and other carotenoids as modifiable risk factors for age-related maculopathy and cataract: the POLA Study. *Invest Ophthalmol Vis Sci* 47:2329-35.

[51] Gale CR, Hall NF, Phillips DI, and Martyn CN (2003) Lutein and zeaxanthin status and risk of age-related macular degeneration. *Invest Ophthalmol Vis Sci* 44:2461-5.

[52] Cho E, Seddon JM, Rosner B, Willett WC, and Hankinson SE (2004) Prospective study of intake of fruits, vegetables, vitamins, and carotenoids and risk of age-related maculopathy. *Arch Ophthalmol* 122:883-92.

[53] Moeller SM, Parekh N, Tinker L, Ritenbaugh C, Blodi B, Wallace RB, and Mares JA (2006) Associations between intermediate age-related macular degeneration and lutein and zeaxanthin in the Carotenoids in Age-related Eye Disease Study (CAREDS): ancillary study of the Women's Health Initiative. *Arch Ophthalmol* 124:1151-62.

[54] Cho E, Hankinson SE, Rosner B, Willett WC, and Colditz GA (2008) Prospective study of lutein/zeaxanthin intake and risk of age-related macular degeneration. *Am J Clin Nutr* 87:1837-43.

[55] Richer S, Stiles W, Statkute L, Pulido J, Frankowski J, Rudy D, Pei K, Tsipursky M, and Nyland J (2004) Double-masked, placebo-controlled, randomized trial of lutein and antioxidant supplementation in the intervention of atrophic age-related macular degeneration: the Veterans LAST study (Lutein Antioxidant Supplementation Trial). *Optometry* 75:216-30.

[56] Bartlett HE and Eperjesi F (2007) Effect of lutein and antioxidant dietary supplementation on contrast sensitivity in age-related macular disease: a randomized controlled trial. *Eur J Clin Nutr* 61:1121-7.

[57] Seddon JM, Reynolds R, and Rosner B (2010) Associations of smoking, body mass index, dietary lutein, and the LIPC gene variant rs10468017 with advanced age-related macular degeneration. *Mol Vis* 16:2412-24.

[58] Neale BM, Fagerness J, Reynolds R, Sobrin L, Parker M, Raychaudhuri S, Tan PL, Oh EC, Merriam JE, Souied E, Bernstein PS, Li B, Frederick JM, Zhang K, Brantley MA, Jr., Lee AY, Zack DJ, Campochiaro B, Campochiaro P, Ripke S, Smith RT, Barile GR, Katsanis N, Allikmets R, Daly MJ, and Seddon JM (2010) Genome-wide association study of advanced age-related macular degeneration identifies a role of the hepatic lipase gene (LIPC). *Proc Natl Acad Sci U S A* 107:7395-400.

[59] Loane E, Kelliher C, Beatty S, and Nolan JM (2008) The rationale and evidence base for a protective role of macular pigment in age-related maculopathy. *Br J Ophthalmol* 92:1163-8.

[60] Dietzel M, Zeimer M, Heimes B, Claes B, Pauleikhoff D, and Hense HW (2011) Determinants of macular pigment optical density and its relation to age-related maculopathy: results from the Muenster Aging and Retina Study (MARS). *Invest Ophthalmol Vis Sci* 52:3452-7.

[61] Weigert G, Kaya S, Pemp B, Sacu S, Lasta M, Werkmeister RM, Dragostinoff N, Simader C, Garhofer G, Schmidt-Erfurth U, and Schmetterer L (2011) Effects of lutein

supplementation on macular pigment optical density and visual acuity in patients with age-related macular degeneration. *Invest Ophthalmol Vis Sci.*

[62] Trumbo PR and Ellwood KC (2006) Lutein and zeaxanthin intakes and risk of age-related macular degeneration and cataracts: an evaluation using the Food and Drug Administration's evidence-based review system for health claims. *Am J Clin Nutr* 84:971-4.

[63] Neelam K, Hogg RE, Stevenson MR, Johnston E, Anderson R, Beatty S, and Chakravarthy U (2008) Carotenoids and co-antioxidants in age-related maculopathy: design and methods. *Ophthalmic Epidemiol* 15:389-401.

[64] Alves-Rodrigues A and Shao A (2004) The science behind lutein. *Toxicol Lett* 150:57-83.

[65] Dagnelie G, Zorge IS, and McDonald TM (2000) Lutein improves visual function in some patients with retinal degeneration: a pilot study via the Internet. *Optometry* 71:147-64.

[66] Shao A and Hathcock JN (2006) Risk assessment for the carotenoids lutein and lycopene. *Regul Toxicol Pharmacol* 45:289-98.

[67] Padayatty SJ, Katz A, Wang Y, Eck P, Kwon O, Lee JH, Chen S, Corpe C, Dutta A, Dutta SK, and Levine M (2003) Vitamin C as an antioxidant: evaluation of its role in disease prevention. *Journal of the American College of Nutrition* 22:18-35.

[68] McGregor GP and Biesalski HK (2006) Rationale and impact of vitamin C in clinical nutrition. *Current opinion in clinical nutrition and metabolic care* 9:697-703.

[69] Alvarez RA, Liou GI, Fong SL, and Bridges CD (1987) Levels of alpha- and gamma-tocopherol in human eyes: evaluation of the possible role of IRBP in intraocular alpha-tocopherol transport. *Am J Clin Nutr* 46:481-7.

[70] Handelman GJ, Machlin LJ, Fitch K, Weiter JJ, and Dratz EA (1985) Oral alpha-tocopherol supplements decrease plasma gamma-tocopherol levels in humans. *J Nutr* 115:807-13.

[71] Mares-Perlman JA, Klein R, Klein BE, Greger JL, Brady WE, Palta M, and Ritter LL (1996) Association of zinc and antioxidant nutrients with age-related maculopathy. *Arch Ophthalmol* 114:991-7.

[72] SanGiovanni JP, Chew EY, Clemons TE, Ferris FL, 3rd, Gensler G, Lindblad AS, Milton RC, Seddon JM, and Sperduto RD (2007) The relationship of dietary carotenoid and vitamin A, E, and C intake with age-related macular degeneration in a case-control study: AREDS Report No. 22. *Arch Ophthalmol* 125:1225-32.

[73] Klein BE, Knudtson MD, Lee KE, Reinke JO, Danforth LG, Wealti AM, Moore E, and Klein R (2008) Supplements and age-related eye conditions the beaver dam eye study. *Ophthalmology* 115:1203-8.

[74] Taylor HR, Tikellis G, Robman LD, McCarty CA, and McNeil JJ (2002) Vitamin E supplementation and macular degeneration: randomised controlled trial. *BMJ* 325:11.

[75] Christen WG, Glynn RJ, Chew EY, and Buring JE (2010) Vitamin E and age-related macular degeneration in a randomized trial of women. *Ophthalmology* 117:1163-8.

[76] Keilin D and Mann T (1940) Carbonic anhydrase. Purification and nature of the enzyme. *The Biochemical journal* 34:1163-76.

[77] Vallee BL and Auld DS (1990) Zinc coordination, function, and structure of zinc enzymes and other proteins. *Biochemistry* 29:5647-59.

[78] Coleman JE (1992) Zinc proteins: enzymes, storage proteins, transcription factors, and replication proteins. *Annual review of biochemistry* 61:897-946.
[79] Berg JM and Shi Y (1996) The galvanization of biology: a growing appreciation for the roles of zinc. *Science* 271:1081-5.
[80] Nriagu J, *Zinc Deficiency in Human Health,* in *Encyclopedia of Environmental Health,* C. Editor in, xA, and O.N. Jerome, Editors. 2011, Elsevier: Burlington. p. 789-800.
[81] Aggett PJ and Comerford JG (1995) Zinc and human health. *Nutr Rev* 53:S16-22.
[82] Galin MA, Nano HD, and Hall T (1962) Ocular zinc concentration. *Investigative ophthalmology* 1:142-8.
[83] Karcioglu ZA (1982) Zinc in the eye. *Surv Ophthalmol* 27:114-22.
[84] Grahn BH, Paterson PG, Gottschall-Pass KT, and Zhang Z (2001) Zinc and the eye. *J Am Coll of Nutr* 20:106-18.
[85] Solomons NW and Russell RM (1980) The interaction of vitamin A and zinc: implications for human nutrition. *Am J Clin Nutr* 33:2031-40.
[86] Wagner PA (1985) Zinc nutriture in the elderly. *Geriatrics* 40:111-3, 117-8, 124-5.
[87] Stur M, Tittl M, Reitner A, and Meisinger V (1996) Oral zinc and the second eye in age-related macular degeneration. *Invest Ophthalmol Vis Sci* 37:1225-35.
[88] Cho E, Stampfer MJ, Seddon JM, Hung S, Spiegelman D, Rimm EB, Willett WC, and Hankinson SE (2001) Prospective Study of Zinc Intake and the Risk of Age-Related Macular Degeneration. *Ann Epidemiol* 11:328-336.
[89] Evans J (2008) Antioxidant supplements to prevent or slow down the progression of AMD: a systematic review and meta-analysis. *Eye* 22:751-60.
[90] Klein ML, Francis PJ, Rosner B, Reynolds R, Hamon SC, Schultz DW, Ott J, and Seddon JM (2008) CFH and LOC387715/ARMS2 genotypes and treatment with antioxidants and zinc for age-related macular degeneration. *Ophthalmology* 115:1019-25.
[91] Ho L, van Leeuwen R, Witteman JC, van Duijn CM, Uitterlinden AG, Hofman A, de Jong PT, Vingerling JR, and Klaver CC (2011) Reducing the genetic risk of age-related macular degeneration with dietary antioxidants, zinc, and omega-3 fatty acids: the Rotterdam study. *Arch Ophthalmol* 129:758-66.
[92] Johnson AR, Munoz A, Gottlieb JL, and Jarrard DF (2007) High dose zinc increases hospital admissions due to genitourinary complications. *J Urol* 177:639-43.
[93] Kishan AU, Modjtahedi BS, Martins EN, Modjtahedi SP, and Morse LS (2011) Lipids and age-related macular degeneration. *Survey of ophthalmology* 56:195-213.
[94] Fliesler SJ and Anderson RE (1983) Chemistry and metabolism of lipids in the vertebrate retina. *Progress in lipid research* 22:79-131.
[95] Rotstein NP, Aveldano MI, Barrantes FJ, and Politi LE (1996) Docosahexaenoic acid is required for the survival of rat retinal photoreceptors in vitro. *J Neurochem* 66:1851-9.
[96] Rotstein NP, Aveldano MI, Barrantes FJ, Roccamo AM, and Politi LE (1997) Apoptosis of retinal photoreceptors during development in vitro: protective effect of docosahexaenoic acid. *J Neurochem* 69:504-13.
[97] Politi L, Rotstein N, and Carri N (2001) Effects of docosahexaenoic acid on retinal development: cellular and molecular aspects. *Lipids* 36:927-35.

[98] Politi LE, Rotstein NP, and Carri NG (2001) Effect of GDNF on neuroblast proliferation and photoreceptor survival: additive protection with docosahexaenoic acid. *Invest Ophthalmol Vis Sci* 42:3008-15.
[99] Litman BJ, Niu SL, Polozova A, and Mitchell DC (2001) The role of docosahexaenoic acid containing phospholipids in modulating G protein-coupled signaling pathways: visual transduction. *J Mol Neurosci* 16:237-42; discussion 279-84.
[100] Gibson NJ and Brown MF (1993) Lipid headgroup and acyl chain composition modulate the MI-MII equilibrium of rhodopsin in recombinant membranes. *Biochemistry* 32:2438-54.
[101] Brown MF (1994) Modulation of rhodopsin function by properties of the membrane bilayer. *Chem Phys Lipids* 73:159-80.
[102] Neuringer M, Connor WE, Van Petten C, and Barstad L (1984) Dietary omega-3 fatty acid deficiency and visual loss in infant rhesus monkeys. *J Clin Invest* 73:272-6.
[103] Neuringer M, Connor WE, Lin DS, Barstad L, and Luck S (1986) Biochemical and functional effects of prenatal and postnatal omega 3 fatty acid deficiency on retina and brain in rhesus monkeys. *Proc Natl Acad Sci U S A* 83:4021-5.
[104] MacDonald IM, Hebert M, Yau RJ, Flynn S, Jumpsen J, Suh M, and Clandinin MT (2004) Effect of docosahexaenoic acid supplementation on retinal function in a patient with autosomal dominant Stargardt-like retinal dystrophy. *Br J Ophthalmol* 88:305-6.
[105] James MJ, Gibson RA, and Cleland LG (2000) Dietary polyunsaturated fatty acids and inflammatory mediator production. *Am J Clin Nutr* 71:343S-8S.
[106] Mares-Perlman JA, Brady WE, Klein R, VandenLangenberg GM, Klein BE, and Palta M (1995) Dietary fat and age-related maculopathy. *Arch Ophthalmol* 113:743-8.
[107] Smith W, Mitchell P, and Leeder SR (2000) Dietary fat and fish intake and age-related maculopathy. *Arch Ophthalmol* 118:401-4.
[108] Cho E, Hung S, Willett WC, Spiegelman D, Rimm EB, Seddon JM, Colditz GA, and Hankinson SE (2001) Prospective study of dietary fat and the risk of age-related macular degeneration. *Am J Clin Nutr* 73:209-18.
[109] Seddon JM, Rosner B, Sperduto RD, Yannuzzi L, Haller JA, Blair NP, and Willett W (2001) Dietary fat and risk for advanced age-related macular degeneration. *Arch Ophthalmol* 119:1191-9.
[110] Chua B, Flood V, Rochtchina E, Wang JJ, Smith W, and Mitchell P (2006) Dietary fatty acids and the 5-year incidence of age-related maculopathy. *Arch Ophthalmol* 124:981-6.
[111] Seddon JM, George S, and Rosner B (2006) Cigarette smoking, fish consumption, omega-3 fatty acid intake, and associations with age-related macular degeneration: the US Twin Study of Age-Related Macular Degeneration. *Arch Ophthalmol* 124:995-1001.
[112] Delcourt C, Carriere I, Cristol JP, Lacroux A, and Gerber M (2007) Dietary fat and the risk of age-related maculopathy: the POLANUT study. *Eur J Clin Nutr* 61:1341-4.
[113] SanGiovanni JP, Chew EY, Clemons TE, Davis MD, Ferris FL, 3rd, Gensler GR, Kurinij N, Lindblad AS, Milton RC, Seddon JM, and Sperduto RD (2007) The relationship of dietary lipid intake and age-related macular degeneration in a case-control study: AREDS Report No. 20. *Arch Ophthalmol* 125:671-9.

[114] Augood C, Chakravarthy U, Young I, Vioque J, de Jong PT, Bentham G, Rahu M, Seland J, Soubrane G, Tomazzoli L, Topouzis F, Vingerling JR, and Fletcher AE (2008) Oily fish consumption, dietary docosahexaenoic acid and eicosapentaenoic acid intakes, and associations with neovascular age-related macular degeneration. *Am J Clin Nutr* 88:398-406.

[115] SanGiovanni JP, Chew EY, Agron E, Clemons TE, Ferris FL, 3rd, Gensler G, Lindblad AS, Milton RC, Seddon JM, Klein R, and Sperduto RD (2008) The relationship of dietary omega-3 long-chain polyunsaturated fatty acid intake with incident age-related macular degeneration: AREDS report no. 23. *Arch Ophthalmol* 126:1274-9.

[116] Tan JS, Wang JJ, Flood V, and Mitchell P (2009) Dietary fatty acids and the 10-year incidence of age-related macular degeneration: the Blue Mountains Eye Study. *Arch Ophthalmol* 127:656-65.

[117] Wang JJ, Rochtchina E, Smith W, Klein R, Klein BE, Joshi T, Sivakumaran TA, Iyengar S, and Mitchell P (2009) Combined effects of complement factor H genotypes, fish consumption, and inflammatory markers on long-term risk for age-related macular degeneration in a cohort. *Am J Epidemiol* 169:633-41.

[118] Chong EW, Kreis AJ, Wong TY, Simpson JA, and Guymer RH (2008) Dietary omega-3 fatty acid and fish intake in the primary prevention of age-related macular degeneration: a systematic review and meta-analysis. *Arch Ophthalmol* 126:826-33.

[119] Hodge WG, Schachter HM, Barnes D, Pan Y, Lowcock EC, Zhang L, Sampson M, Morrison A, Tran K, Miguelez M, and Lewin G (2006) Efficacy of omega-3 fatty acids in preventing age-related macular degeneration: a systematic review. *Ophthalmology* 113:1165-72; quiz 1172-3, 1178.

[120] Collaboration HLT (2005) Dose-dependent effects of folic acid on blood concentrations of homocysteine: a meta-analysis of the randomized trials. *Am J Clin Nutr* 82:806-12.

[121] Heuberger RA, Fisher AI, Jacques PF, Klein R, Klein BE, Palta M, and Mares-Perlman JA (2002) Relation of blood homocysteine and its nutritional determinants to age-related maculopathy in the third National Health and Nutrition Examination Survey. *Am J Clin Nutr* 76:897-902.

[122] Axer-Siegel R, Bourla D, Ehrlich R, Dotan G, Benjamini Y, Gavendo S, Weinberger D, and Sela BA (2004) Association of neovascular age-related macular degeneration and hyperhomocysteinemia. *Am J Ophthalmol* 137:84-9.

[123] Rochtchina E, Wang JJ, Flood VM, and Mitchell P (2007) Elevated serum homocysteine, low serum vitamin B12, folate, and age-related macular degeneration: the Blue Mountains Eye Study. *Am J Ophthalmol* 143:344-6.

[124] Nowak M, Swietochowska E, Wielkoszynski T, Marek B, Kos-Kudla B, Szapska B, Kajdaniuk D, Glogowska-Szelag J, Sieminska L, Ostrowska Z, Koziol H, and Klimek J (2005) Homocysteine, vitamin B12, and folic acid in age-related macular degeneration. *Eur J Ophthalmol* 15:764-7.

[125] Vine AK, Stader J, Branham K, Musch DC, and Swaroop A (2005) Biomarkers of cardiovascular disease as risk factors for age-related macular degeneration. *Ophthalmology* 112:2076-80.

[126] Coral K, Raman R, Rathi S, Rajesh M, Sulochana KN, Angayarkanni N, Paul PG, and Ramakrishnan S (2006) Plasma homocysteine and total thiol content in patients with exudative age-related macular degeneration. *Eye* 20:203-7.

[127] Kamburoglu G, Gumus K, Kadayifcilar S, and Eldem B (2006) Plasma homocysteine, vitamin B12 and folate levels in age-related macular degeneration. *Graefes Arch Clin Exp Ophthalmol* 244:565-9.

[128] Seddon JM, Gensler G, Klein ML, and Milton RC (2006) Evaluation of plasma homocysteine and risk of age-related macular degeneration. *Am J Ophthalmol* 141:201-3.

[129] Domagala TB, Undas A, Libura M, and Szczeklik A (1998) Pathogenesis of vascular disease in hyperhomocysteinaemia. *J Cardiovasc Risk* 5:239-47.

[130] Chambers JC, Obeid OA, and Kooner JS (1999) Physiological increments in plasma homocysteine induce vascular endothelial dysfunction in normal human subjects. *Arterioscler Thromb Vasc Biol* 19:2922-7.

[131] McDowell IF and Lang D (2000) Homocysteine and endothelial dysfunction: a link with cardiovascular disease. *J Nutr* 130:369S-372S.

[132] Christen WG, Glynn RJ, Chew EY, Albert CM, and Manson JE (2009) Folic acid, pyridoxine, and cyanocobalamin combination treatment and age-related macular degeneration in women: the Women's Antioxidant and Folic Acid Cardiovascular Study. *Arch Intern Med* 169:335-41.

[133] Prior RL, Cao G, Martin A, Sofic E, McEwen J, O'Brien C, Lischner N, Ehlenfeldt M, Kalt W, Krewer G, and Mainland CM (1998) Antioxidant Capacity As Influenced by Total Phenolic and Anthocyanin Content, Maturity, and Variety of Vaccinium Species. *Journal of Agricultural and Food Chemistry* 46:2686-2693.

[134] Cao G, Sofic E, and Prior RL (1996) Antioxidant Capacity of Tea and Common Vegetables. *Journal of Agricultural and Food Chemistry* 44:3426-3431.

[135] Wang H, Cao G, and Prior RL (1996) Total Antioxidant Capacity of Fruits. *Journal of Agricultural and Food Chemistry* 44:701-705.

[136] De Rosso VV, Moran Vieyra FE, Mercadante AZ, and Borsarelli CD (2008) Singlet oxygen quenching by anthocyanin's flavylium cations. *Free radical research* 42:885-91.

[137] Liakopoulos G, Nikolopoulos D, Klouvatou A, Vekkos KA, Manetas Y, and Karabourniotis G (2006) The photoprotective role of epidermal anthocyanins and surface pubescence in young leaves of grapevine (Vitis vinifera). *Annals of botany* 98:257-65.

[138] Bagchi D, Sen CK, Bagchi M, and Atalay M (2004) Anti-angiogenic, antioxidant, and anti-carcinogenic properties of a novel anthocyanin-rich berry extract formula. *Biochemistry. Biokhimiia* 69:75-80, 1 p preceding 75.

[139] Bagchi D, Roy S, Patel V, He G, Khanna S, Ojha N, Phillips C, Ghosh S, Bagchi M, and Sen CK (2006) Safety and whole-body antioxidant potential of a novel anthocyanin-rich formulation of edible berries. *Molecular and cellular biochemistry* 281:197-209.

[140] Sadilova E, Carle R, and Stintzing FC (2007) Thermal degradation of anthocyanins and its impact on color and in vitro antioxidant capacity. *Molecular nutrition & food research* 51:1461-71.

[141] Seeram NP (2008) Berry Fruits: Compositional Elements, Biochemical Activities, and the Impact of Their Intake on Human Health, Performance, and Disease. *J Agric Food Chem* 56:627-629.

[142] Chang RC and So KF (2008) Use of anti-aging herbal medicine, Lycium barbarum, against aging-associated diseases. What do we know so far? *Cell Mol Neurobiol* 28:643-52.

[143] Li SY, Yang D, Yeung CM, Yu WY, Chang RC, So KF, Wong D, and Lo AC (2011) Lycium barbarum polysaccharides reduce neuronal damage, blood-retinal barrier disruption and oxidative stress in retinal ischemia/reperfusion injury. *PLoS One* 6:e16380.

[144] Ho YS, So KF, and Chang RC (2010) Anti-aging herbal medicine--how and why can they be used in aging-associated neurodegenerative diseases? *Ageing Res Rev* 9:354-62.

[145] Heuberger RA, Mares-Perlman JA, Klein R, Klein BE, Millen AE, and Palta M (2001) Relationship of dietary fat to age-related maculopathy in the Third National Health and Nutrition Examination Survey. *Arch Ophthalmol* 119:1833-8.

[146] Chiu CJ, Milton RC, Klein R, Gensler G, and Taylor A (2009) Dietary compound score and risk of age-related macular degeneration in the age-related eye disease study. *Ophthalmology* 116:939-46.

11

Two-Photon Excitation Photodynamic Therapy: Working Toward a New Treatment for Wet Age-Related Macular Degeneration

Ira Probodh and David Thomas Cramb
Department of Chemistry, University of Calgary
Canada

1. Introduction

Photodynamic therapy (PDT) exploits the cytotoxic effects of light-activated compounds to achieve spatially selective tissue eradication. It is used in treating a wide range of tumors (Lou et al., 2003), localized infections (Hamblin & Hasan, 2004), and diseases like the wet form of age-related macular degeneration (Bressler & Bressler, 2000). The treatment involves application of a non-toxic photosensitizer that is preferentially taken up by the target cells/tissue. Optical excitation of the photosensitizer produces reactive oxygen species that cause localised, apoptotic cell death. Herein we review the application of a new modality - two-photon excitation-PDT (TPE-PDT) - to the treatment of wet age-related macular degeneration (wet-AMD). We show that the application of TPE-PDT, in conjunction with newly developed photosensitizers, has the potential to greatly improve therapy of wet-AMD.

1.1 Why two-photon photodynamic therapy (TPE-PDT)?

1.1.1 Photodynamic therapy (PDT)

Wet-AMD is characterised by generation of blood vessels in the normally avascular retinal macula. The newly formed blood vessels leak fluid and/or blood under the macula, leading to rapid vision loss through damage to the photoreceptors (Rattner & Nathans, 2006). PDT, using single photon activation of the photosensitizer Verteporfin (trade name Visudyne), has been used for the treatment of wet-AMD since 2000 (Bressler & Bressler, 2000). In the clinic, verteporfin is first administered to patients through systemic injections (Soubrane & Bressler, 2001), and the photosensitizer accumulates in areas of high cellular reproduction like the neovasculature in the retinal tissue. Photo-irradiation of the photosensitizer leads to a localised, Type II photoreaction associated with singlet oxygen generation (Schmidt-Erfurth & Hasan, 2000). The photosensitizer absorbs a photon and is promoted to the excited singlet state that converts to an excited triplet state through intersystem crossing. An energy transfer between the triplet excited state of photosensitizer and naturally occurring triplet oxygen then produces reactive singlet oxygen. While Type I reactions involving radicals are also possible, PDT is generally accepted as occurring predominantly through the singlet oxygen mechanism.

The PDT-induced vessel occlusion, *in vivo*, is generally attributed to singlet oxygen mediated direct vascular damage of blood vessel endothelium. This initiates a cascade of responses which include platelet aggregation, leukocyte adhesion, vascular permeabilization and vasoconstriction (Krammer, 2001). These, in turn, are expected to cause vascular occlusion.

The short lifetime of singlet oxygen (3.5μs in aqueous environment (Pervaiz, 2001)) ensures that the area affected by it is spatially confined to a small volume. It is estimated that singlet oxygen can diffuse to a distance of around 100nm or less (Skovsen et al., 2005) *in vivo*. PDT, thus, offers a relatively selective and non-invasive method to occlude the abnormal vascularization characteristic of wet-AMD. The stages in PDT for treatment of wet-AMD are diagrammed in Figure 1.

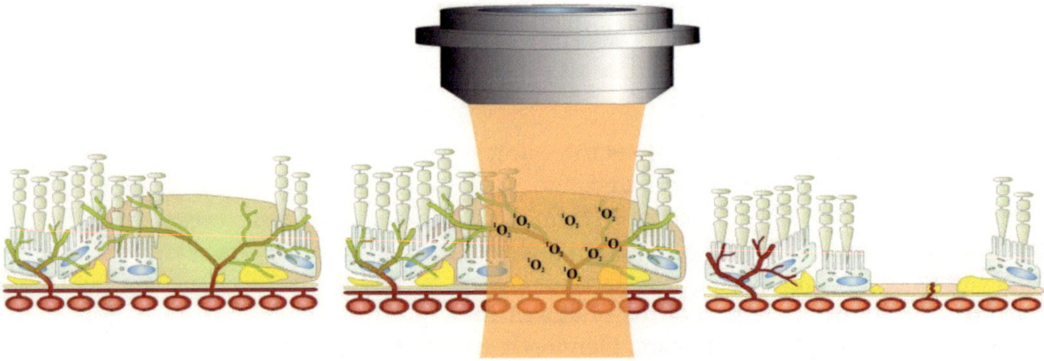

$$\text{Verteporfin} + O_2 + h\nu \longrightarrow {}^1O_2 \longrightarrow \text{Vessel closure}$$

Fig. 1. Visual representation of Verteporfin photodynamic therapy: injected verteporfin accumulates in the retinal neovasculature, where it is activated by illumination with a 680nm laser beam. Laser activation leads to singlet oxygen production that in turn leads to vessel occlusion. [Adapted from PhD thesis of K. S. Samkoe (Samkoe, 2007)]

Currently, clinical PDT treatment involves excitation of Verteporfin with 689nm laser light that excites via a one-photon absorption peak in the so-called Q-band of the photosensitizer. The disadvantage of this treatment regime is that one-photon excitation can damage the over- and underlying tissues adjacent to the treated area, through excitation of photosensitizer present there (Reinke et al., 1999). This deleterious side-effect can be reduced by using two-photon excitation of photosensitizer.

1.1.2 Two-photon excitation PDT (TPE-PDT)

Two-photon excitation (TPE) of fluorophores is extensively utilized in confocal microscopy (Oheim et al., 2006; So et al., 2000). Because two-photon absorption cross-sections are very small, excitation requires high fluxes of light that can be achieved by using a tightly focused femtosecond laser beam as the light source. In TPE, a molecule is excited by simultaneous absorption of two photons of half the energy, or twice the wavelength, of one photon excitation. The first photon excites the molecule from its ground state to a virtual intermediate excited state. A second photon, simultaneously absorbed, promotes the molecule from the virtual intermediate state to the singlet excited state. The probability of this event is very small, and it is proportional to the square of the light intensity. Two-photon absorption, therefore, occurs only at the focal plane of a tightly focused laser beam (Goyan et al., 2001; Oheim et al., 2006). It should be noted that the excited states achieved by one and two-photon absorption are identical. The photophysical and photochemical properties of the photosensitizer are thus, unaffected by the mode of excitation (Goyan & Cramb, 2000; Samkoe et al., 2006).

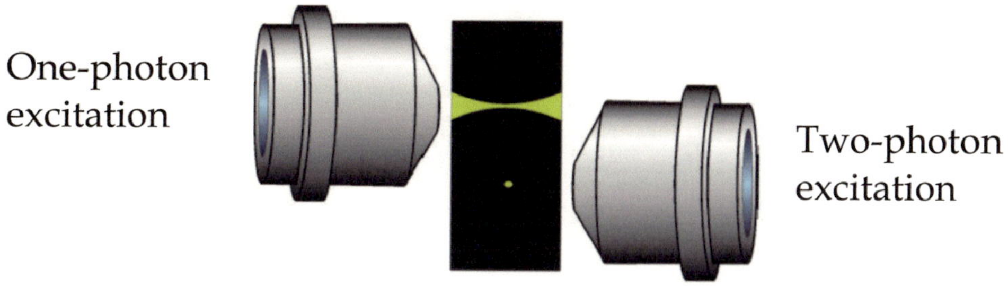

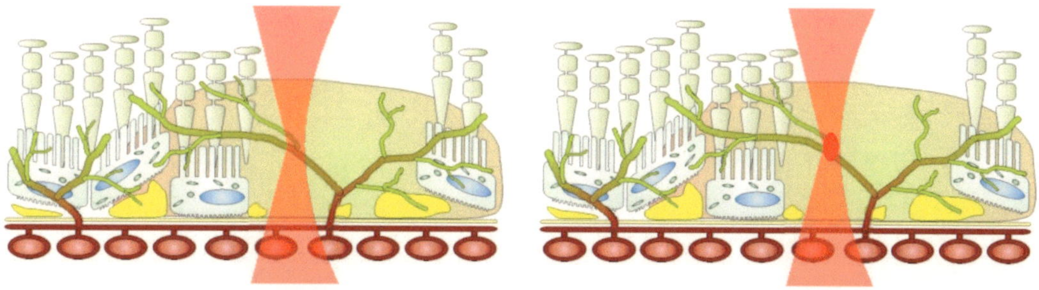

Fig. 2. In one photon excitation, photosensitizer activation occurs throughout the path of the laser beam, but in two-photon excitation, activation occurs only at the focus of the laser beam (red oval in right panel). The localised excitation in TPE-PDT is likely to cause less collateral damage. [Adapted from PhD thesis of K. S. Samkoe (Samkoe, 2007)]

Typically, excitation volumes of a few femtoliters can be achieved with two-photon absorption. This extremely confined excitation volume allows for high spatial selectivity. Use of a TPE treatment modality therefore, has the potential to selectively excite photosensitizer in the neovasculature, leaving the surrounding tissue unaffected (see Figure 2). In the following sections we review the experiments that demonstrate TPE-PDT *in vitro* and vessel occlusion *in vivo* with clinically approved and novel photosensitizers, and discuss the implications of its therapeutic use.

2. TPE-PDT in vitro – Testing photosensitizers in cell-lines

While *in vivo* experiments in animal models are essential to test and demonstrate the efficacy of drugs, it is very useful to quickly pre-screen drugs in cellular models before expending time and effort on laborious animal experiments. Cells can grow faster than animals, are inexpensive to maintain and easier to handle. In the context of PDT, they are particularly useful since cell death post-PDT treatment can be easily quantified.

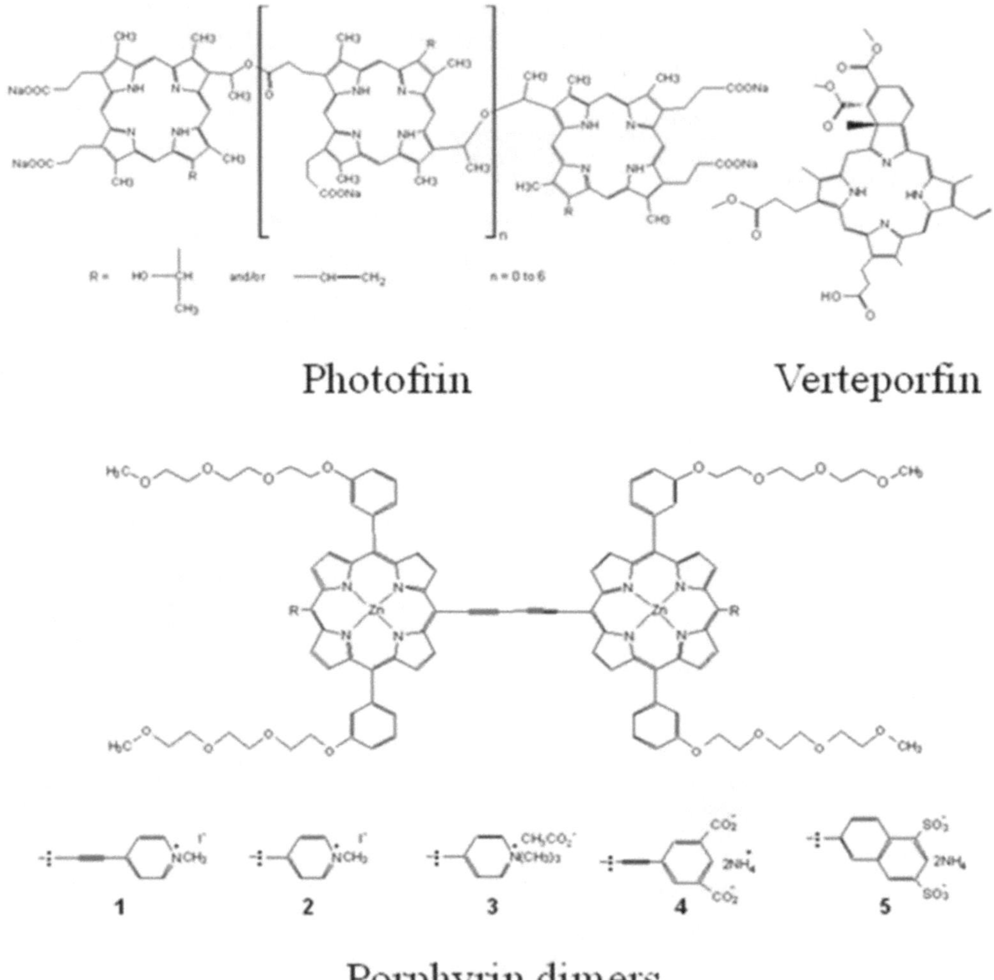

Fig. 3. The photosensitizers [Porphyrin dimers adapted from (Collins et al., 2008)]

Khurana et al (Khurana et al., 2007) have used endothelial cells to assess the TPE-PDT efficacy of photosensitizers approved for one photon PDT - namely, photofrin and verteporfin. They incubated a confluent monolayer of endothelial cells (YPEN-1) with each photosensitizer and performed TPE-PDT by irradiating the cell layer with the 865nm laser line of a femtosecond Ti:Sapphire laser at various output powers. TPE-PDT effect was quantified by using cell permeability stains to assess cell death post-treatment. The authors achieved TPE-PDT induced cell death with both photosensitizers, but Verteporfin was around seven times more effective, consistent with its higher two-photon cross-section. Using verteporfin and by varying the laser dose, they were also able to demonstrate the non-linear dependence of TPE-PDT on light intensity, providing unambiguous support of the involvement of two-photon processes in PDT.

While utilizing clinically approved photosensitizers for TPE-PDT is very attractive, their small two-photon absorption may be limiting in the clinical context. Collins et al (Collins et al., 2008) reported the use of "designer" TPE-PDT drugs - novel porphyrin dimers specifically designed to have high two-photon absorption cross section. The authors tested a series of porphyrin dimers for their PDT-induced cytotoxicity in a cancer cell line and demonstrated the higher TPE-PDT efficiency of dimer 1 (fig. 3) relative to verteporfin. Dimer 1 was then selected for *in vivo* TPE-PDT testing [section 3.2.2] and is a strong candidate for future development as a TPE-PDT photosensitizer.

3. TPE-PDT in vivo

3.1 Complete occlusion of neovasculature in the chicken CAM

3.1.1 The CAM as a model for wet-AMD

The chicken chorioallantoic membrane (CAM) is a transparent extra-embryonic membrane that grows against the inner wall of the developing egg. It is an external lung and waste exchange system for the embryo, and has a wide range of blood vessel sizes - from a few microns to several hundred microns in diameter (Patten, 1971). This makes it easy to find blood vessels that are similar in size to the neovasculature produced in the human eye during AMD (see Figure 4), and like the latter, the blood vessels are undergoing rapid angiogenesis between days 5 to 9 of gestation (Schlatter et al., 1997). The chicken embryo has a short gestation period and is easy to manipulate. It is as such, an inexpensive and useful model for the neovasculature occurring in wet-AMD.

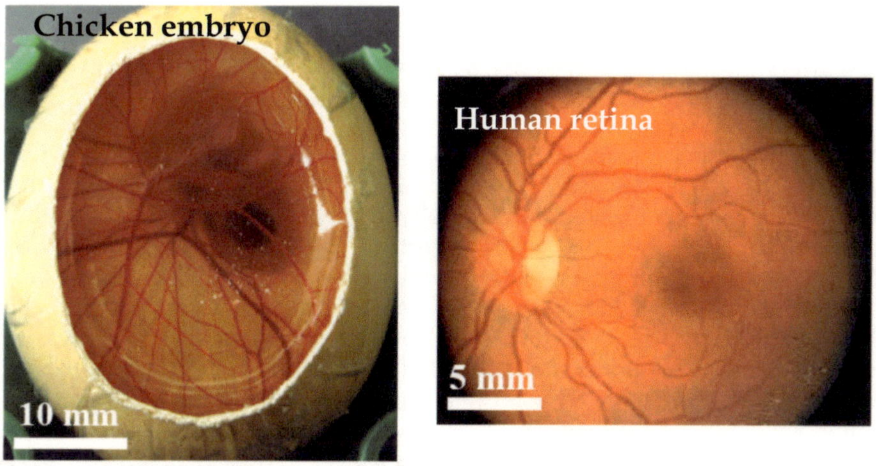

Fig. 4. The chicken chorio-allantoic membrane (CAM) exhibits blood vessels similar in size to those in the human eye, making it a good model for the neovasculature in wet-AMD. [Picture of chicken embryo reproduced with permission from Clancy et al., 2010, *Chemical Physics Letters*, 488, 99-111; picture of human retina reproduced from PhD thesis of K. S. Samkoe (Samkoe, 2007).]

3.1.2 Experimental set-up for PDT in the chicken embryo

The following protocol to prepare the embryo was developed in the Cramb group (Samkoe et al., 2007). Chicken eggs are incubated at 37°C and 60% humidity for 9 days prior to the experiment. On day 4.5, the eggs are "windowed" by first draining 3-4ml of albumen from the blunt end using a syringe, and then cutting a small window in the egg-shell. The window is then covered by cellulose tape for the duration of the incubation, and widened before the experiment to facilitate injection.

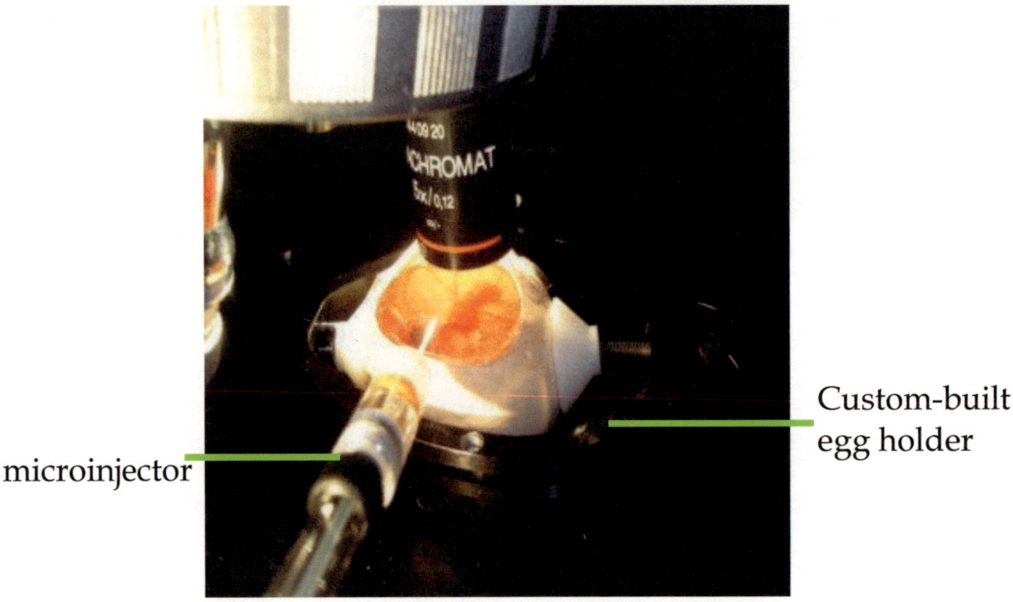

Fig. 5. TPE-PDT in the chicken CAM. Photosensitizer is injected with the microinjector attached to the custom-built stage and TPE-PDT is carried out by focusing the laser beam on the treated artery through the microscope objective. [Picture reproduced from PhD thesis of Y. Gregoriou (Gregoriou, 2011)]

For the TPE-PDT experiments, the embryo was mounted on an upright fluorescence microscope with a custom designed sample stage (Figure 5). Verteporfin was administered as a vesicle preparation, injected intrarterially or intravenously, using a microinjector attached to the sample stage. 10min after injection, PDT was performed by directing the light (780nm) of a Ti:Sapphire laser (pulse duration ~ 100fsec) into the selected artery. Laser power of the incident light, duration of the laser illumination and the number of laser treatments were varied to achieve optimal PDT treatment. Vessel occlusion was monitored by taking video images of the treated areas before and after PDT treatment. For tracking long term occlusion, embryos were monitored for up to 6hrs after TPE-PDT treatment. For the multiple short laser treatments, each treatment was performed by focusing the laser beam on to the upper wall of the blood vessel for the required time, then moving it to another spot, close by, on the same artery.

3.1.3 Vessel occlusion by TPE-PDT in the chicken embryo

The first experiments demonstrating TPE-PDT-induced complete occlusion of blood vessels in the CAM occluded up to 15μm diameter arteries (Samkoe et al., 2007). A laser power of

38mW (corresponding to a fluence of $1.1x10^8 J/cm^2$) and treatment time of 5min achieved complete occlusion of these small arteries immediately after the treatment. As expected, increasing the drug dose, the laser power, and/or the laser treatment time increases the efficacy of occlusion, presumably through increased singlet oxygen generation. By increasing the laser power and treatment times, it was also possible to achieve long-term occlusion of blood vessels. A minimum of 45mW laser power and a laser treatment time of 3min were required for long term occlusion of up to 50μm arteries (Khurana et al., 2009) (fig.6).

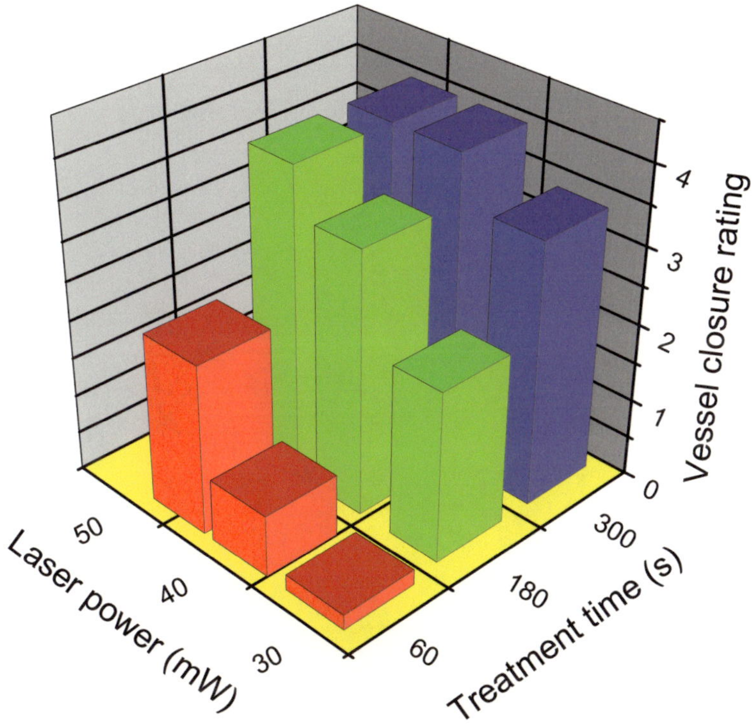

Fig. 6. Optimising laser dosage to occlude 50μm arteries. A vessel closure rating of 4 equals complete occlusion. [Adapted with permission from Khurana et al., (2009) *Journal of Biomedical Optics*, 14, 064006.]

Clearly, increasing the laser power and laser treatment times has the potential to improve occlusion efficacy of TPE-PDT and shut down larger feeder vessels. So is there a glass ceiling? The two major limiting factors are the laser's maximum power output which limits the maximum fluence, and the photosensitizer/oxygen concentration in the excitation volume, which limits the singlet oxygen generated during the treatment. In our experiments, it appears to be the latter, with the TPE-PDT efficacy levelling off at laser powers of 120mW for the highest drug dose tried (2 mg per kg of body weight). The option of increasing the treatment times is not preferred as longer treatment times reduce the long-term viability of the embryo and limit the usefulness of the model in terms of tracking long-term occlusion. Moreover, for patient compliance during TPE-PDT, shorter treatment times are preferred.

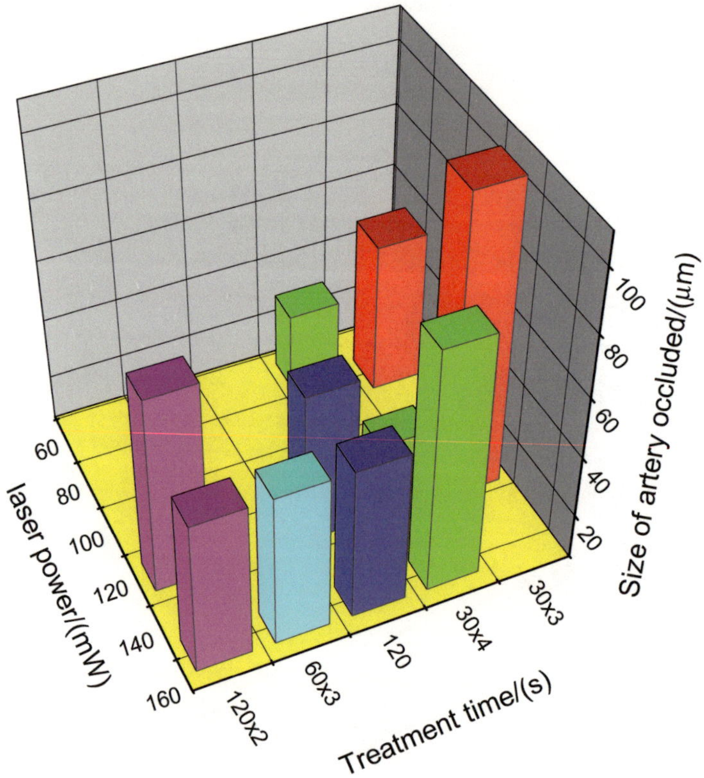

Fig. 7. Varying the laser dosage and treatment regimes to occlude large blood vessels shows that multiple short treatments are more useful than long single treatments in vessel occlusion.

Multiple short laser treatments, interspersed with 'dark' periods, could overcome these limitations by exciting a large number of photosensitizers in a short period, and then allowing the blood flow to replenish the ground state photosensitizer and/or oxygen during the 'dark' period. The examples in Fig. 7 and 8 clearly indicate that multiple short laser treatments are more efficacious than single long treatments to achieve long-term occlusion of large vessels. We were able to completely occlude up to 100μm sized arteries using laser power as low as 70mW with 30sx3 laser treatments, whereas a laser power of 120mW and 120s treatment time only succeeded in occluding up to 60μm arteries. Our data suggest that in the context of clinical verteporfin TPE-PDT treatment, it would be useful to investigate multiple short laser treatments to achieve optimal PDT efficiency and shut down large feeder vessels.

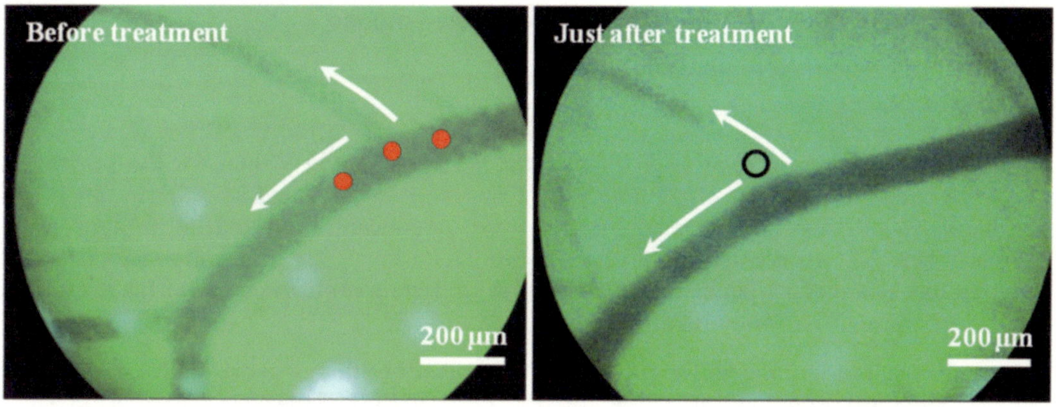

Fig. 8. Blood vessel occlusion after TPE-PDT. 2 mg/kg Verteporfin liposomal solution injected intravenously; 3×30s treatments with 70mW laser achieved almost complete occlusion of a 55μm artery immediately after treatment. (The red dots mark the approximate positions of the laser beam during TPE-PDT treatment)

3.2 Vascular occlusion in the mouse window model

3.2.1 The mouse window chamber model for testing vascular occlusion

Khurana et al (Khurana et al., 2009) have investigated TPE-PDT in a murine chamber window model. Surgical placement of a transparent window (1cm diameter) into the dorsal skin of a mouse allows for direct visualization of skin vasculature and administration of PDT treatment under a confocal laser scanning microscope (see Figure 9). This has the advantage of using a more robust animal model that allows for tracking of vascular occlusion on the long term - up to 25hrs. With the chicken CAM model, it is typically possible to track vessel occlusion only up to 6-7hrs after the treatment. The disadvantage of using the mouse model for wet-AMD is that the blood vessels tested are normal healthy vessels, not leaky neovasculature of the type found in wet-AMD and the chicken CAM.

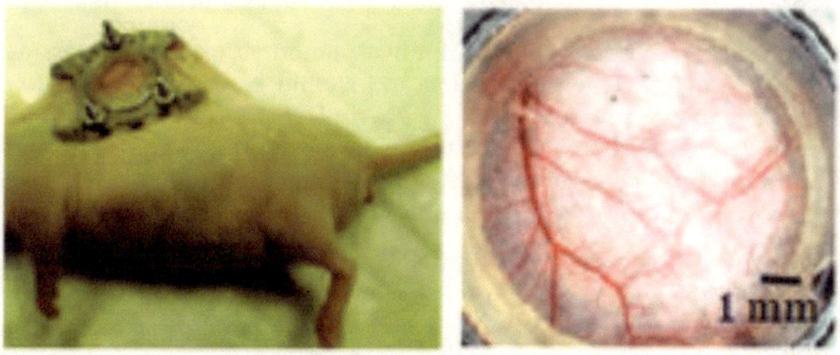

Fig. 9. The murine window chamber model. Nude mouse with surgically implanted window (left), vasculature visible through the window (right) [Reproduced with permission from Khurana et al., (2009) *Journal of Biomedical Optics*, 14, 064006]

3.2.2 Vessel occlusion by TPE-PDT in the windowed mouse

Khurana et al (Khurana et al., 2009) tested two different photosensitizers for TPE-PDT - verteporfin and a novel porphyrin dimer specifically designed for larger two-photon absorption. For TPE-PDT, a small area (80x80μm^2) on the selected blood vessel was raster scanned with the appropriate laser (865nm for verteporfin and 920nm for the porphyrin dimer). A range of photosensitizer and light doses were investigated in order to obtain the optimal value of drug-light product (product of drug concentration and light fluence) and compare TPE-PDT to conventional one photon excitation PDT. The authors focused on complete occlusion of 40-50μm diameter arteries and compared the verteporfin drug-light product of one and two-photon PDT.

The drug-light product for verteporfin TPE-PDT was more than three orders of magnitude higher than the corresponding value for one photon PDT. This was as expected since verteporfin has a much lower absorption cross-section for two-photon excitation. Consequently, a much higher light and drug dose would be necessary to achieve the same vascular occlusion. Interestingly, the corresponding verteporfin TPE-PDT drug-light product in the chicken CAM was ten times higher, suggesting that the CAM vasculature is much less responsive to TPE-PDT. It must be noted that the neovasculature in the CAM is very leaky compared to the mouse vasculature tested. It is quite possible that the higher drug-light product in the CAM is a consequence of lower effective drug concentrations in the excitation volume due to the leaky nature of the vessels.

The porphyrin dimer (dimer 1, fig.3) tested by Khurana et al (Khurana et al., 2009) had a 340-fold higher two-photon absorption cross-section compared to verteporfin, but exhibited only a twenty times lower drug-light product. The lower than expected effectiveness of the photosensitizer is probably due to poorer uptake and/or different localization to PDT-sensitive sites in the vasculature.

4. TPE-PDT: Challenges

For the transition of TPE-PDT from the lab to the clinic, there are still several roadblocks to be met. The main challenges in the development of TPE-PDT are the need for: TPE-specific drugs, inexpensive lasers, adaptive optics to correct for optical aberration in the lens/cornea, and integration of technology into a "point and shoot" package for physicians.

A good TPE-specific drug needs to have high two-photon absorption, low human toxicity, high efficiency for singlet oxygen generation and should be easily targeted to the retinal neovasculature. The previously mentioned Porphyrin Dimer 1 (section 2 and fig. 3) meets at least three of these criteria. It has high two-photon absorption, very high singlet oxygen yield and shows promise for targeting to the neovasculature (Collins et al., 2008). It is, as such, a promising candidate for testing as a TPE-PDT drug.

Currently, TPE-PDT can only be achieved by excitation with expensive, high energy, pulsed lasers that can provide the high energy densities required for two-photon absorption. However, photosensitizers with very high two-photon absorption can potentially be activated by inexpensive low energy lasers, making TPE-PDT an economically viable treatment. Porphyrin dimers, with their large two-photon absorption cross-section and high efficiency of singlet oxygen generation, hold out the promise of inexpensive TPE-PDT treatment (Drobizhev et al., 2005; Kobuke & Ogawa, 2008).

The next challenge would be to develop adaptive optics for localized delivery of laser light into the retinal neovasculature. The laser beam needs to be tightly focused upon the macular neovasculature, and the defocusing effect of the eye-lens as well as the cornea needs to be overcome to achieve this. Research is currently under way at the Campbell laboratory, University of Waterloo, to develop an ophthalmoscope for TPE-PDT.

5. TPE-PDT and anti-VEGF therapy

Photodynamic therapy has proved extremely useful in prohibiting choroidal neovascular leakage and conservation of visual acuity (Arnold et al., 2001; Azab et al., 2004). It does not, however, prevent reoccurrence of retinal leakage, and treatment needs to be repeated at regular intervals (Schmidt-Erfurth et al., 1999). For effective arrest and/or cure of wet-AMD, PDT needs to be complemented by other treatments that prevent the formation of neovasculature. Of these, anti-VEGF therapy shows the greatest promise (Abouammoh & Sharma, 2011; Chiang & Regillo, 2011; Ozkiris, 2010). It targets VEGF-A, the vascular endothelial growth factor (VEGF) that is associated with promoting neovascularisation and angiogenesis. The role of VEGF-A in the pathogenesis of the wet-AMD is well recognized (Ferrara et al., 2003; Kliffen et al., 1997). PDT has also been implicated in the upregulation of VEGF, thereby promoting vascularisation, even as it eradicates the existing neovasculature. A treatment strategy that targets VEGF at the same time as it occludes existing neovasculature is therefore, strongly indicated.

Currently, two anti-VEGF strategies are most commonly used in treatment, both of which involve antibodies to VEGF-A (Abouammoh & Sharma, 2011). Bevacizumab (Avastin, Genentech, San Fransisco, California, USA) is a humanized monoclonal antibody to VEGF-A, while Ranibizumab (Lucentis, Genentech, San Fransisco, California, USA) is a monoclonal antibody fragment derived from Bevacizumab. Both Avastin and Lucentis are administered through intraocular injections and have been shown to significantly improve the visual acuity. In both cases, the treatment requires repeated intraocular injections and neither of them can eradicate pre-existing neovasculature. Combining anti-VEGF therapy with TPE-PDT for treating wet-AMD has the potential to reduce the number of anti-VEGF injections, while still greatly improving the visual acuity by blocking neovascularisation of the retinal macula and destroying pre-existing leakage.

Preliminary investigations of combined Avastin and one-photon PDT treatments suggest that while the combination therapy does not always improve visual acuity, it does reduce the number of retreatments required (Abouammoh & Sharma, 2011; Chiang & Regillo, 2011). Clinical trials are currently under way in North America and Europe to investigate the effects of combined PDT and Lucentis anti-VEGF therapy (Abouammoh & Sharma, 2011; Chiang & Regillo, 2011).

6. Conclusions

Laboratory experiments show that two-photon excitation photodynamic therapy offers potential for better selectivity and lower collateral damage in treating wet age-related macular degeneration. Experiments in the chicken embryo and mouse window models show that it is possible to achieve long-term, complete occlusion of blood vessels using two-photon excitation of verteporfin. Design of photosensitizers with higher two-photon absorption cross sections is likely to improve the efficacy of the TPE-PDT treatment modality in wet-AMD. Pre-clinical and clinical studies on the safety and efficacy of two-photon excitation photodynamic therapy of wet-AMD are needed before two-photon excitation photodynamic therapy is applied for clinical use.

7. References

Abouammoh, M. & Sharma, S., (2011) Ranibizumab versus bevacizumab for the treatment of neovascular age-related macular degeneration. *Current Opinion in Ophthalmology,* 22, 152-158.

Arnold, J., Kilmartin, D., Olson, J., Neville, S., Robinson, K., Laird, A., Richmond, C., Farrow, A., McKay, S., McKechnie, R., Evans, G., Aaberg, T. M., Brower, J., Waldron, R., Loupe, D., Gillman, J., Myles, B., Saperstein, D. A., Schachat, A. P., Bressler, N. M., Bressler, S. B., Nesbitt, P., Porter, T., Hawse, P., Harnett, M., Eager, A., Belt, J., Cain, D., Emmert, D., George, T., Herring, M., McDonald, J., Mones, J., Corcostegui, B., Gilbert, M., Duran, N., Sisquella, M., Nolla, A., Margalef, A., Miller, J. W., Gragoudas, E. S., Lane, A. M., Emmanuel, N., Holbrook, A., Evans, C., Lord, U. S., Walsh, D. K., Callahan, C. D., DuBois, J. L., Moy, J., Kenney, A. G., Milde, I., Platz, E. S., Lewis, H., Kaiser, P. K., Holody, L. J., Lesak, E., Lichterman, S., Siegel, H., Fattori, A., Ambrose, G., Fecko, T., Ross, D., Burke, S., Conway, J., Singerman, L., Zegarra, H., Novak, M., Bartel, M., Tilocco-DuBois, K., Ilc, M., Schura, S., Joyce, S., Tanner, V., Rowe, P., Smith-Brewer, S., Greanoff, G., Daley, G., DuBois, J., Lehnhardt, D., Kukula, D., Fish, G. E., Jost, B. F., Anand, R., Callanan, D., Arceneaux, S., Arnwine, J., Ellenich, P., King, J., Aguado, H., Rollins, R., Anderson, T., Nork, C., Duignan, K., Boleman, B., Jurklies, B., Pauleikhoff, D., Hintzmann, A., Fischer, M., Sowa, C., et al., (2001) Verteporfin therapy of subfoveal choroidal neovascularization in age-related macular degeneration: Two-year results of a randomized clinical trial including lesions with occult with no classic choroidal neovascularization-verteporfin in photodynamic therapy report 2. *American Journal of Ophthalmology,* 131, 541-560.

Azab, M., Benchaboune, M., Blinder, K. J., Bressler, N. M., Bressler, S. B., Gragoudas, E. S., Fish, G. E., Hao, Y., Haynes, L., Lim, J. I., Menchini, U., Miller, J. W., Mones, J., Potter, M. J., Reaves, A., Rosenfeld, P. J., Strong, A., Su, X. Y., Slakter, J. S., Schmidt-Erfurth, U. & Sorenson, J. A., (2004) Verteporfin therapy of subfoveal choroidal neovascularization in age-related macular degeneration: Meta-analysis of 2-year safety results in three randomized clinical trials: Treatment of age-related macular degeneration with photodynamic therapy and verteporfin in photodynamic therapy study report no. 4. *Retina,* 24, 1-12.

Bressler, N. M. & Bressler, S. B., (2000) Photodynamic therapy with verteporfin (visudyne): Impact on ophthalmology and visual sciences. *Investigative Ophthalmology and Visual Science,* 41, 624-628.

Chiang, A. & Regillo, C. D., (2011) Preferred therapies for neovascular age-related macular degeneration. *Current Opinion in Ophthalmology,* 22, 199-204.

Clancy, A. A., Gregoriou, Y., Yaehne, K. & Cramb, D. T., (2010) Measuring properties of nanoparticles in embryonic blood vessels: Towards a physicochemical basis for nanotoxicity. *Chemical Physics Letters,* 488, 99-111.

Collins, H. A., Khurana, M., Moriyama, E. H., Mariampillai, A., Dahlstedt, E., Balaz, M., Kuimova, M. K., Drobizhev, M., Yang, V. X. D., Phillips, D., Rebane, A., Wilson, B. C. & Anderson, H. L., (2008) Blood-vessel closure using photosensitizers engineered for two-photon excitation. *Nature Photonics,* 2, 420-424.

Drobizhev, M., Stepanenko, Y., Dzenis, Y., Karotki, A., Rebane, A., Taylor, P. N. & Anderson, H. L., (2005) Extremely strong near-IR two-photon absorption in conjugated porphyrin dimers: Quantitative description with three-essential-states model. *Journal of Physical Chemistry B,* 109, 7223-7236.

Ferrara, N., Gerber, H. P. & LeCouter, J., (2003) The biology of vegf and its receptors. *Nature Medicine,* 9, 669-676.

Goyan, R., Paul, R. & Cramb, D. T., (2001) Photodynamics of latex nanospheres examined using two-photon fluorescence correlation spectroscopy. *Journal of Physical Chemistry B,* 105, 2322-2330.

Goyan, R. L. & Cramb, D. T., (2000) Near-infrared two-photon excitation of protoporphyrin ix: Photodynamics and photoproduct generation. *Photochemistry and Photobiology,* 72, 821-827.

Gregoriou, Y. (2011) Quantum dot bioaccumulation in angiogenic tissue: Towards a physicochemical basis for nanotoxicity. PhD thesis submitted to the Department of Chemistry, University of Calgary, Calgary, Canada.

Hamblin, M. R. & Hasan, T., (2004) Photodynamic therapy: A new antimicrobial approach to infectious disease? *Photochemical and Photobiological Sciences,* 3, 436-450.

Khurana, M., Collins, H. A., Karotki, A., Anderson, H. L., Cramb, D. T. & Wilson, B. C., (2007) Quantitative in vitro demonstration of two-photon photodynamic therapy using photofrin and visudyne. *Photochemical and Photobiological Sciences,* 83, 1441-1448.

Khurana, M., Moriyama, E. H., Mariampillai, A., Samkoe, K., Cramb, D. & Wilson, B. C., (2009) Drug and light dose responses to focal photodynamic therapy of single blood vessels in vivo. *Journal of Biomedical Optics,* 14, 064006.

Kliffen, M., Sharma, H. S., Mooy, C. M., Kerkvliet, S. & de Jong, P. T., (1997) Increased expression of angiogenic growth factors in age-related maculopathy. *British Journal of Ophthalmology,* 81, 154-162.

Kobuke, Y. & Ogawa, K., (2008) Recent advances in two-photon photodynamic therapy. *Anti-Cancer Agents in Medicinal Chemistry,* 8, 269-279.

Krammer, B., (2001) Vascular effects of photodynamic therapy. *Anticancer Research,* 21, 4271-4277.

Lou, P. J., Jones, L. & Hopper, C., (2003) Clinical outcomes of photodynamic therapy for head-and-neck cancer. *Technology in Cancer Research and Treatment,* 2, 311-317.

Oheim, M., Michael, D. J., Geisbauer, M., Madsen, D. & Chow, R. H., (2006) Principles of two-photon excitation fluorescence microscopy and other nonlinear imaging approaches. *Advanced Drug Delivery Reviews,* 58, 788-808.

Ozkiris, A., (2010) Anti-VEGF agents for age-related macular degeneration. *Expert Opinion on Therapeutic Patents,* 20, 103-118.

Patten, B. M. (1971) *Early embryology of the chick.* McGraw-Hill Book Company, New York.

Pervaiz, S., (2001) Reactive oxygen-dependent production of novel photochemotherapeutic agents. *Faseb Journal,* 15, 612-617.

Rattner, A. & Nathans, J., (2006) Macular degeneration: Recent advances and therapeutic opportunities. *Nature Reviews Neuroscience,* 7, 860-872.

Reinke, M. H., Canakis, C., Husain, D., Michaud, N., Flotte, T. J., Gragoudas, E. S. & Miller, J. W., (1999) Verteporfin photodynamic therapy retreatment of normal retina and choroid in the cynomolgus monkey. *Ophthalmology,* 106, 1915-1923.

Samkoe, K. S., Fecica, M. S., Goyan, R. L., Buchholz, J. L., Campbell, C., Kelly, N. M. & Cramb, D. T., (2006) Photobleaching kinetics of optically trapped multilamellar vesicles containing verteporfin using two-photon excitation. *Photochemistry and Photobiology,* 82, 152-157.

Samkoe, K. S., Clancy, A. A., Karotki, A., Wilson, B. C. & Cramb, D. T., (2007) Complete blood vessel occlusion in the chick chorioallantoic membrane using two-photon excitation photodynamic therapy: Implications for treatment of wet age-related macular degeneration. *Journal of Biomedical Optics,* 12, 034025.

Samkoe, K. S. (2007) Two-photon excitation photodynamic therapy: Progress towards a new treatment for wet age-related macular degeneration. PhD thesis submitted to the Department of Chemistry, University of Calgary, Calgary, Canada.

Schlatter, P., Konig, M. F., Karlsson, L. M. & Burri, P. H., (1997) Quantitative study of intussusceptive capillary growth in the chorioallantoic membrane (cam) of the chicken embryo. *Microvascular Research,* 54, 65-73.

Schmidt-Erfurth, U., Miller, J. W., Sickenberg, M., Laqua, H., Barbazetto, I., Gragoudas, E. S., Zografos, L., Piguet, B., Pournaras, C. J., Donati, G., Lane, A. M., Birngruber, R., van den Berg, H., Strong, H. A., Manjuris, U., Gray, T., Fsadni, M. & Bressler, N. M., (1999) Photodynamic therapy with verteporfin for choroidal neovascularization caused by age-related macular degeneration: Results of retreatments in a phase 1 and 2 study. *Archives of Ophthalmology,* 117, 1177-1187.

Schmidt-Erfurth, U. & Hasan, T., (2000) Mechanisms of action of photodynamic therapy with verteporfin for the treatment of age-related macular degeneration. *Survey of Ophthalmology,* 45, 195-214.

Skovsen, E., Snyder, J. W., Lambert, J. D. & Ogilby, P. R., (2005) Lifetime and diffusion of singlet oxygen in a cell. *Journal of Physical Chemistry B,* 109, 8570-8573.

So, P. T. C., Dong, C. Y., Masters, B. R. & Berland, K. M., (2000) Two-photon excitation fluorescence microscopy. *Annual Review of Biomedical Engineering,* 2, 399-429.

Soubrane, G. & Bressler, N. M., (2001) Treatment of subfoveal choroidal neovascularisation in age related macular degeneration: Focus on clinical application of verteporfin photodynamic therapy. *British Journal of Ophthalmology,* 85, 483-495.

12

Clinical Application of Drug Delivery Systems for Treating AMD

Noriyuki Kuno and Shinobu Fujii
Santen Pharmaceutical Co., Ltd.
Japan

1. Introduction

Due to transparent ocular media, it is relatively easy to observe intraocular tissues such as the vitreous and retina without invasion, and various administration approaches including intravitreal and subretinal injection, or implantation can be applicable. Since the eye-ball is a closed organ, novel therapeutic molecules such as an antisense oligonucleotide for cytomegalovirus retinitis (Fomivirsen; Vitraven®, Isis Pharmaceuticals, Inc., Carlsbad, CA U.S. and Novartis, Basel, Switzerland), an aptamer (e.g. Pegaptanib sodium; Macugen®, Pfizer, Inc., New York, NY, U.S.) or a small interfering RNA for neovascular (wet) age-related macular degeneration (AMD), have been investigated in human eyes before their applications for systemic diseases. In addition, many injectable or implantable drug delivery systems for chronic vitreoretinal diseases including AMD, diabetic macular edema, retinal vein occlusion, uveitis, and retinitis pigmentosa (RP), using polymer technology and/or mechanical engineering, have been developing (Figure 1).

This chapter focuses on drug delivery systems under clinical applications and in late experimental stage for the treatment of both wet and atrophic (dry) AMD (Table 1).

2. Significance of drug delivery systems for AMD

For the treatment of wet AMD, a standard therapy is monthly intravitreal injections of ranibizumab, an anti-vascular endothelial growth factor (VEGF) monoclonal antibody fragment (Lucentis®, Genentech, Inc., South San Francisco, CA, U.S.) (Genentech Inc.) and photodynamic therapy (PDT) by systemic administration of verteporfin (Visudyne®, QLT Ophthalmics, Inc., Menlo Park, CA, U.S.). The monthly cost of Lucentis® is about $2,000 and that means effective treatment by Lucentis® faces a serious social problem (Martin et al., 2010, Gower et al., 2010, Patel et al., 2010). Also frequent intravitreal injections might cause several complications, it has been reported that prevalence of lens damage, endophthalmitis and rhegmatogenous retinal detachment were 0.006% (2 of 32,318 injections) (Meyer, Rodrigues et al., 2010), 0.029% (3 of 10,254 cases) (Pilli et al., 2008) and 0.013% (5 of 35,942 injections) (Meyer, Michels et al., 2010), respectively. In addition, recently sustained elevation of intraocular pressure (IOP) after intravitreal injections of anti-VEGF agents has been reported (Good et al., 2011). Although the mechanism of IOP elevation is unclear, aggregation of proteins and/or leaching of silicone from the syringe barrel and rubber stopper might cause to clog the trabecular meshwork. It has also been demonstrated that aggregated proteins induce a more significant immunological response than non-aggregated proteins (Rosenberg, 2006). Furthermore, a lack of selective targeting of verteporfin to neovascular endothelial cells causes to damage the normal retinal tissues such as the retinal pigment epithelium (RPE) and photoreceptors. Therefore, it is necessary to develop drug delivery systems which can be easily and non-invasively administered, have long-term controlled-release by a single administration, and/or selective-targeting potency to the pathologic tissues for the treatment of AMD to overcome the disadvantages in the current wet AMD therapy.

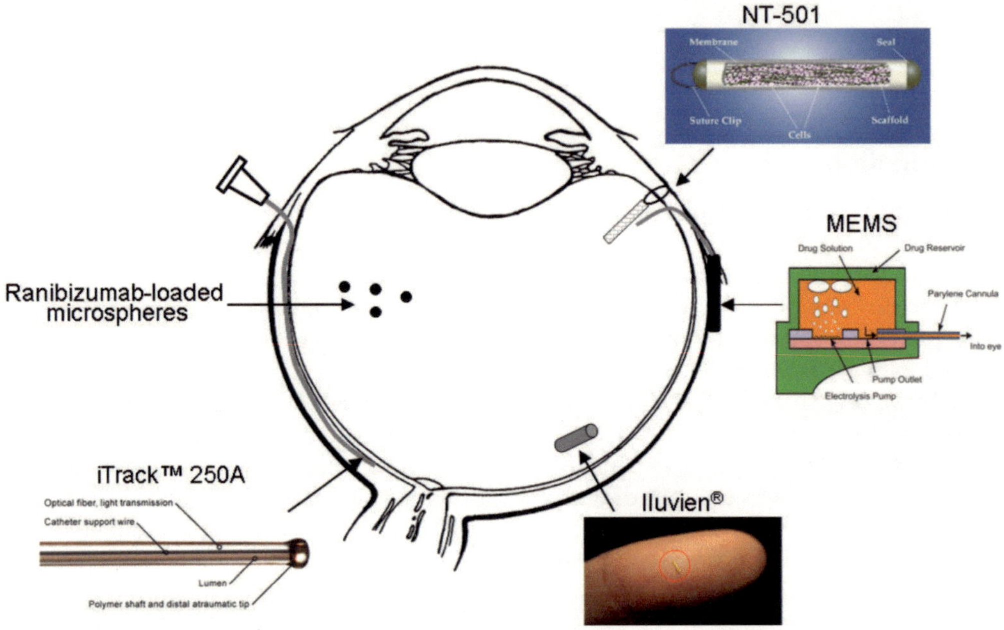

Fig. 1. Example of drug delivery systems for the treatment of AMD

On the other hand, tachyphylaxis is a diminished therapeutic response to a drug after repeated administrations over time. It has been reported that 8.5% (5 of 59 patients) of wet AMD patients who received repeated intravitreal injections of bevacizumab developed tachyphylaxis (Forooghian et al., 2009). The median time to develop tachyphylaxis after the first bevacizumab injection was 100 weeks with a median of 8 injections before tachyphylaxis development. Other groups have also reported that tachyphylaxis with ranibizumab and bevacizumab for wet AMD (Schaal et al., 2008, Keane et al., 2008, Eghoj & Sorensen, 2011) was found. It is thought that the generation of neutralizing antibodies to bevacizumab did not significantly contribute to the development of tachyphylaxis (Forooghian et al., 2011). A combination of bevacizumab and triamcinolone acetonide (TA) improved the reduction of bevacizumab efficacy caused by anti-VEGF tachyphylaxis. Therefore, there is an urgent need to develop drugs and their drug delivery systems targeting other pathways not involving VEGF for patients who develop anti-VEGF tachyphylaxis or non-responders.

In addition to wet AMD, dry AMD is a chronic, progressive retinal degenerative disease, therefore, drug delivery systems are absolutely needed.

Active ingredient	Brand name	Development stage	Mode of action	Administration Route	Excipients/ Carriers
			PEGylation		
Pegaptanib	Macugen®	Launched	Anti-VEGF aptamer	IVT injection	PEG
ARC1905	-	P1 (dAMD) P1 (wAMD)	Anti-C5 aptamer	IVT injection	PEG
E10030	-	P2 (wAMD)	Anti-PDGF aptamer	IVT injection	PEG
			Sustained release		
Fluocinolone acetonide	Iluvien®	P2 (dAMD) P2 (wAMD)	Inhibition of microglial activation	IVT implant	Polyimide/PVA
NT-501	-	P2 (dAMD)	Neurotrophin (CNTF)	IVT implant	Semi-permeable membrane
Brimonidine	-	P2 (dAMD)	α2 adrenergic agonist	IVT implant	PLGA
			Targeting		
Verteporfin	Visudyne®	Launched	PDT	IV injection	Negatively-charged liposome
WST-11	Stakel®	P2 (wAMD)	PDT	IV injection	-
I-con1	-	P1/2a (wAMD)	NK cell-mediated apoptosis	IVT injection	-
VEGFR epitope peptide	-	P1 (wAMD)	CTLs-mediated apoptosis	SC injection	-
			Gene induction		
PEDF	-	P1 (wAMD)	Antiangiogenesis by PEDF	IVT injection	Ad
sFLT01	-	P1 (wAMD)	VEGF decoy	IVT injection	AAV2
Endstatin Angiostatin	RetinoStat®	P1 (wAMD)	Antiangiogenesis by endostatin, angiostatin	SRT injection	EIAV

Ad, adenovirus; AAV2, adeno-associated virus serotype 2; AMD, age-related macular degeneration; C5, complement factor 5; CNTF, ciliary neurotrophic factor; CTLs, cytotoxic T lymphocytes; EIAV, equine infectious anaemia virus; IV, intravenous; IVT, intravitreal; NK, natural killer; PDGF, platelet-derived growth factor; PDT, photodynamic therapy; PEDF, pigment epithelium-derived factor; PEG, poly(ethylene gycol); PLGA, poly(lactide-co-glycolide); PVA, poly(vinyl alcohol); SC, subcutaneous; SRT, subretinal; VEGF, vascular endothelial growth factor

Table 1. Promising drug candidates for wet/dry AMD in clinical trials

3. Traditional formulation

An eye-drop, irrespective of the instilled volume, often eliminates rapidly within 5 to 6 minutes after an administration, and only a small amount (1–3%) of an eye-drop actually reaches the intraocular tissue. Therefore, it is difficult to provide and maintain an adequate concentration of drug in the precorneal area. More than 75% of applied ophthalmic solution is lost via nasolachrymal drainage and absorbed systemically via conjunctiva, then ocular drug availability is very low (Kuno & Fujii, 2011b). Generally topical applied drugs do not reach the posterior segment of the eye, thus, some additives or carriers to enhance the retention time and intraocular absorption are needed. Several eye-drops formulations are challenged to treat for AMD under clinical trials.

3.1 Pazopanib

Some studies have suggested that inhibition of VEGF signalling alone is sufficient to suppress choroidal neovascularization (CNV), however, others have demonstrated a more potent suppression of angiogenesis by inhibiting multiple tyrosine kinase receptors (Bergers et al., 2003, Erber et al., 2004, Kwak et al., 2000). It may be a more desirable therapeutic approach that drugs inhibit multiple angiogenic pathways. Pazopanib is a multi-tyrosine kinase inhibitor of VEGF receptor (VEGFR)-1, VEGFR-2, VEGFR-3, platelet-derived growth factor receptor (PDGFR)-α and -β, fibroblast growth factor receptor (FGFR) -1 and -3, cytokine receptor (Kit), interleukin-2 receptor inducible T-cell kinase (Itk), leukocyte-specific protein tyrosine kinase (Lck), and transmembrane glycoprotein receptor tyrosine kinase (c-Fms). *In vitro*, pazopanib inhibited ligand-induced autophosphorylation of VEGFR-2, Kit and PDGFR-β receptors. *In vivo*, pazopanib inhibited VEGF-induced VEGFR-2 phosphorylation in mouse lungs, angiogenesis in a mouse model, and the growth of some human tumor xenografts in mice (GlaxoSmithKline plc.). Pazopanib is currently prescribed for advanced renal cell carcinoma.

Yafai et al. have demonstrated that eye-drop formulation of pazopanib complexed with cyclodextrin significantly inhibited CNV in laser-induced CNV rat model (Yafai et al., 2011). Since this effect was obtained by overdose of eye-drops (30 μL/eye), it is doubtful whether this effective inhibition of CNV resulted from a topical absorption of pazopanib. A phase II clinical study of pazopanib eye-drops for the treatment of wet AMD is currently underway (ClinicalTrials.gov. NCT01134055). Unfortunately, actual formulation of pazopanib eye-drops used in clinical study is not disclosed.

3.2 Tandospirone

Serotonin (5-hydroxytryptamine; 5-HT) and its multiple receptors regulate various physiological functions. 5-HT_{1A} receptor plays an important role for the control of sleep, feeding and anxiety. 5-HT_{1A} receptor agonists have also neuroprotective effects in animal models including central nervous system ischemia (Saruhashi et al., 2002, Mauler & Horvath, 2005, Ramos et al., 2004, Kukley et al., 2001, Torup et al., 2000, Piera et al., 1995), acute subdermal hematoma (Fournier et al., 1993), traumatic brain injury (Alessandri et al., 1999, Kline et al., 2002), excitotoxicity (Oosterink et al., 2003, Cosi et al., 2005), a Parkinson's disease model animal induced by 1-methyl-4-phenyl-1,2,3,6-tetrahydropyridine (Bibbiani et al., 2001, Bezard et al., 2006), and sciatic nerve crush (Fournier et al., 1993). Additionally, it was reported that the 5-HT_{1A} agonists delayed the progression of motor neuron degeneration in pmn mice (Duong et al., 1998) and reduced lipid peroxidation in a rat epilepsy model (de Freitas et al., 2010). Such neuroprotective effects are considered to be caused by neuronal membrane hyperpolarization via G protein-coupled K^+ channels, decreasing glutamate release, blocking Ca^{2+} channels or Na^+ channels, activation of MAPK (mitogen-actiated protein kinase)/ERK (extracellular signal-regulated kinase) signalling pathway resulting expression of anti-apoptotic proteins and inhibition of caspase, and an expression of brain derived neurotrophic factor (BDNF) mRNA, S100β and nerve growth factor. Also 5-HT_{1A} was expressed in rats and rabbits retina (Kusol & Brunken, 2000).

Recently, it has been reported that tandospirone, 5-HT_{1A} agonist, which is widely used for the treatment of anxiety disorders, has a neuroprotective effect for retinal lesions due to light-damage (Collier et al., 2009, Rhoades et al., 2009, Wang et al., 2009, Collier et al., 2010). The studies have also suggested tandospirone increases of MEK (mitogen-activated extracellular signal regulated kinase) 1/2 and ERK 1/2 phosphorylation, leading to the subsequent upregulation of anti-oxidant and anti-apoptotic proteins, including superoxide dismutase (SOD)-1, SOD-2, B-cell lymphoma (Bcl)-2 and Bcl-$_{XL}$ (Rhoades et al., 2009), or a decrease complement factors (C3, CFB, CFH) and membrane attack complex (MAC) deposition in the outer retina (Wang et al., 2009) (Figure 2). Currently, an eye-drops formulation of tandospirone (AL-8309B, Alcon Laboratories, Inc., Fort Worth, TX, U.S.) is under a Phase III study for the treatment of dry AMD (ClinicalTrials.gov. NCT00890097). Actual eye-drop formulation of tandospirone currently conducted in clinical study is not also disclosed.

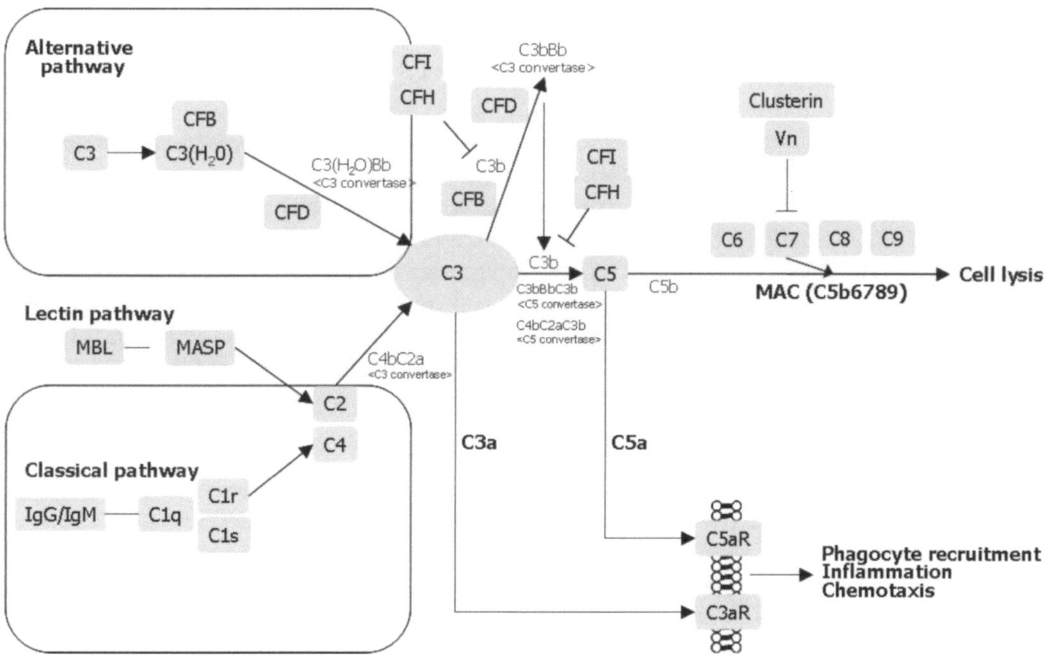

Fig. 2. Complement cascade

In the classical pathway, the cascade is initiated by the binding of C1q to antibody-antigen complex. The lectin pathway is initiated by the binding of carbohydrates associated with microbes to lectin proteins such as mannose-binding lectin (MBL). C1q and MBL form complexes with mannose-binding lectin-associated serine protease (MASP), which cleave C4 into C4a and C4b,C2 into C2a and C2b. C4b binds to C2a (C4bC2a), work as a C3 convertase resulting degradation of C3 into C3a and C3b. C3b binds with C4bC2a to form C4bC2aC3b work as a C5 convertases.

In the alternative pathway, C3 convertase is formed via a spontaneous hydrolysis of an internal C3 thioester into C3(H2O). C3(H2O) binds to factor B and D and forms soluble C3 convertase; C3(H2O)Bb and subsequently formed membrane-bound C3 convertase; C3bBb resulting cleavage of C3 into C3a and C3b. C3b binds C3bBb to form C3bBbC3b (C5 convertase).

In all pathways, C5 convertases cleaves C5 to C5a and C5b. C5b initiates the formation of the membrane attack complex (MAC) consisting of C5b, C6, C7, C8, and C9. The MAC creates a pore in the cell membrane of its targets (microbes, damaged cells) leading to cell lysis and death. The anaphylatoxins C3a and C5a work to increase vascular permeability, initiate degranulation of mast cells and neutrophils, induce cytokine release from macrophages, and mediate leukocyte chemotaxis.

Complement factor H (CFH) inhibits C3b through complement factor I (CFI) binding. Clusterin and vitronection (Vn) inhibits MAC formation by binding with a complex of C5b-7.

4. PEGylation

Covalent bonding of drug molecules to poly(ethylene glycol) (PEG), referred to as PEGylation, is a popular approach to modify and enhance the water solubility and pharmacokinetic and pharmacodynamic properties of biological and small-molecule drugs. In general, PEGs are inert water-soluble polymers, but recently it has been reported that a subretinal injection of PEG induced CNV with dose-dependency via complement activation in mice (Lyzogubov et al., 2011). PEGs can be attached to proteins and other therapeutic molecules, leading to increase the hydrodynamic volume of the therapeutic molecules. In addition, PEGs can shield drugs from interactions with enzymes and from inactivation by the immune system. As a result, PEGylated drugs can exhibit prolonged half-life, higher stability, increased water solubility, and reduced immunogenicity. It is thought that conjugates bearing branched chain PEG show increased thermal stability and higher resistance to enzymatic degradation compared to bearing linear PEG (Hamidi et al., 2008).

4.1 Macugen®

Pegaptanib sodium is a chemically-modified oligonucleotide of 28 nucleotides which linked with 40 kDa branched PEG (two arms of 20 kDa linear PEG units), which binds to $VEGF_{165}$. Pegaptanib was approved by FDA in 2004, and was both the first approved aptamer-based drug and the first approved pharmacotherapy for wet AMD. In rabbit eyes at 24 hours after an intravitreal injection, radiolabeled pegaptanib could be penetrated and distributed in the retina (Eyetech Inc.). In a monkey pharmacokinetics study, pegaptanib was eliminated from the vitreous with a half-life of 94 hours (Drolet et al., 2000), which has been increased by 3.91

times compared to the parent drug (non-PEGylated aptamer) (Simone Fishburn, 2008). After an intravitreal injection, pegaptanib is absorbed intact into the systemic circulation, but the concentration in plasma was 800-several thousand-fold lower than that in the vitreous. In addition, the elimination half-life was 9.3 hours after a single intravenous injection in rhesus monkeys (1 mg/kg). This "flip-flop" kinetics might cause to estimate the vitreous humor half-life in the vitreous from the plasma half-life in human. In clinical situation, pegaptanib is used as intravitreal injections of 0.3 mg once every 6 weeks.

4.2 ARC1905

ARC1905 (Ophthotech Corp., Princeton, NJ, U.S.) is a chemically-modified oligonucleotide of 39 nucleotides bound to branched PEG (two arms of 20 kDa linear PEG units), and binds to complement factor C5, leading to prevent the formation of key terminal fragments C5a and MAC (C5b-9). C5a is an important inflammatory activator inducing vascular permeability, recruitment and activation of phagocytes. MAC is involved to initiate cell lysis. Therefore, by inhibiting these C5-mediated inflammation and RPE death leading to geographic atrophy (GA), ARC1905 might be promising for both wet and dry AMD (Kuno & Fujii, 2011a). A phase I study to evaluate the safety, tolerability, and pharmacokinetic profile of multiple doses of intravitreal ARC1905 in combination with multiple doses of Lucentis® is currently in progress. In addition, it has been demonstrated by histopathological examination human dry AMD lesions strongly stained for C5a and MAC at key pathology sites (Anderson et al., 2002). A Phase I clinical trial to evaluate of an intravitreal ARC1905 in patients with GA is undergoing (ClinicalTrials.gov. NCT00950638).

4.3 E10030

E10030 (Ophthotech Corp.) is a chemically-modified oligonucleotide of 29 nucleotides linked with branched PEG (two arms of 20 kDa linear PEG units), and binds to PDGF-B, which is known to play a role of in the recruitment and maturation of pericytes that can increase resistance to the anti-VEGF treatment for wet AMD. PDGF and its receptor (PDGFR) do not act on vascular endothelial cells, but on pericytes. Therefore, inhibition of PDGF signalling might cause to achieve regression of neovascular vessels. Jo et al. have demonstrated that a combination therapy with anti-VEGF aptamer (Pegaptanib sodium) and anti-PDGFR-β antibody is more effective for CNV prevention and regression compared to monotherapy in the laser-induced CNV model (Jo et al., 2006). In an open-label Phase I clinical study conducted by Ophthotech, 59% of patients treated with E10030 and Lucentis® gained significant vision (3-line gain or better) at 12 weeks after the start of therapy. Interestingly, there was a mean decrease of 86% in the area of CNV at 12 weeks (Ophthotech Corporation). A randomized, controlled, Phase II study of E10030 in combination with Lucentis® for the treatment of wet AMD is currently underway (ClinicalTrials.gov. NCT01089517).

5. Sustained-release systems

To reduce the frequency of administration, many controlled drug delivery systems have been investigated by using biodegradable or non-biodegradable polymeric devices for the treatment of various retinal diseases as well as AMD (Kuno & Fujii, 2010). In general, drug release from biodegradable matrices consisting of poly(lactide-co-glycolide) (PLGA) is degradation-controlled, in contrast, diffusion-controlled drug release is obtained from non-biodegradable matrices such as silicone and ethylene-vinyl acetate copolymers (EVA). Some sustained-release formulations with constant drug release properties are currently under late clinical stage, but stimuli-responsive formulations with drug release triggered by pathophysiological condition do not exist in developmental stage yet.

5.1 Iluvien®

It has been reported that activated microglia was accumulated in the degenerative retinas including light-damage mouse (Zhang et al., 2005), rd mouse (Zeiss & Johnson, 2004), Royal College of Surgeons (RCS) rat (Thanos, 1992, Roque et al., 1996), and human eyes of RP and AMD (Gupta et al., 2003). Activated microglia is mainly accumulated within outer nuclear layer and adjacent to the RPE. In contrast, resting microglia shows a downregulated phenotype and a low level of membrane receptors expression; however, it quickly transforms into phagocyte when stimulated by infectious agents, cellular debris, and membrane fragments, such as lipopolysaccharides (Kreutzberg, 1996, Gehrmann, 1996, Pawate et al., 2004, Whitton, 2007). Within 24 hours of activation, microglial cells enlarge, acquire an ameboid macrophage-like shape, leading to increased microglial IgG reactivity and upregulation of complement receptors, and intercellular adhesion molecules (Orr et al., 2002). Activated microglia releases cytotoxic molecules, including tumor necrosis factor (TNF)-α, interleukin (IL)-1β, IL-10, interferon (IFN)-γ, hydrogen peroxide, and superoxide anion (Orr et al., 2002, Boje & Arora, 1992, Banati et al., 1993, Kreutzberg, 1995, Kim & de Vellis, 2005), which may induce apoptosis in otherwise healthy cells such as photoreceptors, RPE, and vascular endothelial cells. Once the activating stimulus is eliminated, microglia quickly returns to their resting state. While the stimulus continues, however, microglial cells express major histocompatibility complex (MHC) class I and II (Kreutzberg, 1995, Nakanishi, 2003) and inflammatory glycoproteins (Aloisi, 2001), which are self-stimulating and stimulate/recruit other immune cells. Microglia then clusters around neurons, adheres to their surfaces, continually produces cytotoxins that leads to neuronal death, and consequently recruit and activate additional microglia (Kreutzberg, 1996, Banati et al., 1993, Klegeris & McGeer, 2000) via chemokines such as CCL-5 (RANTES), macrophage inflammation protein (MIP)-1α and MIP-1β, monocyte chemoattractant protein (MCP)-1 and MCP-3 (Boje & Arora, 1992, Banati et al., 1993, McGeer et al., 1993, Min et al., 2004).

Recently, a retinal neuroprotective effect of sustained-release of a corticosteroid, fluocinolone acetonide (FA) for progressive retinal degeneration has been demonstrated in RCS rat (Glybina et al., 2009) and S334ter mutant rhodopsin transgenic rats (Glybina et al., 2010). In both animal models, FA treatment was associated with significant decrease in the number of microglial cells in both the outer and inner nuclear layer. In addition, corticosteroids have a genomic neuroprotective effect via Trk activation, leading to a trophic effect (Jeanneteau et al., 2008). An injectable, rod-shaped intravitreal implant with FA (Iluvien®; length: 3.5 mm, diameter: 0.37 mm, formerly Medidur™) has been developed by Alimera Sciences (Alpharetta, GA, U.S.) for the treatment of dry AMD under Phase II study (ClinicalTrials.gov. NCT00695318). Furthermore, the feasibility study of Medidur™ as a maintenance therapy for wet AMD patients who have been treated with Lucentis® for at least 6 months and have reached a plateau is currently in a pilot Phase II (ClinicalTrials.gov. NCT00605423).

5.2 Ranibizumab-loaded microspheres

Despite the remarkable effectiveness for treating wet AMD and other retinal diseases by Lucentis®, patients and physicians have been hoping for an alternative to the frequent intravitreal injections. SurModics, Inc. (Eden Prairie, MN, U.S.) and Genentech, Inc. have been developing a biodegradable microparticles incorporated ranibizumab currently under preclinical stage (SurModics Inc). It is hoped that ranibizumab-loaded microparticles can deliver ranibizumab over a period of approximately 4 to 6 months (Helzner, 2010).

5.3 NT-501

Neuroprotective effect of ciliary neurotrophic factor (CNTF) has been confirmed in various animal models of retinal degeneration including light-damaged rats, mutant rhodopsin transgenic mice, and a dog model. In addition, the long-term effect of CNTF has been shown by repeated intravitreal injections of CNTF in an autosomal dominant feline model of rod-cone dystrophy or an intravitreal injection of adeno-associated viral (AAV) vectors incorporated CNTF-cDNA in mutant rhodopsin transgenic rats. Neurotech Pharmaceuticals, Inc. (Lincoln, RI, U.S.) has been developing "Encapsulated Cell Technology", which provides an extracellular delivery of CNTF through long-term and stable intraocular release at constant doses through a device implanted in the vitreous. It contains human RPE cell line (ARPE-19) genetically modified to secrete recombinant human CNTF. The device (NT-501) consists of a sealed semi-permeable membrane capsule surrounding a scaffold of 6 strands of polyethylene terephthalate yarn, which can be loaded with cells (length; 6 mm, diameter; 1 mm). The device is surgically implanted in the vitreous through a tiny scleral incision and is anchored by a single suture through a titanium loop at one end of the device. The semi-permeable membrane allows the outward diffusion of CNTF and other cellular metabolites and the inward diffusion of nutrients necessary to support the cell survival in the vitreous cavity while protecting the contents from host cellular immunologic attack.

A Phase I clinical trial for RP has been completed and demonstrated well tolerated for 6 months implantation (Sieving et al., 2006). Eighteen-month results in a Phase II study for patients with GA with dry AMD were reported (Jaffe et al., 2010) (Zhang et al., 2011); participants were randomized in a 2:1:1 ratio to receive a high (20 ng/day) or low dose (5 ng/day) NT-501, or to sham surgery, respectively. Among eyes with baseline best corrected visual acuity (BCVA) 20/63, the mean BCVA in the high dose group was 10.5 and 10.0 letters greater than the low dose/sham group at 12 months ($p=0.03$) and 18 months, respectively. Stabilized visual acuity was accompanied by the corresponding structural changes; NT-501 treatment resulted in a dose-dependent increase of retinal thickness as early as 4 months after implantation and this increase was maintained through 6, 12 and 18 months ($p<0.001$). The growth rate of GA area was reduced in treated eyes compared to fellow eyes at 12 and 18 months. In addition, NT-501 also prevented secondary cone degeneration in RP patients (Talcott et al., 2011).

5.4 Brimonidine-loaded intravitreal implant

Brimonidine is an $\alpha 2$ adrenergic agonist, which can release various neurotrophins including BDNF, CNTF (Lonngren et al., 2006, Kim et al., 2007), and b-FGF (Lai et al., 2002). These neurotrophins have potential to prevent apoptosis of photoreceptors and/or RPE (Azadi et al., 2007, Zhang et al., 2009). A biodegradable, rod-shaped PLGA intravitreal implant containing brimonidine tartrate is now in a Phase II clinical study for dry AMD (ClinicalTrials.gov. NCT00658619) by Allergan Inc. (Irvine, CA, U.S.).

6. Targeting systems

Selective targeting to the neovascular lesions is desired for the improvement of therapeutic efficacy and the reduction of normal tissue damage. Active targeting to neovascular endothelial cells using highly-expressed specific molecules on endothelial cells has been widely investigated for the treatment of CNV. In addition, immunotherapy in conjunction with active targeting is also developing for regression of CNV.

6.1 Visudyne®

Visudyne® (QLT Ophthalmics, Inc., Menlo Park, CA, U.S.) is an intravenous liposomal formulation containing a photosensitizer, verteporfin in PDT for predominantly classic subfoveal CNV due to wet AMD, pathologic myopia or presumed ocular histoplasmosis (QLT Ophthalmics). Plasma lipoproteins, such as low-density lipoprotein (LDL), have been proposed to enhance the delivery of hydrophobic verteporfin to malignant tissue since tumor cells have increased the number of LDL receptors (Allison et al., 1994). In addition, liposomes composed of negatively charged phospholipids such as phosphatidylglycerol are taken up into tumor cells by LDL receptor-mediated endocytosis (Amin et al., 2002). It is thought that verteporfin released into the blood stream from liposomes is associated with LDL and is taken up into neovascular tissue, on the other hand, un-dissociated verteporfin, which is still encapsulated in the liposomes, is selectively accumulated in neovascular endothelial cells via LDL receptor-mediated endocytosis, since phosphatidylglycerol is the major constituent of Visudyne®.

Since LDL receptors are also expressed in RPE as well as endothelial cells (Hayes et al., 1989), verteporfin PDT causes damage to RPE associated with photoreceptor lesions. Indeed, adverse effects by verteporfin PDT have been reported (Tzekov et al., 2006, Ozdemir et al., 2006, Oner et al., 2005a, 2005b) in clinical situation. To enhance PDT effects and minimize damage of normal tissues, highly selective targeting might be necessary.

6.2 WST-11 (Stakel®)

Serum albumin has the unique ability to reversibly or covalently bind various endogenous or exogenous ligands with high affinity, resulting in working as a transporter and depot protein for various compounds (Kragh-Hansen, 1990). The cellular uptake of serum albumin via receptor (albondin)-mediated endocytosis (Schnitzer & Oh, 1994, John et al., 2001) might cause highly efficient intracellular trafficking. WST-11 (Stakel®, Steba Biotech S.A., Toussus-Le-Noble, France) is a negatively charged, water-soluble bacteriochlorophyll derivative with maximum absorption wavelength in the near infrared (753 nm) and rapid clearance from the body (Mazor et al., 2005, Brandis et al., 2005). WST-11 binds to serum albumin and has potent anti-neovascularization via the generation of hydroxyl radicals when stimulated by the proper light wavelength. Berdugo et al. have demonstrated that WST-11 PDT, which selectively occludes CNV, could be achieved in laser-induced CNV model of rats without the damages to the retinal tissues such as RPE and photoreceptors unlike verteporfin PDT.

Steba Biotech S.A. currently conducts a Phase II study for WST-11 PDT in wet AMD patients (ClinicalTrials.gov. NCT01021956).

6.3 I-con1

Tissue factor (TF) acts as a primary cellular initiator of blood coagulation, and has following additional biological functions involving neovascularization. TF can induce angiogenesis by upregulating VEGF and also promote angiogenesis via TF-initiated coagulation pathways. Thrombin stimulation of platelets, which is a major VEGF transporter, releases VEGF (Mohle et al., 1997), leading to stimulate endothelial cells to induce and expose more TF, following further thrombin formation. In addition, TF expressed in surgically excited CNV membrane and AMD eyes was related to active inflammation site accompanied by an accumulation of macrophages and fibrin deposition (Grossniklaus et al., 2002). It has been reported that TF mRNA expression in AMD was 32-fold higher than in the non-AMD (Cho et al., 2011) and TF was expressed only on neovascular endothelial cells not normal vascular endothelial cells (Contrino et al., 1996). Therefore, TF might be a specific target for neovascular tissues.

hI-con1 (Iconic Therapeutics, Inc., Atlanta, GA, U.S.) is a chimeric IgG-like homodimeric protein composed of a targeting-domain (mutated, inactivated factor VIIa, which is a ligand for TF) fused to an effector-domain (human IgG Fc) with an intact hinge region (Iconic Therapeutics). Once hI-con1 binds to TF on the surface of neovascular endothelial cells, the effector-domain mobilizes natural killer (NK) cells mediated via the Fc receptor, leading to activating the complement cascade (Wang et al., 1999, Hu & Li, 2010) and inducing the selective apoptosis of TF-expressing cells. Consequently, NK cells do not induce apoptosis of other cells including normal vascular tissue and RPE and neural retina. Bora et al. have demonstrated that intravitreal mouse factor VII-human IgG1 Fc chimeric conjugate inhibited CNV in a laser-induced CNV model in mice (Bora et al., 2003). In addition, Tezel et al. reported that this immunoprotein could selectively regress already-established CNV in laser-induced pig model (Tezel et al., 2007). A Phase I/IIa study of intravitreal hI-con1 for wet AMD is currently underway (Iconic Therapeutics).

6.4 Anti-VEGFR vaccine

VEGFR2 (Flk-1) plays a pivotal role in endothelial cell proliferation and migration (Millauer et al., 1993, Risau, 1997), and is upregulated during CNV formation (Wada et al., 1999). VEGFR2 vaccination therapy has been progressed in the cancer field (Niethammer et al., 2002, Wada et al., 2005, Pan et al., 2008). The strategy of VEGFR vaccination therapy for wet AMD is to induce apoptosis of neovascular endothelial cells, and inhibition and regression of CNV by cytotoxic T lymphocytes (CTLs). Takahashi et al. have demonstrated that vaccination with human VEGFR2-derived epitope peptide (VEGFR2-773) significantly inhibited CNV in laser-induced A2/Kb transgenic mice, which express chimeric human-mouse MHC class I molecule, and this chimeric molecule shows 71% concordance with the human CTL repertoire (Vitiello et al., 1991). VEGFR2 peptide induces CTLs in the histocompatibility leukocyte antigen (HLA) class I-restricted manner (Wada et al., 2005).

It is thought that the advantage of VEGFR2 vaccination is long-lasting therapeutic effect on the vascular endothelial cells since endothelial cells are genetically stable and do not show the downregulation of HLA class I molecules (Niethammer et al., 2002). It has been reported that, 60.8% and 19.9% in Japanese population share a common HLA-A*2402 allele and HLA-A*0201 allele, respectively (Date et al., 1996). HLA-A*2402 restricted VEGFR1- and VEGFR2-derived peptide vaccination therapy for wet AMD is conducted under a Phase I study in Japan (ClinicalTrials.gov. NCT00791570).

7. Gene therapy

Adenoviral (Ad) and AAV vectors are non-integrating and transduce both dividing and non-dividing cells. However, Ad and AAV elicit CTLs-mediated immune responses resulting in limitation of duration of transgene expression (McConnell & Imperiale, 2004). Helper-dependent Ad can extend the duration of ocular expression from less than 3 months to up to 1 year (Lamartina et al., 2007). Lentiviral vectors can induce stable, long-term transgene expression in the retinal (Balaggan et al., 2006). Lentivirus, which are integrating vectors, have the risk of insertional oncogenesis. Highly deleted (Molina et al., 2004), self-inactivating (Berkowitz et al., 2001) and non-integrating (Yanez-Munoz et al., 2006) lentiviral vectors have been developed as safer vectors. In general, subretinal injections are conducted in the operating room and are more invasive than intravitreal injections. If a single subretinal injection of a vector to provide prolonged suppression of CNV, it might be reasonable and feasible to substitute for repeated intravitreal injections of Lucentis®.

7.1 Pigment epithelium-derived factor

AdPEDF.11D is E1-, partial E3-, and E4-deleted Ad vector, which is replication-deficient, expressing pigment epithelium-derived factor (PEDF). A Phase I study of intravitreal AdPEDF.11D conducted by GenVec, Inc. (Gaithersburg, MD, U.S.) has completed. The results have shown that several complications such as mild inflammation, corneal edema, and elevated IOP were observed in some patients, but systemic hematogenous vector spread and systemic immune responses were not observed. Although hyperpermeability appeared to resolve in some patients received high-dose AdPEDF.11D, unfortunately, patients received high-dose (10^{8}-$10^{9.5}$ particle units) had no change in visual acuity compared to low-dose (10^{6}-$10^{7.5}$ particle units) patients whose visual acuity appeared to worsen over the course of study (Campochiaro et al., 2006). Further clinical trials have not progressed after the completion of a Phase I study in 2006.

7.2 sFLT01

sFLT01 is an antiangiogenic fusion protein consisting of the VEGF/placental growth factor (PlGF) binding domain of human Flt-1 (hVEGFR1) fused to the Fc portion of human IgG1 through a polyglycine linker (Bagley et al., 2011). Therefore, sFLT01 acts as a VEGF decoy. It has been reported that an intravitreal injection of AAV serotype 2 (AAV2) vector coding for sFLT01 (AAV2-sFLT01) significantly inhibited CNV in laser-induced CNV model of mice and monkeys (Lukason et al., 2011) and retinal neovascularization in mouse oxygen-induced retinopathy model (Pechan et al., 2009). Interestingly, sFLT01 expression in the retina continued for up to 12 months after an intravitreal injection (Pechan et al., 2009). A Phase I clinical trial of AAV2-sFLT01 is currently conducted by Genzyme (Cambridge, MA, U.S.) (ClinicalTrials.gov. NCT01024998).

7.3 RetinoStat®

RetinoStat® (Oxford Biomedica, Oxford, UK) is an equine infectious anaemia virus (EIAV)-based lentiviral vector expressing human endostatin and angiostatin, which are endogenous angiostatic factors. EIAV can transduce both dividing and non-dividing cells. Endostatin is an internal fragment of collagen XVIII, and downregulates the expression of the antiapoptotic proteins such as Bcl-2 and Bcl-$_{XL}$ (Dhanabal et al., 1999), and may interact with endothelial cell surface receptors and integrins leading to apoptosis of endothelial cells in active neovascularization, but not mature vasculature. In addition, endostatin blocks VEGF signalling via a direct interaction with VEGFR2 (Kim et al., 2002). Angiostatin is a cleavage product of plasminogen, which has the kringle domains, and promotes apoptosis of proliferating vascular endothelial cells similar to endostatin (Claesson-Welsh et al., 1998, Hari et al., 2000). Also, angiostatin downregulates VEGF expression (Hajitou et al., 2002, Sima et al., 2004). RetinoStat® incorporates RPE-specific vitelliform macular dystrophy gene (VMD2) promoter, leading to limited transgene expression to RPE after a subretinal injection (Kan et al., 2009). Kachi et al. have demonstrated that a subretinal injection of RetinoStat® significantly inhibited CNV in laser-induced CNV model of mice (Kachi et al., 2009). A Phase I study of subretinal RetinoStat® in wet AMD patients is currently ongoing (ClinicalTrials.gov. NCT01301443).

8. Devices

Mechanical devices have been developing for the purpose of more selective drug targeting, chronic infusion, or stimuli-responsive drug release.

8.1 Microcatheter

A microcatheter, iTrack™ 250A (iScience Interventional™, Menlo Park, CA, U.S.) is originally designed for canaloplasty (iScience Interventional™), which is a new treatment for glaucoma (Lewis et al., 2009, 2011). The iTrack™ 250A consists of an optical fiber to allow transmission of light to the microcannula tip for surgical illumination and guidance. Recently, this microcatheter is challenged to use for suprachoroidal drug delivery (Olsen, 2007, Rizzo et al., 2010). The pharmacokinetic study of suprachoroidal delivery of TA in pigs has shown that TA remained in the ocular tissues for at least 120 days, and the systemic exposure was very low (Olsen et al., 2006). In contrast, the study to compare the pharmacokinetics of bevacizumab between intravitreal and suprachoroidal injections to pigs (Olsen et al., 2011) reported that the profile of intravitreal injections of bevacizumab was more sustained than that of suprachoroidal injections at the same dosage level. Intravitreal injected bevacizumab distributed more to the inner retina, whereas suprachoroidal injected bevacizumab distributed primarily to the choroid, RPE, and photoreceptor outer segments. Scharioth et al. have tried to conduct suprachoroidal injections of bevacizumab in the wet AMD patients who were non-responder of intravitreal anti-VEGF therapy and/or initial BCVA < 0.05 (Scharioth et al., 2011). In the case of the patient who had a history of 21 intravitreal anti-VEGF injections with poor response to this therapy, and BCVA was 0.1, a significant reduction of pigment epithelial detachment was observed at 4 weeks after a suprachoroidal injection of bevacizumab, BCVA slightly improved to 0.16 and the subfoveal membrane totally disappeared at 8 weeks. During 6 months of follow-up, no signs of recurrence were observed.

8.2 Micropump™ system

A microelectromechanical systems (MEMS) drug delivery device is investigated for the treatment of chronic and refractory ocular diseases (Lo et al., 2009, Saati et al., 2010). MEMS device can be re-filled with the drug solution, giving long-term drug therapy which avoids repeated surgeries. The first generation of MEMS is a manually-controlled system limited by variations in the drug-release duration and force applied for depressing of the reservoir. To resolve this problem, the next generation device consists of an electrolysis chamber with electrolysis actuation to precisely delivery the desired dosage volume, a drug reservoir with refill port, battery and electronics. Biocompatible and flexible parylene is used to construct the MEMS. Battery and wireless inductive power transfer can be used to drive electrolysis. Electrolysis is a low power process in which the electrochemically-induced phase change of water to hydrogen and oxygen gas generates pressure in the reservoir forcing the drug through the cannula (Saati et al., 2010). The reservoir is implanted in the subconjunctival space and flexible cannula is inserted through incision into the anterior or posterior segment. Gonzalez-Soto et al. have demonstrated that a slower prolonged infusion of the same volume and concentration of intravitreal ranibizumab is equivalent to a bolus intravitreal injection of ranibizumab to human VEGF-induced retinal hyperpermeability model of rabbits (Gonzalez-Soto et al., 2011).

Replenish, Inc. (Pasadena, CA, U.S.) plans to enter clinical trials for a refillable and programmable pump that would be implanted in the eye to feed medicine for glaucoma or AMD. The Replenish device can last more than 5 years before needing replacement, much longer than current treatments (Flanigan, 2009).

8.3 ODTx

On Demand Therapeutics, Inc. (Menlo Park, CA, U.S.) has been developing a multi-reservoir implantable device for laser-activated drug delivery to the posterior segment of the eye (RetinaToday, 2010) (On Demand Therapeutics Inc). The injectable, biocompatible, non-resorbable device (ODTx) contains reservoirs designed for drug release in optimized doses. The reservoirs are capable of storing small- or large-molecule drugs that can be released via a standard, non-invasive laser activation procedure. The multiple reservoir system allows for ophthalmologists to control drug delivery by activating specific reservoirs, while unactivated reservoirs remain intact. Unfortunately, clinical trials of ODTx have not progressed yet.

9. Conclusion

Recent advances in drug delivery systems under clinical situation and in the late experimental stages are described in this chapter. AMD is chronic, progressive and refractory retinal degenerative disease, and induced by complex pathophysiological conditions. It is necessary to consider further the most efficacious combinations of optimal drugs, doses, routes, and drug release patterns (sustained-release, pulsatile-release, or controlled-release by responding to a trigger) based on the pathophysiology and progressive courses of the targeted disease.

10. References

Alessandri, B., Tsuchida, E. & Bullock, R. M. (1999). The neuroprotective effect of a new serotonin receptor agonist, BAY X3702, upon focal ischemic brain damage caused by acute subdural hematoma in the rat. *Brain Res*, Vol.845, No.2, 232-235

Allison, B. A., Pritchard, P. H. & Levy, J. G. (1994). Evidence for low-density lipoprotein receptor-mediated uptake of benzoporphyrin derivative. *Br J Cancer*, Vol.69, No.5, 833-839

Aloisi, F. (2001). Immune function of microglia. *GLIA*, Vol.36, No.2, 165-179

Amin, K., Wasan, K. M., Albrecht, R. M. & Heath, T. D. (2002). Cell association of liposomes with high fluid anionic phospholipid content is mediated specifically by LDL and its receptor, LDLr. *J Pharm Sci*, Vol.91, No.5, 1233-1244

Anderson, D. H., Mullins, R. F., Hageman, G. S. & Johnson, L. V. (2002). A role for local inflammation in the formation of drusen in the aging eye. *Am J Ophthalmol*, Vol.134, No.3, 411-431

Azadi, S., Johnson, L. E., Paquet-Durand, F., Perez, M. T., Zhang, Y., Ekstrom, P. A. & van Veen, T. (2007). CNTF+BDNF treatment and neuroprotective pathways in the rd1 mouse retina. *Brain Res*, Vol.1129, No.1, 116-129

Bagley, R. G., Kurtzberg, L., Weber, W., Nguyen, T. H., Roth, S., Krumbholz, R., Yao, M., Richards, B., Zhang, M., Pechan, P., Schmid, S., Scaria, A., Kaplan, J. & Teicher, B. A. (2011). sFLT01: A novel fusion protein with antiangiogenic activity. *Molecular Cancer Therapeutics*, Vol.10, No.3, 404-415

Balaggan, K. S., Binley, K., Esapa, M., Iqball, S., Askham, Z., Kan, O., Tschernutter, M., Bainbridge, J. W. B., Naylor, S. & Ali, R. R. (2006). Stable and efficient intraocular gene transfer using pseudotyped EIAV lentiviral vectors. *Journal of Gene Medicine*, Vol.8, No.3, 275-285

Banati, R. B., Gehrmann, J., Schubert, P. & Kreutzberg, G. W. (1993). Cytotoxicity of microglia. *GLIA*, Vol.7, No.1, 111-118

Bergers, G., Song, S., Meyer-Morse, N., Bergsland, E. & Hanahan, D. (2003). Benefits of targeting both pericytes and endothelial cells in the tumor vasculature with kinase inhibitors. *Journal of Clinical Investigation*, Vol.111, No.9, 1287-1295

Berkowitz, R., Ilves, H., Wei Yu, L., Eckert, K., Coward, A., Tamaki, S., Veres, G. & Plavec, I. (2001). Construction and molecular analysis of gene transfer systems derived from bovine immunodeficiency virus. *Journal of Virology*, Vol.75, No.7, 3371-3382

Bezard, E., Gerlach, I., Moratalla, R., Gross, C. E. & Jork, R. (2006). 5-HT1A receptor agonist-mediated protection from MPTP toxicity in mouse and macaque models of Parkinson's disease. *Neurobiol Dis*, Vol.23, No.1, 77-86

Bibbiani, F., Oh, J. D. & Chase, T. N. (2001). Serotonin 5-HT1A agonist improves motor complications in rodent and primate parkinsonian models. *Neurology*, Vol.57, No.10, 1829-1834

Boje, K. M. & Arora, P. K. (1992). Microglial-produced nitric oxide and reactive nitrogen oxides mediate neuronal cell death. *Brain Res*, Vol.587, No.2, 250-256

Bora, P. S., Hu, Z., Tezel, T. H., Sohn, J. H., Kang, S. G., Cruz, J. M. C., Bora, N. S., Garen, A. & Kaplan, H. J. (2003). Immunotherapy for choroidal neovascularization in a laser-induced mouse model simulating exudative (wet) macular degeneration. *Proc Natl Acad Sci U S A*, Vol.100, No.5, 2679-2684

Brandis, A., Mazor, O., Neumark, E., Rosenbach-Belkin, V., Salomon, Y. & Scherz, A. (2005). Novel water-soluble bacteriochlorophyll derivatives for vascular-targeted photodynamic therapy: Synthesis, solubility, phototoxicity and the effect of serum proteins. *Photochemistry and Photobiology*, Vol.81, No.4, 983-993

Campochiaro, P. A., Nguyen, Q. D., Shah, S. M., Klein, M. L., Holz, E., Frank, R. N., Saperstein, D. A., Gupta, A., Stout, J. T., Macko, J., DiBartolomeo, R. & Wei, L. L. (2006). Adenoviral vector-delivered pigment epithelium-derived factor for neovascular age-related macular degeneration: Results of a phase I clinical trial. *Human Gene Therapy*, Vol.17, No.2, 167-176

Cho, Y., Cao, X., Shen, D., Tuo, J., Parver, L. M., Rickles, F. R. & Chan, C. C. (2011). Evidence for enhanced tissue factor expression in age-related macular degeneration. *Laboratory Investigation*, Vol.91, No.4, 519-526

Claesson-Welsh, L., Welsh, M., Ito, N., Anand-Aptei, B., Soker, S., Zetter, B., O'Reilly, M. & Folkman, J. (1998). Angiostatin induces endothelial cell apoptosis and activation of focal adhesion kinase independently of the integrin-binding motif RGD. *Proc Natl Acad Sci U S A*, Vol.95, No.10, 5579-5583

ClinicalTrials.gov. NCT00950638, A study of ARC1905 (Anti-C5 aptamer) in subjects with dry age-related macular degeneration, Available from: <http://clinicaltrials.gov/ct2/show/NCT00950638?term=ARC1905&rank=1>

ClinicalTrials.gov. NCT00605423, The MAP Study: Fluocinolone acetonide (FA)/Medidur™ for age related macular degeneration (AMD) Pilot, Available from: <http://clinicaltrials.gov/ct2/show/NCT00605423?term=Iluvien&rank=12>

ClinicalTrials.gov. NCT00890097, Geographic atrophy treatment evaluation (GATE), Accessed January 26, 2011, Available from: <http://clinicaltrials.gov/ct2/show/NCT00890097?term=AL-8309B&rank=1>

ClinicalTrials.gov. NCT01301443, Phase I dose escalation safety study of RetinoStat in advanced age-related macular degeneration (AMD) (GEM), Available from: <http://clinicaltrials.gov/ct2/show/NCT01301443?term=RetinoStat&rank=1>

ClinicalTrials.gov. NCT01024998, Safety and tolerability study of AAV2-sFLT01 in patients with neovascular age-related macular degeneration, Available from: <http://clinicaltrials.gov/ct2/show/NCT01024998?term=sFLT01&rank=1>

ClinicalTrials.gov. NCT00695318, Fluocinolone acetonide intravitreal inserts in geographic atrophy, Available from: <http://clinicaltrials.gov/ct2/show/NCT00695318?term=Iluvien&rank=15>

ClinicalTrials.gov. NCT01134055, Dose ranging study of pazopanib to treat neovascular age-related macular degeneration, Available from: <http://clinicaltrials.gov/ct2/show/NCT01134055?term=pazopanib+and+eye+drop&rank=3>

ClinicalTrials.gov. NCT01021956, Safety and preliminary efficacy study of WST11 (Stakel®)-mediated VTP therapy in subjects with CNV associated with AMD, Available from: <http://clinicaltrials.gov/ct2/show/NCT01021956?term=WST11&rank=6>

ClinicalTrials.gov. NCT00791570, Anti-VEGFR vaccine therapy in treating patients with neovascular maculopathy, Available from: <http://clinicaltrials.gov/ct2/show/NCT00791570?term=Osaka+University&rank=5>

ClinicalTrials.gov. NCT00658619, Safety and efficacy of brimonidine intravitreal implant in patients with geographic atrophy due to age-related macular degeneration (AMD), 26.01.2011, Available from: <http://clinicaltrials.gov/ct2/show/NCT00658619>

ClinicalTrials.gov. NCT01089517, A safety and efficacy study of E10030 (Anti-PDGF pegylated aptamer) plus Lucentis for neovascular age-related macular degeneration, Available from: <http://clinicaltrials.gov/ct2/show/NCT01089517?term=E10030&rank=2>

Collier, R. J., Martin, E. A., Cully-Adams, C., Dembinska, O., Hoang, H., Hellberg, M., Krueger, S., Kapin, M. & Romano, C. (2009). Serotonin 5-HT$_{1A}$ agonists protect against blue light-induced phototoxicity. *ARVO Meeting Abstracts*, 675

Collier, R. J., Patel, Y., Martin, E. A., Dembinska, O., Hellberg, M., Krueger, D. S., Kapin, M. A. & Romano, C. (2010). Agonists at the serotonin receptor (5HT$_{1A}$) protect the retina from severe photo-oxidative stress. *Invest Ophthalmol Vis Sci*, doi:10.1167/iovs.1110-6304

Contrino, J., Hair, G., Kreutzer, D. L. & Rickles, F. R. (1996). In situ detection of tissue factor in vascular endothelial cells: Correlation with the malignant phenotype of human breast disease. *Nature Medicine*, Vol.2, No.2, 209-215

Cosi, C., Waget, A., Rollet, K., Tesori, V. & Newman-Tancredi, A. (2005). Clozapine, ziprasidone and aripiprazole but not haloperidol protect against kainic acid-induced lesion of the striatum in mice, in vivo: role of 5-HT$_{1A}$ receptor activation. *Brain Res*, Vol.1043, No.1-2, 32-41

Date, Y., Kimura, A., Kato, H. & Sasazuki, T. (1996). DNA typing of the HLA-A gene: Population study and identification of four new alleles in Japanese. *Tissue Antigens*, Vol.47, No.2, 93-101

de Freitas, R. L., Santos, I. M., de Souza, G. F., Tome Ada, R., Saldanha, G. B. & de Freitas, R. M. (2010). Oxidative stress in rat hippocampus caused by pilocarpine-induced seizures is reversed by buspirone. *Brain Res Bull*, Vol.81, No.4-5, 505-509

Dhanabal, M., Ramchandran, R., Waterman, M. J. F., Lu, H., Knebelmann, B., Segal, M. & Sukhatme, V. P. (1999). Endostatin induces endothelial cell apoptosis. *Journal of Biological Chemistry*, Vol.274, No.17, 11721-11726

Drolet, D. W., Nelson, J., Tucker, C. E., Zack, P. M., Nixon, K., Bolin, R., Judkins, M. B., Farmer, J. A., Wolf, J. L., Gill, S. C. & Bendele, R. A. (2000). Pharmacokinetics and safety of an anti-vascular endothelial growth factor aptamer (NX1838) following injection into the vitreous humor of rhesus monkeys. *Pharmaceutical Research*, Vol.17, No.12, 1503-1510

Duong, F., Fournier, J., Keane, P. E., Guenet, J. L., Soubrie, P., Warter, J. M., Borg, J. & Poindron, P. (1998). The effect of the nonpeptide neurotrophic compound SR 57746A on the progression of the disease state of the pmn mouse. *Br J Pharmacol*, Vol.124, No.4, 811-817

Eghoj, M. S. & Sorensen, T. L. (2011). Tachyphylaxis during treatment of exudative age-related macular degeneration with ranibizumab. *British Journal of Ophthalmology*, doi:10.1136/bjo.2011.203893

Erber, R., Thurnher, A., Katsen, A. D., Groth, G., Kerger, H., Hammes, H. P., Menger, M. D., Ullrich, A. & Vajkoczy, P. (2004). Combined inhibition of VEGF and PDGF signaling enforces tumor vessel regression by interfering with pericyte-mediated endothelial cell survival mechanisms. *The FASEB journal*, Vol.18, No.2, 338-340

Eyetech Inc. Macugen® (pegapranib sodium injection), Available from: <http://www.macugen.com/macugenUSPI.pdf>

Flanigan, J. (2009). Biotech tries to shrug off setbacks, The New York Times.

Forooghian, F., Chew, E. Y., Meyerle, C. B., Cukras, C. & Wong, W. T. (2011). Investigation of the role of neutralizing antibodies against bevacizumab as mediators of tachyphylaxis. *Acta Ophthalmologica*, Vol.89, No.2, e206-e207

Forooghian, F., Cukras, C., Meyerle, C. B., Chew, E. Y. & Wong, W. T. (2009). Tachyphylaxis after intravitreal bevacizumab for exudative age-related macular degeneration. *Retina*, Vol.29, No.6, 723-731

Fournier, J., Steinberg, R., Gauthier, T., Keane, P. E., Guzzi, U., Coude, F. X., Bougault, I., Maffrand, J. P., Soubrie, P. & Le Fur, G. (1993). Protective effects of SR 57746A in central and peripheral models of neurodegenerative disorders in rodents and primates. *Neuroscience*, Vol.55, No.3, 629-641

Gehrmann, J. (1996). Microglia: a sensor to threats in the nervous system? *Res Virol*, Vol.147, No.2-3, 79-88

Genentech Inc. Lucentis®, Available from: <http://www.gene.com/gene/products/information/pdf/lucentis-prescribing.pdf>

GlaxoSmithKline plc. Votrient (pazopanib) tablets, Available from: <http://us.gsk.com/products/assets/us_votrient.pdf>

Glybina, I. V., Kennedy, A., Ashton, P., Abrams, G. W. & Iezzi, R. (2009). Photoreceptor neuroprotection in RCS rats via low-dose intravitreal sustained-delivery of fluocinolone acetonide. *Invest Ophthalmol Vis Sci*, Vol.50, No.10, 4847-4857

Glybina, I. V., Kennedy, A., Ashton, P., Abrams, G. W. & Iezzi, R. (2010). Intravitreous delivery of the corticosteroid fluocinolone acetonide attenuates retinal degeneration in S334ter-4 rats. *Invest Ophthalmol Vis Sci*, Vol.51, No.8, 4243-4252

Gonzalez-Soto, R., Brant-Fernandes, R. A., Humayun, M. S., Varma, R., Journey, M. & Caffey, S. (2011). Intravitreal infusion of ranibizumab with an infusion pump in rabbits. *ARVO Meeting Abstracts*, 3246

Good, T. J., Kimura, A. E., Mandava, N. & Kahook, M. Y. (2011). Sustained elevation of intraocular pressure after intravitreal injections of anti-VEGF agents. *British Journal of Ophthalmology*, Vol.95, No.8, 1111-1114

Gower, E. W., Cassard, S. D., Bass, E. B., Schein, O. D. & Bressler, N. M. (2010). A cost-effectiveness analysis of three treatments for age-related macular degeneration. *Retina*, Vol.30, No.2, 212-221

Grossniklaus, H. E., Ling, J. X., Wallace, T. M., Dithmar, S., Lawson, D. H., Cohen, C., Elner, V. M., Elner, S. G. & Sternberg Jr, P. (2002). Macrophage and retinal pigment epithelium expression of angiogenic cytokines in choroidal neovascularization. *Molecular Vision*, Vol.8, 119-126

Gupta, N., Brown, K. E. & Milam, A. H. (2003). Activated microglia in human retinitis pigmentosa, late-onset retinal degeneration, and age-related macular degeneration. *Exp Eye Res*, Vol.76, No.4, 463-471

Hajitou, A., Grignet, C., Devy, L., Berndt, S., Blacher, S., Deroanne, C. F., Bajou, K., Fong, T., Chiang, Y., Foidart, J. M. & Noel, A. (2002). The antitumoral effect of endostatin and angiostatin is associated with a down-regulation of vascular endothelial growth factor expression in tumor cells. *The FASEB journal*, Vol.16, No.13, 1802-1804

Hamidi, M., Rafiei, P. & Azadi, A. (2008). Designing PEGylated therapeutic molecules: Advantages in ADMET properties. *Expert Opinion on Drug Discovery*, Vol.3, No.11, 1293-1307

Hari, D., Beckett, M. A., Sukhatme, V. P., Dhanabal, M., Nodzenski, E., Lu, H., Mauceri, H. J., Kufe, D. W. & Weichselbaum, R. R. (2000). Angiostatin induces mitotic cell death of proliferating endothelial cells. *Molecular Cell Biology Research Communications*, Vol.3, No.5, 277-282

Hayes, K. C., Lindsey, S., Stephan, Z. F. & Brecker, D. (1989). Retinal pigment epithelium possesses both LDL and scavenger receptor activity. *Invest Ophthalmol Vis Sci*, Vol.30, No.2, 225-232

Helzner, J. (2010). Progress on sustained-delivery Lucentis, Retinal Physicians.

Hu, Z. & Li, J. (2010). Natural killer cells are crucial for the efficacy of Icon (factor VII/human IgG1 Fc) immunotherapy in human tongue cancer. *BMC immunology*, Vol.11, 49

Iconic Therapeutics Plans for clinical studies, Available from: <http://www.iconictherapeutics.com/rdprograms.html>

Iconic Therapeutics hI-con1™, Available from: <http://www.iconictherapeutics.com/icon1.html>

iScience Interventional™ Interventional Ophthalmology, Available from: <http://www.iscienceinterventional.com/US/interventional.htm>

Jaffe, G. J., Tao, W. & Group, C. S. (2010). A Phase 2 study of encapsulated CNTF-secreting cell implant (NT-501) in patients with geographic atrophy associated with dry AMD-18 month results. *ARVO Meeting Abstracts*, 6415

Jeanneteau, F., Garabedian, M. J. & Chao, M. V. (2008). Activation of Trk neurotrophin receptors by glucocorticoids provides a neuroprotective effect. *Proc Natl Acad Sci U S A*, Vol.105, No.12, 4862-4867

Jo, N., Mailhos, C., Ju, M., Cheung, E., Bradley, J., Nishijima, K., Robinson, G. S., Adamis, A. P. & Shima, D. T. (2006). Inhibition of platelet-derived growth factor B signaling enhances the efficacy of anti-vascular endothelial growth factor therapy in multiple models of ocular neovascularization. *American Journal of Pathology*, Vol.168, No.6, 2036-2053

John, T. A., Vogel, S. M., Minshall, R. D., Ridge, K., Tiruppathi, C. & Malik, A. B. (2001). Evidence for the role of alveolar epithelial gp60 in active transalveolar albumin transport in the rat lung. *Journal of Physiology*, Vol.533, No.2, 547-559

Kachi, S., Binley, K., Yokoi, K., Umeda, N., Akiyama, H., Muramatu, D., Iqball, S., Kan, O., Naylor, S. & Campochiaro, P. A. (2009). Equine infectious anemia viral vector-mediated codelivery of endostatin and angiostatin driven by retinal pigmented epithelium-specific VMD2 promoter inhibits choroidal neovascularization. *Human Gene Therapy*, Vol.20, No.1, 31-39

Kan, O., Widdowson, P., Hamirally, S., Binley, K., Nork, M., Miller, P., Bantseev, V., Christian, B., Iqball, S., Mitrophanous, K. A. & Naylor, S. (2009). Ocular tolerance of a lentiviral vector-based angiostatic gene therapy product (RetinoStat®) in rodent, rabbit, and nonhuman primate models. *Human Gene Therapy*, Vol.20, No.4, 403

Keane, P. A., Liakopoulos, S., Ongchin, S. C., Heussen, F. M., Msutta, S., Chang, K. T., Walsh, A. C. & Sadda, S. R. (2008). Quantitative subanalysis of optical coherence tomography after treatment with ranibizumab for neovascular age-related macular degeneration. *Invest Ophthalmol Vis Sci*, Vol.49, No.7, 3115-3120

Kim, H. S., Chang, Y. I., Kim, J. H. & Park, C. K. (2007). Alteration of retinal intrinsic survival signal and effect of alpha2-adrenergic receptor agonist in the retina of the chronic ocular hypertension rat. *Vis Neurosci*, Vol.24, No.2, 127-139

Kim, S. U. & de Vellis, J. (2005). Microglia in health and disease. *J Neurosci Res*, Vol.81, No.3, 302-313

Kim, Y. M., Hwang, S., Pyun, B. J., Kim, T. Y., Lee, S. T., Gho, Y. S. & Kwon, Y. G. (2002). Endostatin blocks vascular endothelial growth factor-mediated signaling via direct interaction with KDR/Flk-1. *Journal of Biological Chemistry*, Vol.277, No.31, 27872-27879

Klegeris, A. & McGeer, P. L. (2000). Interaction of various intracellular signaling mechanisms involved in mononuclear phagocyte toxicity toward neuronal cells. *J Leukoc Biol*, Vol.67, No.1, 127-133

Kline, A. E., Yu, J., Massucci, J. L., Zafonte, R. D. & Dixon, C. E. (2002). Protective effects of the 5-HT1A receptor agonist 8-hydroxy-2-(di-n-propylamino)tetralin against traumatic brain injury-induced cognitive deficits and neuropathology in adult male rats. *Neurosci Lett*, Vol.333, No.3, 179-182

Kragh-Hansen, U. (1990). Structure and ligand binding properties of human serum albumin. *Danish medical bulletin*, Vol.37, No.1, 57-84

Kreutzberg, G. W. (1995). Microglia, the first line of defence in brain pathologies. *Arzneimittel-Forschung*, Vol.45, No.3 A, 357-360

Kreutzberg, G. W. (1996). Microglia: A sensor for pathological events in the CNS. *Trends in Neurosciences*, Vol.19, No.8, 312-318

Kukley, M., Schaper, C., Becker, A., Rose, K. & Krieglstein, J. (2001). Effect of 5-hydroxytryptamine 1A receptor agonist BAY X 3702 on BCL-2 and BAX proteins level in the ipsilateral cerebral cortex of rats after transient focal ischaemia. *Neuroscience*, Vol.107, No.3, 405-413

Kuno, N. & Fujii, S. (2010). Biodegradable intraocular therapies for retinal disorders: Progress to date. *Drugs and Aging*, Vol.27, No.2, 117-134

Kuno, N. & Fujii, S. (2011a). Dry age-related macular degeneration: Recent progress of therapeutic approaches. *Curr Mol Pharmacol*, in press

Kuno, N. & Fujii, S. (2011b). Recent advances in ocular drug delivery systems. *Polymers*, Vol.3, No.1, 193-221

Kusol, K. & Brunken, W. J. (2000). 5-HT(1A) and 5-HT7 receptor expression in the mammalian retina. *Brain Res*, Vol.875, No.1-2, 152-156

Kwak, N., Okamoto, N., Wood, J. M. & Campochiaro, P. A. (2000). VEGF is major stimulator in model of choroidal neovascularization. *Invest Ophthalmol Vis Sci*, Vol.41, No.10, 3158-3164

Lai, R. K., Chun, T., Hasson, D., Lee, S., Mehrbod, F. & Wheeler, L. (2002). Alpha-2 adrenoceptor agonist protects retinal function after acute retinal ischemic injury in the rat. *Vis Neurosci*, Vol.19, No.2, 175-185

Lamartina, S., Cimino, M., Roscilli, G., Dammassa, E., Lazzaro, D., Rota, R., Ciliberto, G. & Toniatti, C. (2007). Helper-dependent adenovirus for the gene therapy of proliferative retinopathies: Stable gene transfer, regulated gene expression and therapeutic efficacy. *Journal of Gene Medicine*, Vol.9, No.10, 862-874

Lewis, R. A., von Wolff, K., Tetz, M., Koerber, N., Kearney, J. R., Shingleton, B. J. & Samuelson, T. W. (2009). Canaloplasty: Circumferential viscodilation and tensioning of Schlemm canal using a flexible microcatheter for the treatment of open-angle glaucoma in adults. Two-year interim clinical study results. *Journal of Cataract and Refractive Surgery*, Vol.35, No.5, 814-824

Lewis, R. A., Von Wolff, K., Tetz, M., Koerber, N., Kearney, J. R., Shingleton, B. J. & Samuelson, T. W. (2011). Canaloplasty: Three-year results of circumferential viscodilation and tensioning of Schlemm canal using a microcatheter to treat open-angle glaucoma. *Journal of Cataract and Refractive Surgery*, Vol.37, No.4, 682-690

Lo, R., Li, P. Y., Saati, S., Agrawal, R. N., Humayun, M. S. & Meng, E. (2009). A passive MEMS drug delivery pump for treatment of ocular diseases. *Biomed Microdevices*, 959-970

Lonngren, U., Napankangas, U., Lafuente, M., Mayor, S., Lindqvist, N., Vidal-Sanz, M. & Hallbook, F. (2006). The growth factor response in ischemic rat retina and superior colliculus after brimonidine pre-treatment. *Brain Res Bull*, Vol.71, No.1-3, 208-218

Lukason, M., Dufresne, E., Rubin, H., Pechan, P., Li, Q., Kim, I., Kiss, S., Flaxel, C., Collins, M., Miller, J., Hauswirth, W., MacLachlan, T., Wadsworth, S. & Scaria, A. (2011). Inhibition of choroidal neovascularization in a nonhuman primate model by intravitreal administration of an AAV2 vector expressing a novel anti-VEGF molecule. *Molecular Therapy*, Vol.19, No.2, 260-265

Lyzogubov, V. V., Tytarenko, R. G., Liu, J., Bora, N. S. & Bora, P. S. (2011). Polyethylene glycol (PEG)-induced mouse model of choroidal neovascularization. *Journal of Biological Chemistry*, Vol.286, No.18, 16229-16237

Martin, D. F., Maguire, M. G. & Fine, S. L. (2010). Identifying and eliminating the roadblocks to comparative-effectiveness research. *New England Journal of Medicine*, Vol.363, No.2, 105-107

Mauler, F. & Horvath, E. (2005). Neuroprotective efficacy of repinotan HCl, a 5-HT1A receptor agonist, in animal models of stroke and traumatic brain injury. *J Cereb Blood Flow Metab*, Vol.25, No.4, 451-459

Mazor, O., Brandis, A., Plaks, V., Neumark, E., Rosenbach-Belkin, V., Salomon, Y. & Scherz, A. (2005). WST11, A novel water-soluble bacteriochlorophyll derivative; cellular uptake, pharmacokinetics, biodistribution and vascular-targeted photodynamic activity using melanoma tumors as a model. *Photochemistry and Photobiology*, Vol.81, No.2, 342-351

McConnell, M. J. & Imperiale, M. J. (2004). Biology of adenovirus and its use as a vector for gene therapy. *Human Gene Therapy*, Vol.15, No.11, 1022-1033

McGeer, P. L., Kawamata, T., Walker, D. G., Akiyama, H., Tooyama, I. & McGeer, E. G. (1993). Microglia in degenerative neurological disease. *GLIA*, Vol.7, No.1, 84-92

Meyer, C. H., Michels, S., Rodrigues, E. B., Hager, A., Mennel, S., Schmidt, J. C., Helb, H. M. & Farah, M. E. (2010). Incidence of rhegmatogenous retinal detachments after intravitreal antivascular endothelial factor injections. *Acta Ophthalmologica*, Vol.89, No.1, 70-75

Meyer, C. H., Rodrigues, E. B., Michels, S., Mennel, S., Schmidt, J. C., Helb, H. M., Hager, A., Martinazzo, M. & Farah, M. E. (2010). Incidence of damage to the crystalline lens during intravitreal injections. *Journal of Ocular Pharmacology and Therapeutics*, Vol.26, No.5, 491-495

Millauer, B., Wizigmann-Voos, S., Schnurch, H., Martinez, R., Moller, N. P. H., Risau, W. & Ullrich, A. (1993). High affinity VEGF binding and developmental expression suggest Flk-1 as a major regulator of vasculogenesis and angiogenesis. *Cell*, Vol.72, No.6, 835-846

Min, K.-J., Pyo, H.-K., Yang, M.-S., Ji, K.-A., Jou, I. & Joe, E.-H. (2004). Gangliosides activate microglia via protein kinase C and NADPH oxidase. *GLIA*, Vol.48, No.3, 197-206

Mohle, R., Green, D., Moore, M. A. S., Nachman, R. L. & Rafii, S. (1997). Constitutive production and thrombin-induced release of vascular endothelial growth factor by human megakaryocytes and platelets. *Proc Natl Acad Sci U S A*, Vol.94, No.2, 663-668

Molina, R. P., Ye, H. Q., Brady, J., Zhang, J., Zimmerman, H., Kaleko, M. & Luo, T. (2004). A synthetic rev-independent bovine immunodeficiency virus-based packaging construct. *Human Gene Therapy*, Vol.15, No.9, 865-877

Nakanishi, H. (2003). Microglial functions and proteases. *Mol Neurobiol*, Vol.27, No.2, 163-176

Niethammer, A. G., Xiang, R., Becker, J. C., Wodrich, H., Pertl, U., Karsten, G., Eliceir, B. P. & Reisfeld, R. A. (2002). A DNA vaccine against VEGF receptor 2 prevents effective angiogenesis and inhibits tumor growth. *Nature Medicine*, Vol.8, No.12, 1369-1375

Olsen, T. W. (2007). Drug delivery to the suprachoroidal space shows promise. *Retina Today*, Vol.March, 36-39

Olsen, T. W., Feng, X., Wabner, K., Conston, S. R., Sierra, D. H., Folden, D. V., Smith, M. E. & Cameron, J. D. (2006). Cannulation of the suprachoroidal space: A novel drug delivery methodology to the posterior segment. *Am J Ophthalmol*, Vol.142, No.5, 777-787

Olsen, T. W., Feng, X., Wabner, K., Csaky, K., Pambuccian, S. & Cameron, J. D. (2011). Pharmacokinetics of pars plana intravitreal injections versus microcannula suprachoroidal injections of bevacizumab in a porcine model. *Invest Ophthalmol Vis Sci*, Vol.52, No.7, 4749-4756

On Demand Therapeutics Inc The ODTx solution, Available from: <http://www.ondemandtx.com/the-odtx-solution.aspx>

Oner, A., Karakucuk, S., Mirza, E. & Erkilic, K. (2005a). Electrooculography after photodynamic therapy. *Documenta Ophthalmologica*, Vol.111, No.2, 83-86

Oner, A., Karakucuk, S., Mirza, E. & Erkilic, K. (2005b). The changes of pattern electroretinography at the early stage of photodynamic therapy. *Documenta Ophthalmologica*, Vol.111, No.2, 107-112

Oosterink, B. J., Harkany, T. & Luiten, P. G. M. (2003). Post-lesion administration of 5-HT1A receptor agonist 8-OH-DPAT protects cholinergic nucleus basalis neurons against NMDA excitotoxicity. *NeuroReport*, Vol.14, No.1, 57-60

Ophthotech Corporation E10030 - Anti-PDGF Aptamer, Available from: <http://www.ophthotech.com/products/e10030/>

Orr, C. F., Rowe, D. B. & Halliday, G. M. (2002). An inflammatory review of Parkinson's disease. *Prog Neurobiol*, Vol.68, No.5, 325-340

Ozdemir, H., Karacorlu, S. A. & Karacorlu, M. (2006). Early optical coherence tomography changes after photodynamic therapy in patients with age-related macular degeneration. *Am J Ophthalmol*, Vol.141, No.3, 574-576

Pan, J., Jin, P., Yan, J. & Kabelitz, D. (2008). Anti-angiogenic active immunotherapy: A new approach to cancer treatment. *Cancer Immunology, Immunotherapy*, Vol.57, No.8, 1105-1114

Patel, J. J., Mendes, M. A., Bounthavong, M., Christopher, M. L., Boggie, D. & Morreale, A. P. (2010). Cost-utility analysis of bevacizumab versus ranibizumab in neovascular age-related macular degeneration using a Markov model. *J Eval Clin Pract*, doi: 10.1111/j.1365-2753.2010.01546.x.

Pawate, S., Shen, Q., Fan, F. & Bhat, N. R. (2004). Redox regulation of glial inflammatory response to lipopolysaccharide and interferongamma. *J Neurosci Res*, Vol.77, No.4, 540-551

Pechan, P., Rubin, H., Lukason, M., Ardinger, J., DuFresne, E., Hauswirth, W. W., Wadsworth, S. C. & Scaria, A. (2009). Novel anti-VEGF chimeric molecules delivered by AAV vectors for inhibition of retinal neovascularization. *Gene Therapy*, Vol.16, No.1, 10-16

Piera, M. J., Beaughard, M., Michelin, M. T. & Massingham, R. (1995). Effects of the 5-hydroxytryptamine1A receptor agonists, 8-OH-DPAT, buspirone and flesinoxan, upon brain damage induced by transient global cerebral ischaemia in gerbils. *Arch Int Pharmacodyn Ther*, Vol.329, No.3, 347-359

Pilli, S., Kotsolis, A., Spaide, R. F., Slakter, J., Freund, K. B., Sorenson, J., Klancnik, J. & Cooney, M. (2008). Endophthalmitis associated with intravitreal anti-vascular endothelial growth factor therapy injections in an office setting. *Am J Ophthalmol*, Vol.145, No.5, 879-882

QLT Ophthalmics Visudyne® Available from: <http://www.visudyne.com/>

Ramos, A. J., Rubio, M. D., Defagot, C., Hischberg, L., Villar, M. J. & Brusco, A. (2004). The 5HT1A receptor agonist, 8-OH-DPAT, protects neurons and reduces astroglial reaction after ischemic damage caused by cortical devascularization. *Brain Res*, Vol.1030, No.2, 201-220

RetinaToday (2010). Laser-activated, on-Demand drug delivery technology tested in vivo, Available from: <http://bmctoday.net/retinatoday/2010/06/article.asp?f=laser-activated-on-demand-drug-delivery-technology-tested-in-vivo>

Rhoades, K. L., Patel, Y., Collier, R. J. & Romano, C. (2009). AL-8309, A Serotonin 5-HT1A Agonist, Protects RPE Cells From Oxidative Damage. *ARVO Meeting Abstracts*, Vol.50, No.5, 677

Risau, W. (1997). Mechanisms of angiogenesis. *Nature*, Vol.386, No.6626, 671-674

Rizzo, S., Augustin, A. J., Tetz, M., Genovesi-Ebert, F. & Di Bartolo, E. (2010). Suprachoroidal drug delivery for the treatment of advanced, exudative age-related macular degeneration. *ARVO Meeting Abstracts*, Vol.51, No.5, 1256

Roque, R. S., Imperial, C. J. & Caldwell, R. B. (1996). Microglial cells invade the outer retina as photoreceptors degenerate in Royal College of Surgeons rats. *Invest Ophthalmol Vis Sci*, Vol.37, No.1, 196-203

Rosenberg, A. S. (2006). Effects of protein aggregates: An Immunologic perspective. *AAPS Journal*, Vol.8, No.3, E501-E507

Saati, S., Lo, R., Li, P. Y., Meng, E., Varma, R. & Humayun, M. S. (2010). Mini drug pump for ophthalmic use. *Curr Eye Res*, Vol.35, No.3, 192-201

Saruhashi, Y., Matsusue, Y. & Hukuda, S. (2002). Effects of serotonin 1A agonist on acute spinal cord injury. *Spinal Cord*, Vol.40, No.10, 519-523

Schaal, S., Kaplan, H. J. & Tezel, T. H. (2008). Is there tachyphylaxis to intravitreal anti-vascular endothelial growth factor pharmacotherapy in age-related macular degeneration? *Ophthalmology*, Vol.115, No.12, 2199-2205

Scharioth, G. B., Raak, P. & Pavlidis, M. (2011). Suprachoroidal bevacizumab delivery for neovascular AMD treatment, Retinal Physician.

Schnitzer, J. E. & Oh, P. (1994). Albondin-mediated capillary permeability to albumin. Differential role of receptors in endothelial transcytosis and endocytosis of native and modified albumins. *Journal of Biological Chemistry*, Vol.269, No.8, 6072-6082

Sieving, P. A., Caruso, R. C., Tao, W., Coleman, H. R., Thompson, D. J., Fullmer, K. R. & Bush, R. A. (2006). Ciliary neurotrophic factor (CNTF) for human retinal degeneration: phase I trial of CNTF delivered by encapsulated cell intraocular implants. *Proc Natl Acad Sci U S A*, Vol.103, No.10, 3896-3901

Sima, J., Zhang, S. X., Shao, C., Fant, J. & Ma, J. X. (2004). The effect of angiostatin on vascular leakage and VEGF expression in rat retina. *FEBS Letters*, Vol.564, No.1-2, 19-23

Simone Fishburn, C. (2008). The pharmacology of PEGylation: Balancing PD with PK to generate novel therapeutics. *Journal of Pharmaceutical Sciences*, Vol.97, No.10, 4167-4183

SurModics Inc News Release: SurModics enters ophthalmic lisence and development agreement with Roche and Genentech includes development and commercialization of a sustained drug delivery formulation of Lucentis and potential other Genentech compounds, Available from:
<http://phx.corporate-ir.net/phoenix.zhtml?c=80353&p=irol-newsArticle&ID=1339001&highlight=genentech>

Talcott, K. E., Ratnam, K., Sundquist, S. M., Lucero, A. S., Lujan, B. J., Tao, W., Porco, T. C., Roorda, A. & Duncan, J. L. (2011). Longitudinal study of cone photoreceptors during retinal degeneration and in response to ciliary neurotrophic factor treatment. *Invest Ophthalmol Vis Sci*, Vol.52, No.5, 2219-2226

Tezel, T. H., Bodek, E., Sonmez, K., Kaliappan, S., Kaplan, H. J., Hu, Z. & Garen, A. (2007). Targeting tissue factor for immunotherapy of choroidal neovascularization by intravitreal delivery of factor VII-Fc chimeric antibody. *Ocular Immunology and Inflammation*, Vol.15, No.1, 3-10

Thanos, S. (1992). Sick photoreceptors attract activated microglia from the ganglion cell layer: a model to study the inflammatory cascades in rats with inherited retinal dystrophy. *Brain Res*, Vol.588, No.1, 21-28

Torup, L., Moller, A., Sager, T. N. & Diemer, N. H. (2000). Neuroprotective effect of 8-OH-DPAT in global cerebral ischemia assessed by stereological cell counting. *Eur J Pharmacol*, Vol.395, No.2, 137-141

Tzekov, R., Lin, T., Zhang, K. M., Jackson, B., Oyejide, A., Orilla, W., Kulkarni, A. D., Kuppermann, B. D., Wheeler, L. & Burke, J. (2006). Ocular changes after photodynamic therapy. *Invest Ophthalmol Vis Sci*, Vol.47, No.1, 377-385

Vitiello, A., Marchesini, D., Furze, J., Sherman, L. A. & Chesnut, R. W. (1991). Analysis of the HLA-restricted influenza-specific cytotoxic T lymphocyte response in transgenic mice carrying a chimeric human-mouse class I major histocompatibility complex. *Journal of Experimental Medicine*, Vol.173, No.4, 1007-1015

Wada, M., Ogata, N., Otsuji, T. & Uyama, M. (1999). Expression of vascular endothelial growth factor and its receptor (KDR/flk-1) mRNA in experimental choroidal neovascularization. *Curr Eye Res*, Vol.18, No.3, 203-213

Wada, S., Tsunoda, T., Baba, T., Primus, F. J., Kuwano, H., Shibuya, M. & Tahara, H. (2005). Rationale for antiangiogenic cancer therapy with vaccination using epitope peptides derived from human vascular endothelial growth factor receptor 2. *Cancer Research*, Vol.65, No.11, 4939-4946

Wang, B., Chen, Y. B., Ayalon, O., Bender, J. & Garen, A. (1999). Human single-chain Fv immunoconjugates targeted to a melanoma-associated chondroitin sulfate proteoglycan mediate specific lysis of human melanoma cells by natural killer cells and complement. *Proc Natl Acad Sci U S A*, Vol.96, No.4, 1627-1632

Wang, Y., Martin, E., Hoang, H., Rector, R., Morgan, S., Romano, C. & Collier, R. (2009). Inhibition of complement deposition by AL-8309A, a 5-HT1a agonist, in the rat photic-induced retinopathy model. *ARVO Meeting Abstracts*, 685

Whitton, P. S. (2007). Inflammation as a causative factor in the aetiology of Parkinson's disease. *Br J Pharmacol*, Vol.150, No.8, 963-976

Yafai, Y., Yang, X. M., Niemeyer, M., Nishiwaki, A., Lange, J., Wiedemann, P., King, A. G., Yasukawa, T. & Eichler, W. (2011). Anti-angiogenic effects of the receptor tyrosine kinase inhibitor, pazopanib, on choroidal neovascularization in rats. *European Journal of Pharmacology*, Vol.666, No.1-3, 12-18

Yanez-Munoz, R. J., Balaggan, K. S., MacNeil, A., Howe, S. J., Schmidt, M., Smith, A. J., Buch, P., MacLaren, R. E., Anderson, P. N., Barker, S. E., Duran, Y., Bartholomae, C., Von Kalle, C., Heckenlively, J. R., Kinnon, C., Ali, R. R. & Thrasher, A. J. (2006). Effective gene therapy with nonintegrating lentiviral vectors. *Nature Medicine*, Vol.12, No.3, 348-353

Zeiss, C. J. & Johnson, E. A. (2004). Proliferation of Microglia, but not Photoreceptors, in the Outer Nuclear Layer of the rd-1 Mouse. *Invest Ophthalmol Vis Sci*, Vol.45, No.3, 971-976

Zhang, C., Shen, J. K., Lam, T. T., Zeng, H. Y., Chiang, S. K., Yang, F. & Tso, M. O. (2005). Activation of microglia and chemokines in light-induced retinal degeneration. *Mol Vis*, Vol.11, 887-895

Zhang, K., Hopkins, J. J., Heier, J. S., Birch, D. G., Halperin, L. S., Albini, T. A., Brown, D. M., Jaffe, G. J., Taoj, W. & Williams, G. A. (2011). Ciliary neurotrophic factor delivered by encapsulated cell intraocular implants for treatment of geographic atrophy in age-related macular degeneration. *Proc Natl Acad Sci U S A*, Vol.108, No.15, 6241-6245

Zhang, M., Mo, X., Fang, Y., Guo, W., Wu, J., Zhang, S. & Huang, Q. (2009). Rescue of photoreceptors by BDNF gene transfer using in vivo electroporation in the RCS rat of retinitis pigmentosa. *Curr Eye Res*, Vol.34, No.9, 791-799

13

Use of OCT Imaging in the Diagnosis and Monitoring of Age Related Macular Degeneration

Simona-Delia Țălu[1] and Ştefan Țălu[2]
[1]*"Iuliu Hațieganu" University of Medicine and Pharmacy, Cluj-Napoca/Ophthalmology*
[2]*Technical University, Cluj-Napoca/Descriptive Geometry and Engineering Graphics, Faculty of Mechanics*
Romania

1. Introduction

Optical Coherence Tomography (OCT) is a non-invasive, high-resolution imaging technique that has been introduced in the clinical practice at the beginning of the last decade. The first application of this method has been recorded in the field of ophthalmology (Osiac et al., 2011). Retinal diseases such as Age-related Macular Degeneration (AMD), central serous chorio-retinopathy, macular hole, vitreo-macular interface syndrome and diabetic maculopathy have taken advantage of this relatively new imaging method. Among these, AMD is by far, the ocular condition that has benefited the most from the enormous advantages offered by OCT, in terms of diagnosis, response to treatment and monitoring. Future progress in OCT techniques is expected to improve the knowledge in the pathophysiology of this devastating disease. In order to better understand the role of OCT in the management of AMD, a concise review of the physical principles and mathematical equations that sustain this method is provided. The progress in the OCT techniques over the past decade is emphasized, from Time Domain - OCT (TD-OCT) to Spectral Domain - OCT (SD-OCT) and future directions, with implications in the clinical practice. The comparative contribution of TD-OCT and SD-OCT in the different forms of AMD is revealed. The limits of OCT are presented with their possible solutions. After the description of the theoretical data for OCT interpretation, the impact of OCT in the diagnosis is illustrated with examples of various aspects that AMD can display. The role of OCT in the monitoring of AMD is revealed by the response of the wet form of the disease to the anti-VEGF intravitreal injections.

2. OCT imaging in the diagnosis and monitoring of AMD

The development of the retinal imaging was dued to three major events. The first one was represented by the invention of the direct ophthalmoscope by Hermann von Helmholtz in 1851: it opened the field of ocular imaging, by allowing the physicians to examine the retina in vivo. The second one took place in 1961, when Novotny and Davis used fluorescein dye to visualize the retinal circulation, inventing the technique named fluorescein angiography. The third major breakthrough happened in the 1990s, when OCT was invented, providing a fast, non-invasive, radiation-free examination technique, able to visualize precisely the retinal layers - something done before only on pathology slides. It's easy to understand why OCT has become soon an irreplaceable tool in most of the retina practices (Khaderi et al., 2011).

2.1 Theoretical considerations on OCT

Tomography is based on the reconstruction of cross-sectional images of an object using its projections. The concept of optical coherence tomography (OCT) was developed at Massachusetts Institute of Technology in the early 1990s and the first commercial version of OCT was made available by Carl Zeiss (Jena, Germany) in 1996. OCT is an extension of optical coherence domain reflectometry (OCDR). OCT is a modern noninvasive imaging technique with a high depth resolution, based on low coherence interferometry (LCI), that is able to reconstruct (tomographic) sectional images of the object under study. The first application of LCI in ophthalmology was to measure the eye length. OCT is similar to ultrasound imaging, but as an optical echo technique has much higher resolution. The key benefits of OCT are: live sub-surface images at near-microscopic resolution; instant, direct imaging of tissue morphology; no preparation of the sample or subject; no ionizing radiation. OCT is useful in situations where biopsy can't be performed, where sampling areas with conventional biopsies are likely, and that involve guiding surgical / microsurgical procedures.

The most important advantage of OCT as a diagnostic tool in ophthalmology is the obtain of fast, non-contact images of the ocular structures such as cornea, lens, retina and the optic nerve with depth resolutions better than 3 μm. Thus it is used to obtain a cross section of the retina based on the reflectivity on different layers within the retina, allowing detection of morphologic and micrometric modifications in retinal tissue. The ability to measure thickness of retinal layers has potential for early detection of pathologies and disease diagnosis (Talu et al., 2009).

2.2 OCT methods

OCT is applied by two main methods: Time domain OCT (TD-OCT) and Spectral domain OCT (SD-OCT). Each method has its own advantages and limitations.

TD-OCT produces two-dimensional images of the sample internal structure. In TD-OCT, tissue-reflectance information in depth (an A-scan represents a reflectivity profile in depth) is gradually built up over time by moving a mirror in the reference arm of the interferometer. OCT B-scans (a B-scan represents a cross-section image, a lateral x depth map) are generated by collecting many A-scans (Walther et al., 2011).

SD-OCT can be implemented in two formats, Fourier domain (FD-OCT) and swept source (SS-OCT). SD-OCT units acquire entire A-scans in reflected light at a given point in tissue. Information on depth is transformed from the frequency domain to the time domain, without using a moving reference mirror to obtain complete A-scans. The absence of moving parts allows the image to be acquired rapidly - about 60 times faster than with TD-OCT (Walther et al., 2011). The SD-OCT units allow the improvement of the detection and monitoring of retinal diseases, because these ones have ultra high-speed scan rate, superior axial and lateral resolution, cross-sectional (2D) scan, 3D raster scanning and a higher imaging sensitivity than the traditional TD-OCT units. The SD-OCT software permits many operations with 3D data compared with traditional TD-OCT. The great number of scans done per time unit also allows SD-OCT systems to generate 3D reconstructions, which can be further manipulated. Visualization of this data in 3D demonstrates subtle pathology not evident with conventional 2D images (Talu et al., 2009).

2.2.1 Time-domain OCT (TD-OCT) or conventional OCT

A superluminiscent diode emits a light beam which is split into two beams: a beam that enters the eye and is reflected back by the ocular media and a beam reflected by a reference mirror. The two beams meet, generating interferences that are intercepted by a light detector (fig. 1). By displacing the reference mirror, different structures, located at various depths, can be analyzed, thus obtaining an A-scan. The transverse scanning of the retina in a predefined axis (horizontal, vertical or oblique) is generating the B-scan of the retina, composed by the A-scan sequences. There are two important specifications concerning the quality of the image obtained: it depends on the number of retinal scans and partly, on the degree of light absorption by various retinal and subretinal structures. The time which is required in order to get the sections is the main determinant of the quality of the signal, justifying the name of Time Domain which is given to this OCT method. Time domain OCT (TD-OCT) is a technique that produces two-dimensional images of the sample internal structure. In standard TD-OCT two different scanning procedures are used in order to obtain an image: a depth scan using time-domain low coherence interferometry and a lateral scan addressing laterally adjacent positions to obtain the location of light scattering bodies in the sample (Talu et al., 2009).

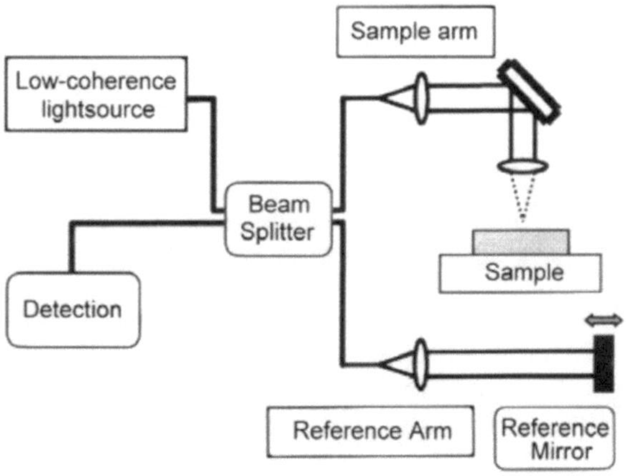

Fig. 1. A simplified schematic of Time domain (TD-OCT)

In TD-OCT, light from the low-coherence light source is divided evenly by the beam splitter. Half the light from the beam splitter is directed toward the sample and half the light toward a moving mirror. Light reflects off the mirror and from within the sample. The light beams reflected back are recombined by the beam splitter and directed into a detector. If the pathlengths match within a coherence length, interference will occur. OCT measures the intensity of interference and uses it to represent back-reflection intensity; the unwanted background light is suppressed by filtering. The OCT signal contains the oscillating term of the intensity, that is the integral of the contribution of the light reflected back from the biological tissue at all depths. TD-OCT uses light to map the layers within the retina in a cross-sectional image. Each image is made up of a series of A-scans scanned through the depth of the tissue and when aligned side by side, creates a B-scan two dimensional cross-sectional image. Each A-scan is acquired by moving a reference mirror to correspond to each point along the depth of the A-scan, and the signals from the reference arm and from the retina are interfered to determine the signal at that point in the A-scan. A TD-OCT system has two major spatial resolutions: axial and transversal resolution. The axial resolution depends on two laser characteristics: coherence length of the light source and pulse duration. The transversal resolution is determined by the focused spot size of the optical beam. The capability of TD-OCT system to produce images with good quality is characterized by the value of the signal to noise ratio (SNR) (Talu et al., 2009).

2.2.2 Spectral-domain OCT (SD-OCT)

The development of the SD-OCT is originating in the Fourier mathematical equation (1807) that can sum a periodic function into a series of sinusoidal functions. When applied to the OCT, the Fourier transformation replaces the sequential measurement of the reflected beam (by moving a mirror in front of the reference beam), with the simultaneous measurement of the light reflection. Subsequently, the image resolution in SD-OCT is 1 μm, as compared to 10 μm in TD-OCT. The practical impact of this improvement in resolution is the early detection of small cystic changes associated with the wet form of AMD. The early diagnosis is followed by the early treatment and the better preservation of the visual function. In SD-OCT, a spectrometer is used in order to analyze simultaneously all the frequencies. Therefore, all echoes of light from the various layers of the retina can be measured simultaneously, making the image acquisition much more rapid: SD-OCT is 50 times faster than the conventional TD-OCT and 100 times faster than the first ultrahigh-resolution OCT (UHR-OCT). The axial depth depends mainly on the bandwidth of the light source. With UHR-OCT, the resolution is 2 – 3 μ (the standard is of 10 μ). This ultrahigh resolution is comparable with the one obtained in histopathology, which makes possible the earlier diagnosis in AMD, better guidance of treatment and improvement of knowledge in the pathogenesis of this disease (Coscas et al., 2009).

Given the possibility to simultaneously get images in various planes, the 3D reconstruction is possible with SD-OCT, allowing the obtaining of hundreds of high-resolution images per second. The reduction of the examination time considerably decreases the artifacts related to patient movements. The SD-OCT images have proven to be clearer and with higher quality as compared to the ones obtained by the successive TD-OCT systems (OCT1, OCT3, stratus). The SD-OCT systems are continuously improving, by adding complementary functions: fundus photography, angiography, microperimetry. The 3D evaluation permits the accurate measurement of the macula (total volume) in various conditions (edema, fluid, drusen, CNV) with implications in the follow up and treatment of AMD (Luviano et al., 2009). The ultra-high resolution images obtained by SD-OCT allow a better differentiation between the retinal and subretinal layers. Further research has led to another significant improvement in resolution and speed: the novel frequency-domain OCT devices (FD-OCT), which are not yet available for widespread use. The difference between SD-OCT and FD-OCT resides in the light source. As explained above, the SD-OCT devices use a broadband light source and a spectrometer, generating readout rates of 40 kHz. FD-OCT utilizes a wavelength-swept laser source, which allows the obtaining of repetition rates as high as 370 kHz. The clinical potential of FD-OCTs is vast, given to their wide fields of view: for instance, they reach the coronary arteries and esophageal epithelium (Khaderi et al., 2011).

Feature	TD-OCT	SD-OCT
Basis	An interferometer measures **sequentially** the echo delay time of light that is reflected by the retinal microstructures.	The Fourier transformation allows the **simultaneous** measurement of the light reflection with a spectrometer
Modality of sampling	It samples one point at the time	It samples all the points simultaneously 60 times faster than TD-OCT
Scanned area	6 radial scans, 20 μ wide and 6 mm long (the area between the 6 scans is not imaged)	65.000 scans in a 6-mm area, without excluding areas
Rate of acquisition	400 scans/second	20.000 - 40.000 scans/second
Result	Two-dimensional images of the sample internal structure	3D reconstruction possible
Image resolution and quality	10 μ	1 μ, clearer

Table 1. Comparison of TD-OCT vs. SD-OCT

2.3 Clinical applications of OCT in AMD

The antero-posterior sections on OCT reveal the succession of the retinal layers and of the Retinal Pigmented Epithelium (RPE), as well as the presence of any spaces between these layers. The information offered by OCT is detailed, simple and easily interpretable.

2.3.1 Basis of OCT interpretation

The OCT signs in AMD are extremely valuable for the ophthalmologist.

Retinal thickening (the thickness of the retina is measured between the internal limiting membrane and the RPE) is determined by the exudation from the choroidal new vessels.

The occult Choroidal Neovascularization (CNV) is revealed by the constant presence of the elevation or detachment of the RPE band. Frequently, the occult CNV is suggested by various alteration of the RPE: irregularities, fragmentation, thickening, thinning.

The subretinal fluid appears as diffuse infiltration or as the constitution of cystic spaces in the macular area.

The classic CNV is translated on OCT as hyper-reflective zones adjacent to or away from the RPE. They must be differentiated from other hyper-reflective structures: fibrous tissue, exudate, pigment, pseudo-vitelliform material.

Other signs of prognostic value can be visualized at the level of the outer retinal layers (outer nuclear layer and external limiting membrane): hyper-reflective spots and areas of densification. They prove the progression of the disease (Coscas et al., 2009).

2.3.2 Technological parameters

Axial resolution (depth) refers to the capability to measure the morphological architecture of each retinal layer.

The depth of penetration depends mainly on two parameters: the optical properties of the tissues and the imaging wavelength that is used. Studies are conducted in order to find a possibility to visualize the choroid.

Transverse resolution of the image could reach a level allowing to distinguish cells.

The sensitivity of detection is a measure of the ease to obtain good quality OCT images in case of ocular media opacities.

The data acquisition time settles the number of transverse pixels of the OCT image.

Image contrast is an additional parameter meant to improve the visualization of various structures.

Functional extensions of OCT have the purpose to offer an optical biopsy of the retina, simultaneously with functional and metabolic data on its activity (Coscas et al., 2009).

2.3.3 Macula

The most frequent application of OCT in retinal disease is the measurement and monitoring of the retinal thickness.

The TD - OCT system (Stratus) gives a macular thickness map which is calculated from 6 radial B-scans crossing at the fovea. By interpolating data from these scans, the average macular thickness is calculated in 9 subfields centered on the fovea. Similarly, the total macular volume is obtained.

The SD-OCT provides images with much higher resolution. Given the differences between the measurements with the two types of OCT (TD and SD), algorithms are necessary in order to establish correlations between them.

Various studies compared the retinal thickness measured with TD-OCT and SD-OCT. For instance, the comparative measurements of the retinal thickness performed with Cirrus HD-OCT and Stratus TD-OCT in healthy individuals revealed that the average retinal thickness measured with SD-OCT has been significantly higher as with TD-OCT: 60 µm thicker (Kakinoki et al., 2009). This is explained by the difference in defining the retinal thickness between the two machines. In TD-OCT, the outer segments of the photoreceptors are not differentiated from the RPE, thus being excluded from the retinal thickness evaluation. The high resolution scans obtained in SD-OCT allows the separation of the outer photoreceptor segments from the RPE and subsequently, their inclusion in the calculation of the retinal thickness (Coscas et al., 2009).

In another recent study, it has been shown an increased measurement in retinal thickness of 65 - 70 µm as measured by Spectralis OCT compared with Stratus OCT which corresponds to the inclusion of the outer segment-RPE-Bruch's membrane complex by Spectralis OCT (Grover et al., 2010). Other studies proved the superiority of SD-OCT versus TD-OCT in quantifying the retinal thickness and evaluating the activity of the CNV membranes in wet AMD (Sayanagi et al, 2009; Mylonas et al, 2009). The differences between the macular thickness and volume measured with TD-OCT and SD-SLO (Scanning Laser Ophthalmoscopy)/OCT have been evaluated in eyes with macular edema and in normal eyes. The SD-SLO/OCT produced fewer artefacts than Stratus TD-OCT in normal and oedematous retina. Retinal thickness measured with SD-SLO/OCT has been significantly higher than retinal thickness obtained with TD-OCT. Therefore, it is advisable to follow the patient with the same OCT device, otherwise a correcting value of 1.1 should be considered when extrapolating the values from TD-OCT to SD-OCT. Retinal volume measurements were strongly reproducible and could be used to compare examinations with Stratus TD-OCT and SD-SLO/OCT (Forte et al., 2009).

The interchangeability of retinal thickness measurements resulting from different protocols of Spectralis OCT (which combines the OCT with the confocal laser ophthalmoscopy) has been evaluated in healthy eyes. It showed good protocol interchangeability for all tested protocols, which is important as it allows the selection of a more rapid and simpler protocol, especially in less cooperative patients. Higher number of measurements might influence negatively the results due to corneal dryness and loss of attentiveness (Wenner et al., 2011).

2.3.4 The segmentation of the retinal layers

TD-OCT can measure the thickness of the entire retina (from the vitreo-retinal interface to the RPE), but the only structure that can be isolated and measured individually is the nerve fiber layer. The TD-OCT conventional software does not allow the measurement of the structures that are external to the RPE: Pigment Epithelial Detachments (PED), CNV. Because the evolution in time of the subretinal space is extremely important for the monitoring and decision making in AMD, they are measured with custom programs or manually.

SD-OCT, by facilitating the image segmentation, makes it possible to individualize certain layers of the retina: plexiform layer, subretinal space, subretinal pigment epithelial space. The segmentation of the retina into two components (neurosensory and subretinal space) is also a promising option for the follow up of AMD (Coscas et al., 2009).

2.3.5 Drusen

The evaluation of drusen is important for the prediction of AMD risk for progression, despite the differences in agreement between observers. Whereas with TD-OCT the imaging of drusen is limited because of artifacts, the SD-OCT is capable to provide its detailed structure, thanks to the segmentation techniques. The internal structure of the drusen, that can now be specified, seems to be an indirect indicator of the complement-related activity which is associated with the risk of progression. However, this observation needs to be validated by clinical studies. The possibility to precisely measure the drusen volume with the support of the computer-assisted techniques offers a very useful tool to monitor the disease and to assess the risk of AMD progression (Coscas et al., 2009).

2.3.6 Choroidal neovascularization

Conventional TD-OCT represents a reference moment in the retinal imaging by having made it possible to: quantify the retinal response to CNV (macular edema, subretinal fluid); establish a correlation between the morphological (cystoid macular edema) and functional (visual acuity) parameters and between the OCT measurements and the response to treatment; visualize the fibro-vascular membranes in the subretinal and sub-RPE space.

The advantages of SD-OCT are represented by: the possibility to generate 3D images of the fibro-vascular complexes and to correlate them with fluorescein angiography and microperimetry; the easier detection of small PED, CNV and subretinal fluid. These advantages are particularly important for the identification of the chorio-retinal anastomoses and for the management of higher precision clinical studies (Coscas et al., 2009).

2.3.7 Geographic atrophy

Areas of geographic atrophy are evaluated in clinical studies by color photographs and autofluorescence. In TD-OCT, the RPE atrophy can be revealed by the increased choroidal hyper-reflectivity. In SD-OCT, the improved transverse resolution differentiates more clearly the limits between the normal and abnormal RPE and the segmentation techniques allow the correlations of the RPE changes with the photoreceptor layer (Coscas et al., 2009).

2.3.8 Therapeutical impact of OCT

Besides its contribution in the diagnosis of AMD, OCT examination is extremely useful in establishing the indication of the modern treatments in wet AMD (intravitreal injections with anti-VEGF agents) and in the monitoring of the response to treatment. The clinical experience has set up an algorithm of follow-up and treatment, although the number of injections is not yet established. However, it seems that the recurrence rate decreases with time (Coscas et al., 2009).

2.3.9 Limits of OCT

OCT cannot precisely describe a CNV network, nor can it define its nature: active or pre-fibrotic. Therefore, the OCT scan must be interpreted in correlation with the fundus photography, direction of scan and ideally, the angiography (Coscas et al., 2009).

Another limitation of OCT is revealed in evaluating the extension of the geographic atrophy (GA). In a recent study, the GA areas identified in SLO scans were significantly larger than the ones detected on the OCT maps. Spectralis OCT showed significantly more mild and severe segmentation errors than 3D and Cirrus OCT. Taking into account the fact that GA is a frequent form of AMD, this limitation should be resolved in order to identify and document RPE loss in a realistic manner (Schutze et al., 2011).

2.3.10 Future developments of OCT

One of the most recent innovations is the possibility to deliver simultaneously data offered by various examination methods: OCT, red-free photography, autofluorescence, angiography, SLO, Eye -Tracking systems, microperimetry (Marschall et al., 2011). The use of various wavelengths would create the possibility to penetrate deeper and examine the choroid. The improvement of the possibilities to process the 3D images will allow the more detailed and precise evaluation of a certain structure (Coscas et al., 2009).

2.4 Personal experience with OCT imaging in the diagnosis and monitoring of AMD

The contribution of OCT in the daily practice is illustrated by several examples of various AMD modifications.

2.4.1 Fourier Domain-OCT (FD-OCT) in the diagnosis of AMD

FD-OCT imaging was performed with a Topcon 3D OCT-1000 instrument (TOPCON, Japan, model 2007) that uses a monochromatic light source of 840 nm wave length. The Topcon 3D OCT-1000 combines FD-OCT system with a color non-mydriatic retinal camera.

In fig. 2a appears the image of a normal fundus, showing the optic nerve head, the macular region and the retinal vessels (arteries and veins). Fig. 2b displays the 2D FD-OCT image of the macula, showing (from the surface to the deep layers): the foveolar depression, the neurosensory retina and the RPE (the red layer). Fig. 2c illustrates the 3D FD-OCT image of the macula, revealing the architecture of the normal macular region, tridimensionally - a true "live biopsy" of the tissues. The tissues with high reflectivity appear more red on the OCT. For instance, on the normal OCT, the RPE band has the highest reflectivity (red color).

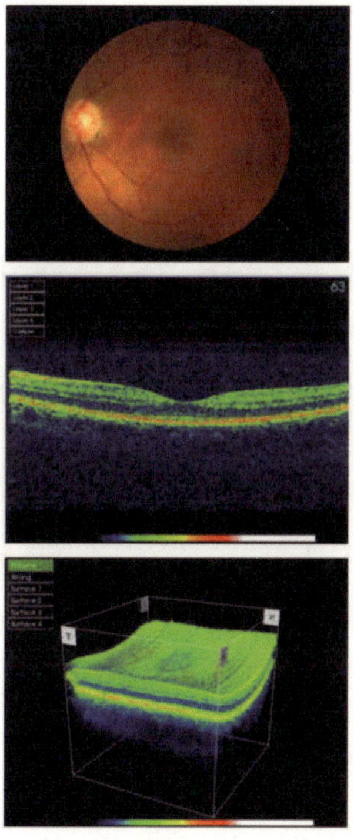

Fig. 2. The normal macula: a) ocular fundus; b) 2D scan; c) 3D scan (courtesy of Dr. F. Balta, Eye Hospital, Bucharest, Romania)

In fig. 3a, the ophthalmoscopic aspect of a wet form of AMD is illustrated: subfoveal neovascular membrane, elevating the retina, on average 1,5 disc diameters in surface. Fig. 3b depicts the 2D FD-OCT image of the macula in wet AMD: elevation of the macular retina, the space under the neurosensory retina is occupied by an irregular, opaque structure; the retinal pigmented epithelium is thickened. The 3D FD-OCT image of the macula in wet AMD (fig. 3c) offers a tridimensional view: elevation of the macular retina, better depiction of the retinal topography, thus improving the visualization of RPE irregularities. The advantage of FD-OCT in AMD is revealed by the fact that because it more densely samples the macula, it will be more likely to diagnose the presence of fluid in its nascent stages, meaning treatment can be introduced early and before it causes limitations to vision. FD-OCT can also capture macular hemorrhaging. While TD-OCT would also theoretically show fluid and blood at the macula, it would not be able to depict with the same accuracy at what retinal layer the buildup occurs.

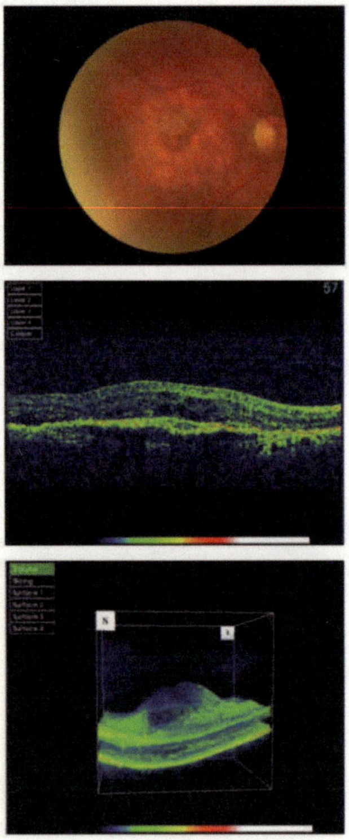

Fig. 3. Age-related macular degeneration: a) ocular fundus; b) 2D scan; c) 3D scan (courtesy of Dr. F. Balta, Eye Hospital, Bucharest, Romania)

2.4.2 Cirrus High Definition-OCT (HD-OCT) in the diagnosis of AMD

Cirrus HD-OCT (Carl Zeiss Meditec) provides detailed maps and quantifies the retinal thickness and volume.The 5-line raster, with over 4.000 A-scans per line, offers such high definition images that differences in fluid are identifiable, thus helping to indicate the specific disease process. The representation of the macula is useful for layer identification, segmentation, and the quantitative and qualitative analysis.

RPE detachment is characterized by the accumulation of fluid between the highly reflective RPE (red line) and the moderately reflective choriocapillaris. Blister-like elevation of the retina and RPE are evident on the OCT image. Figures 4 and 5 depict the PEDs: the red line representing the RPE is irregular and present focal elevations. Fig. 4 also shows the fluid accumulation in the retina in a region adjacent to the RPE detachment.

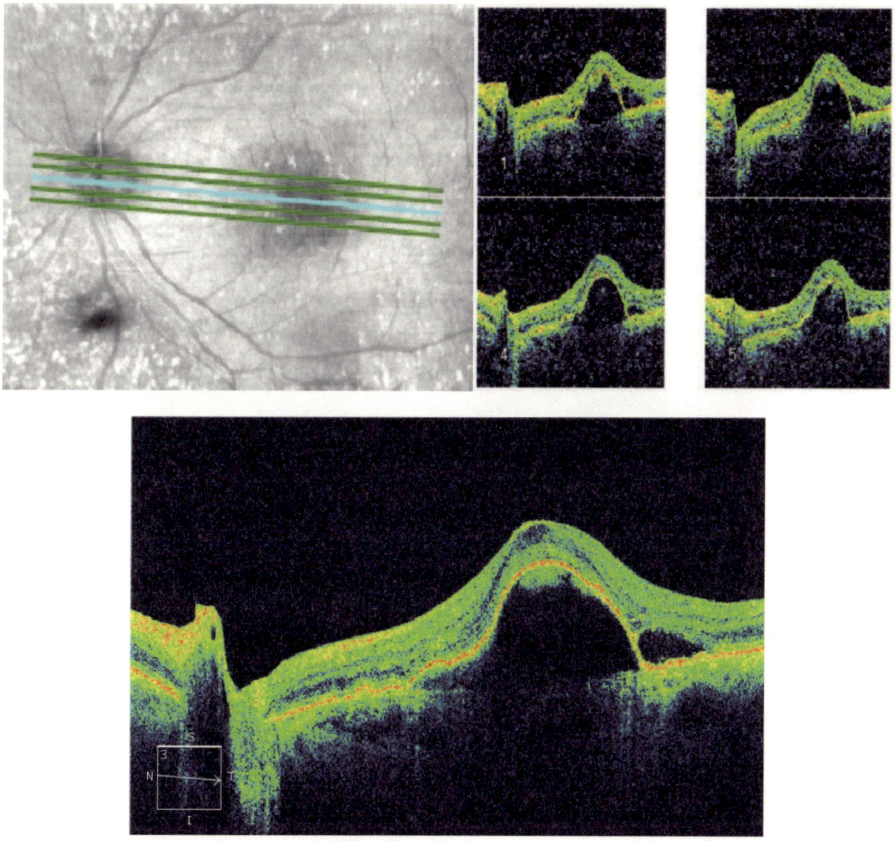

Fig. 4. HD-5 line raster: Drusen and PEDs
(courtesy of Dr. H. Shah, Midland, Texas, USA)

Occult CNV is a term given to a specific „blothcy" appearance on the angiogram. The occult CNV in fig. 6 is suggested by the irregularities and thickening of the RPE layer and the CME appears like small, cystic spaces within the macula. In the figure above, the occult CNV is not accompanied by PED, therefore it is cathegorized as type 2 occult CNV. The type 1 occult CNV associates PEDs and is also named vascularized PED. The occult CNV might be an early phase of the classic CNV and therefore its identification is important for the early diagnosis of the wet AMD.

When the choroidal new vessels that have grown under the macula are seen on the angiogram, this condition is named classic CNV. The classic CNV appears on OCT as a hyper-reflective structure that elevates the RPE. This aspect is easily demonstrated in fig. 7, 8, and 9.

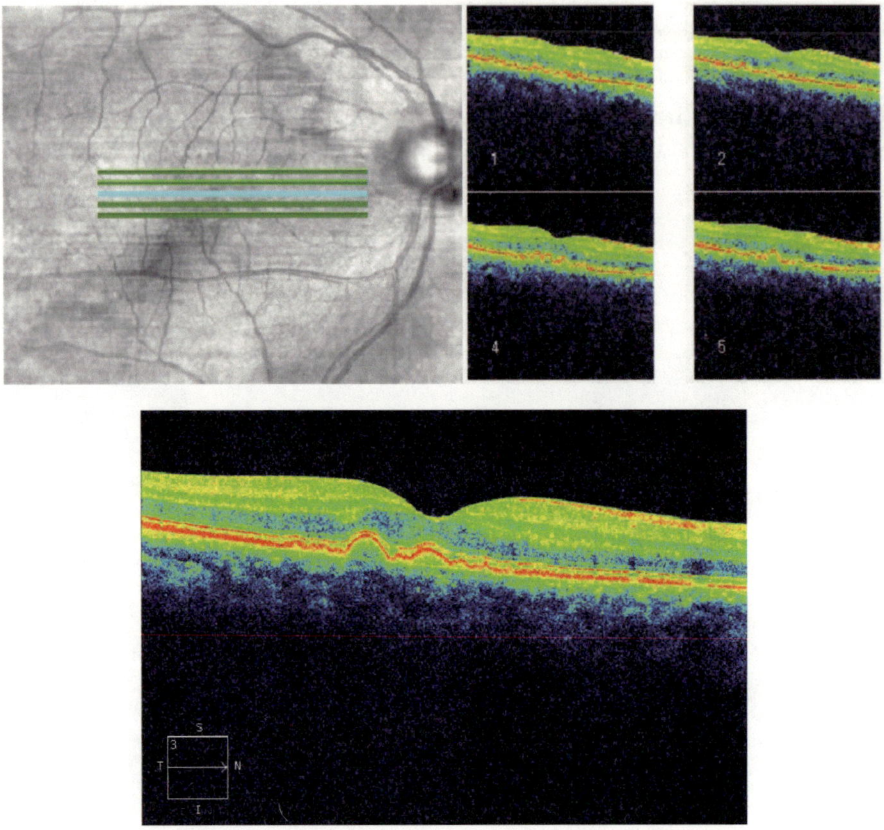

Fig. 5. HD-5 line raster: PEDs (courtesy of Dr. H. Shah, Midland, Texas, USA)

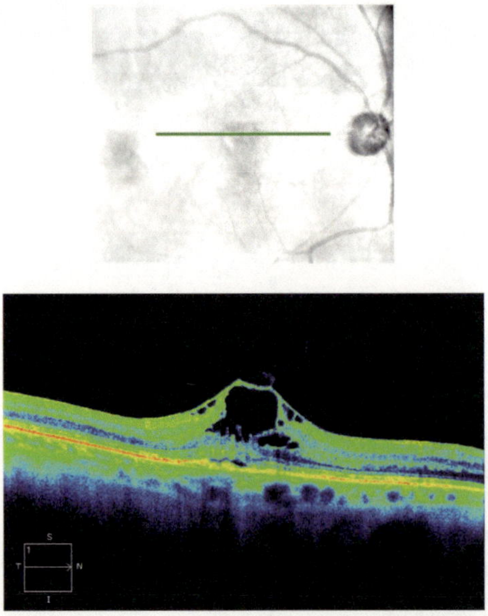

Fig. 6. Occult CNV with CME (courtesy of Dr. H. Shah, Midland, Texas, USA)

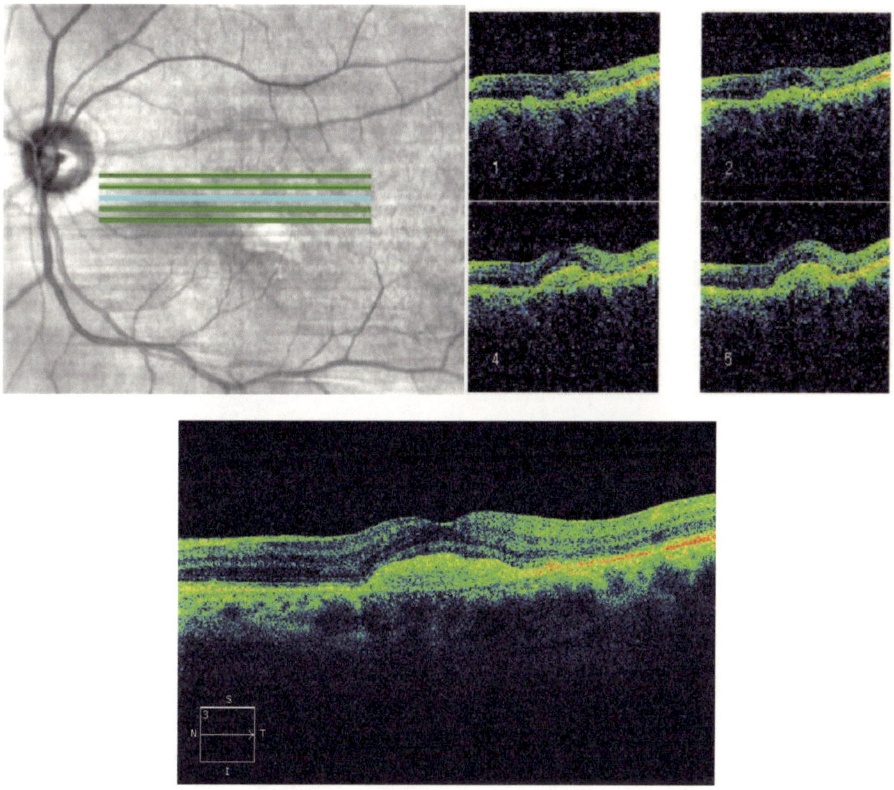

Fig. 7. HD-5 line raster: Classic CNV (courtesy of Dr. H. Shah, Midland, Texas, USA)

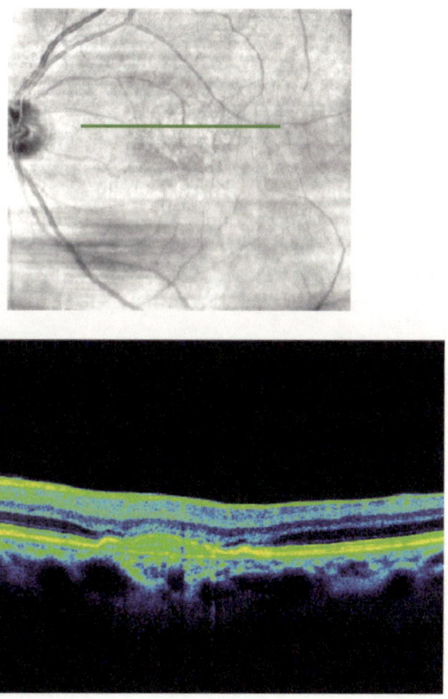

Fig. 8. Classic CNV (courtesy of Dr. H. Shah, Midland, Texas, USA)

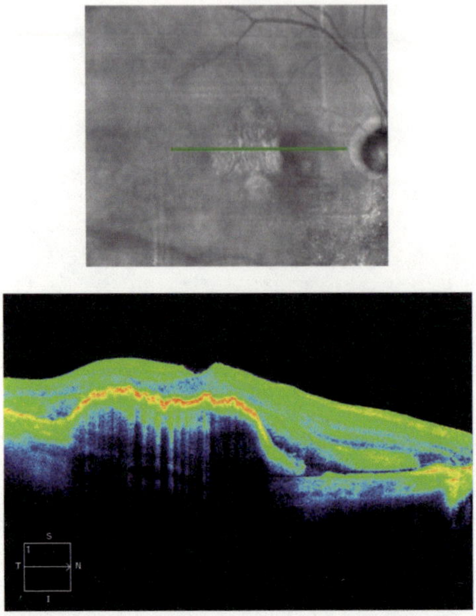

Fig. 9. Classic CNV (courtesy of Dr. H. Shah, Midland, Texas, USA)

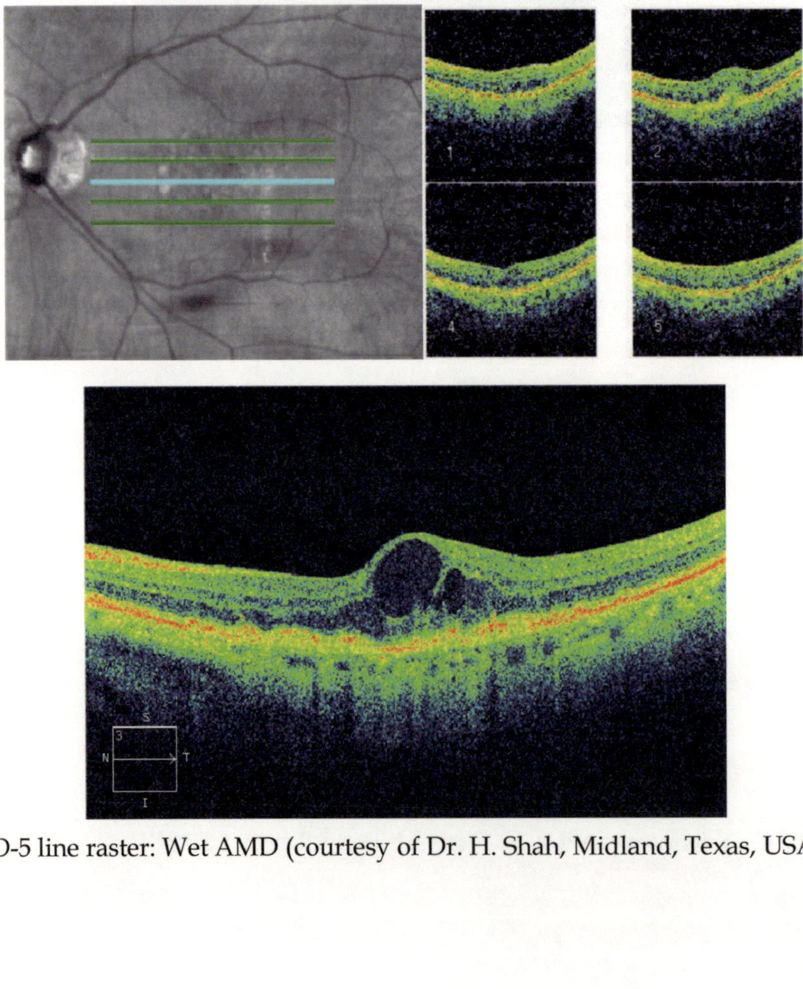

Fig. 10. HD-5 line raster: Wet AMD (courtesy of Dr. H. Shah, Midland, Texas, USA)

In fig. 10 the RPE appears irregular and thickened (suggesting an occult CNV) and under the RPE line there is a hyper-reflective structure slightly elevating the RPE on line 2 of the raster (classic CNV). On the same line, the RPE line appears interrupted. The structure of the neurosensory retina is disorganized by the cystic fluid accumulation within the retinal layers.

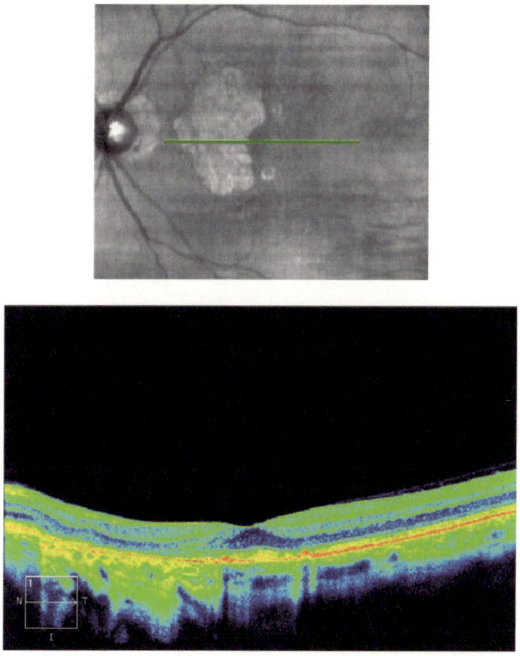

Fig. 11. Choroidal atrophy (courtesy of Dr. H. Shah, Midland, Texas, USA)

Geographic atrophy is the end stage of the dry AMD. The reflectivity of the RPE and underlying choroid is increased (fig. 11). There have been defined spectral-domain OCT patterns that are correlated with a higher risk of atrophy's extension: the irregular margin of the lesion on OCT is significantly associated with increased fundus autofluorescence and a higher risk of progression. The smooth margin of the lesion has been significantly associated with normal fundus autofluorescence and a lower risk of atrophy's progression (Brar M. et al., 2009). In our example (fig. 11), the margins of the choroidal atrophy appear pretty irregular. We can speculate that because it reveals structural changes, the spectral - domain OCT is a better predictor for geographic atrophy's extension, as compared to fundus autofluorescence, but this hasn't been proved yet.

2.4.3 TD-OCT (Stratus) in monitoring AMD

The TD-OCT imaging was performed using a Stratus OCT 2006 commercial instrument (Carl Zeiss Meditec, Dublin, California, USA). The Stratus TD-OCT provides real-time cross-sectional images and quantitative analysis of retinal features to optimize the diagnosis and monitoring of retinal disease and for enhanced pre-and post-therapy assessment. Sensor captures 1 image at a time

In figure 12, the comparation of the macular thickness before and 3 months after Bevacizumab injection revealed no significant modification, which led us to stop the anti-VEGF intravitreal injections.

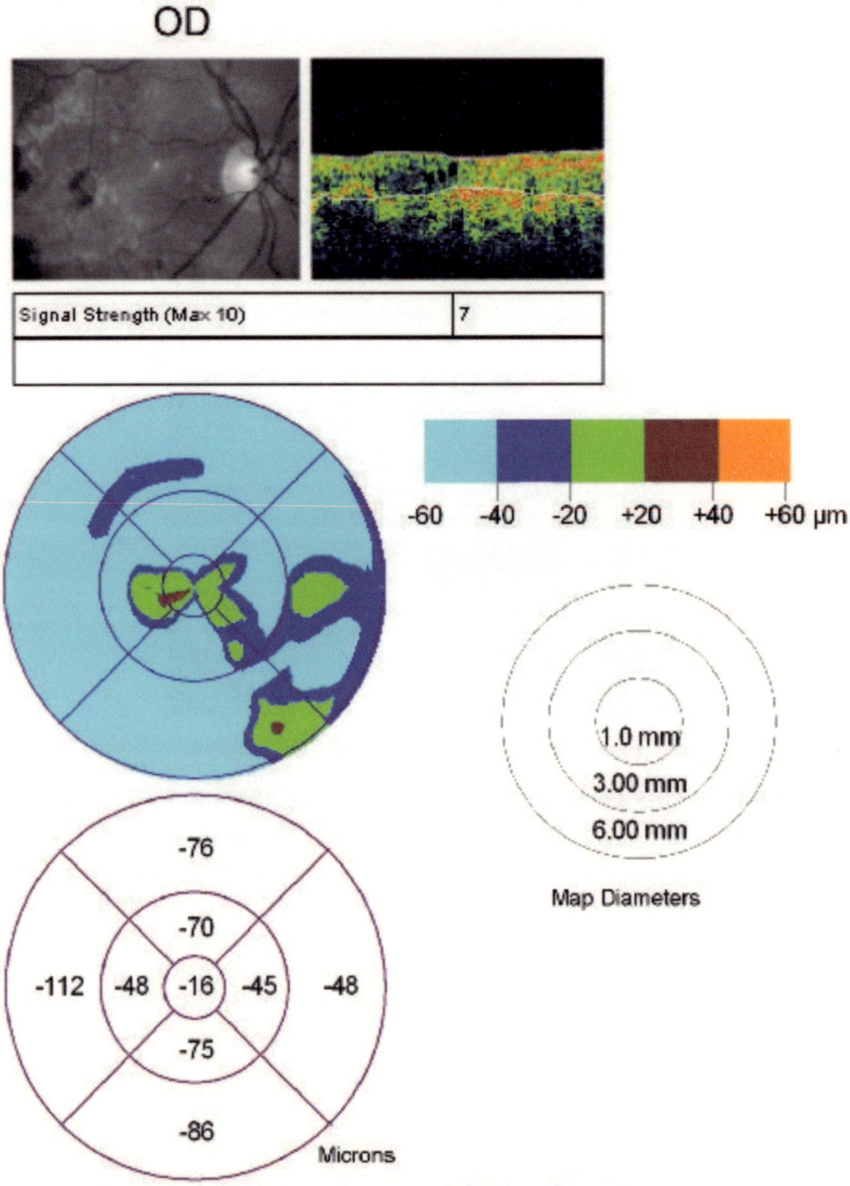

OD	Scans used	1, 2, 3, 4, 5, 6
	Scans used	1, 2, 3, 4, 5, 6

Fig. 12. RTM: comparation of the macular thickness before and 3 months after Bevacizumab injection (courtesy of dr. H. Demea, Review Centre, Cluj-Napoca, Romania)

The next case (figure 13) showed a slight improvement in the right eye, 3 months after 3 Bevacizumab injections. The fibrotic nature of the submacular tissue in the left eye kept us from performing the anti-VEGF intravitreal injections.

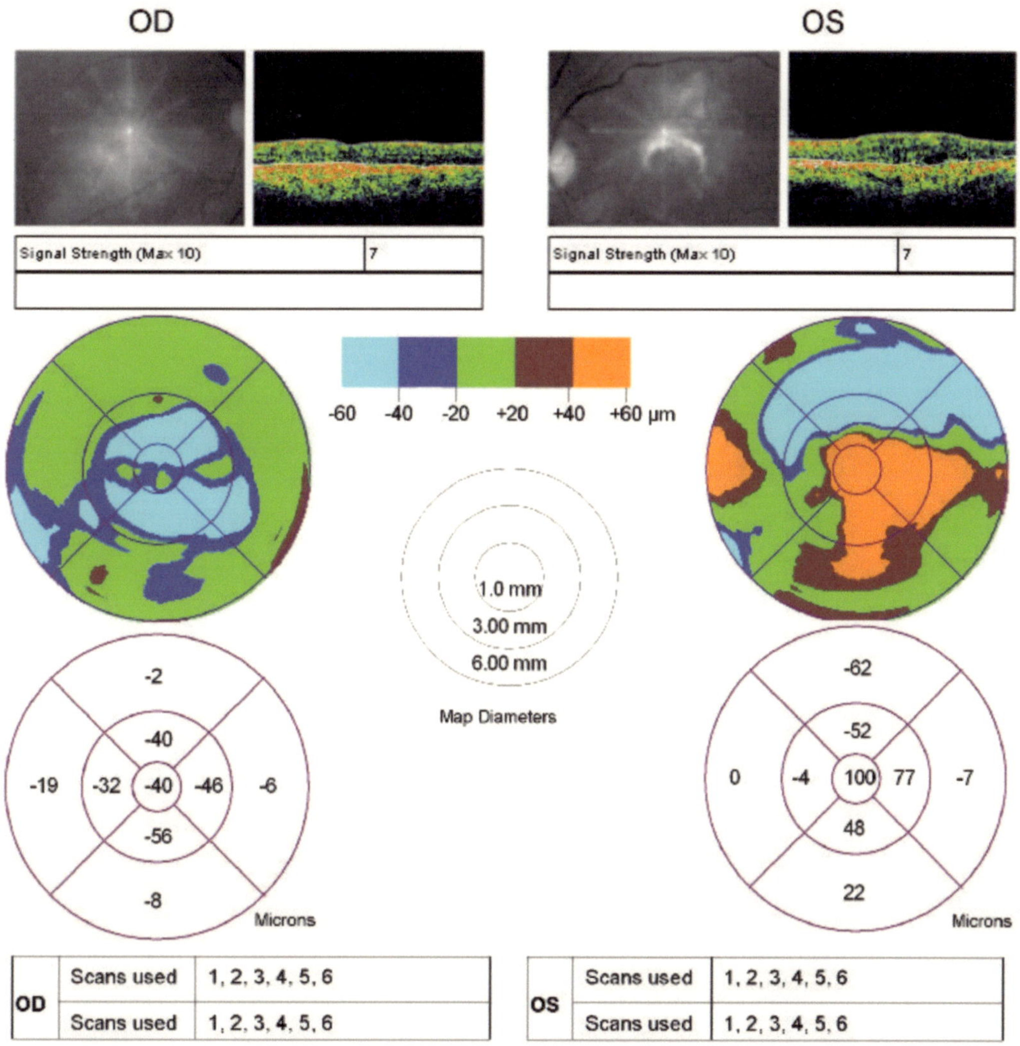

Fig. 13. RTM: comparation of the macular thickness before and 3 months after Bevacizumab injection (courtesy of dr. H. Demea, Review Centre, Cluj-Napoca, Romania)

Figure 14 illustrates the decrease of the macular thickness 3 months after 3 Bevacizumab injections.

In all the cases with favorable outcome, the most spectacular improvement, both in vision and in the anatomical aspect, has been obtained after the first injection. The better results are directly correlated with the early stage of the disease. Even if the vision has not changed from the quantitative point of view, all the patients with a better anatomical aspect of the macula on OCT have also experienced a significant improvement in the quality of vision, translated by the diminishing of the central scotoma, both in surface and in density (Talu et al., 2010).

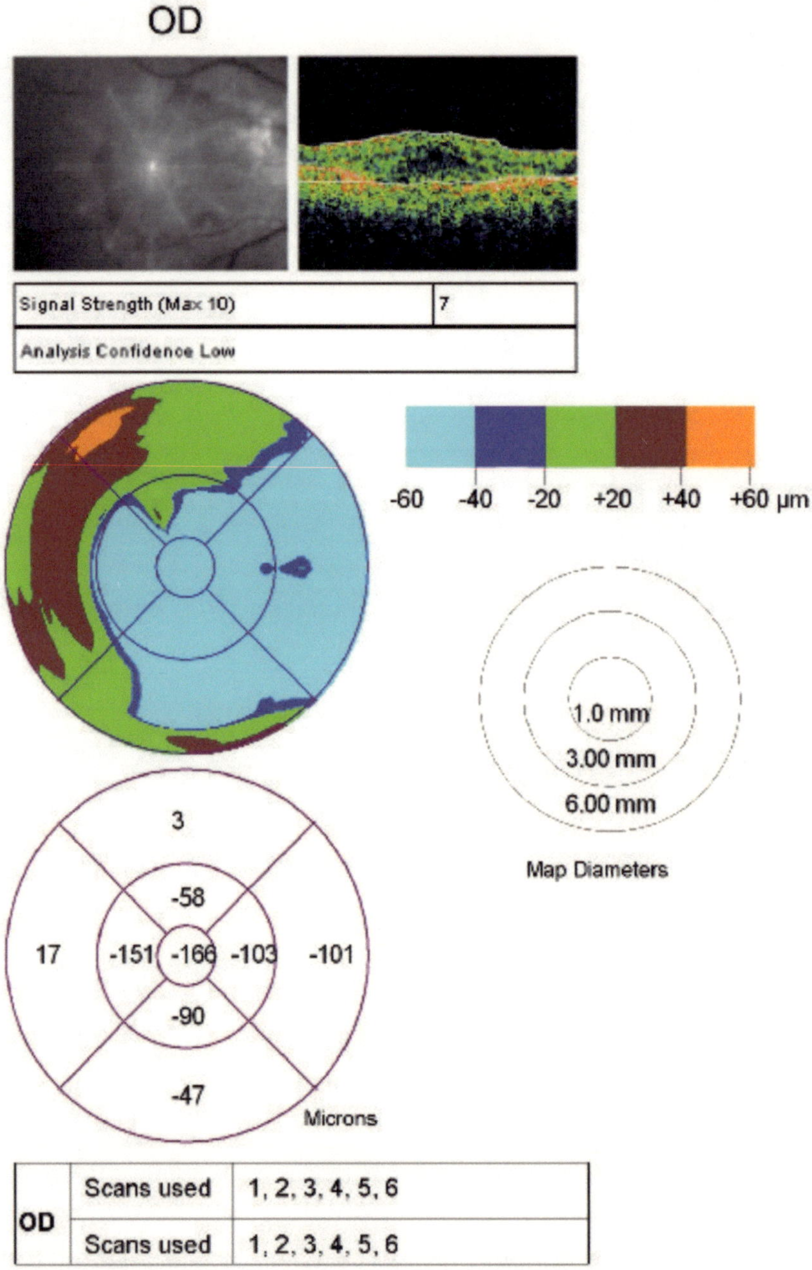

Fig. 14. RTM: comparison of the macular thickness before and 3 months after Bevacizumab injection (courtesy of dr. H. Demea, Review Centre, Cluj-Napoca, Romania)

3. Conclusion

The invention of OCT in the 1990s is a major breakthrough in ocular imaging, as it represents a fast, non-invasive, radiation-free examination technique, able to visualize precisely the retinal layers - something done before only on pathology slides. The information offered by OCT is detailed, simple and easily interpretable. AMD is by far, the ocular condition that has benefited the most from the enormous advantages offered by OCT, in terms of diagnosis, response to treatment and monitoring. OCT is applied by two main methods: Time domain OCT (TD-OCT) and Spectral domain OCT (SD-OCT). TD-OCT produces two-dimensional images of the sample internal structure. SD-OCT can be implemented in two formats, Fourier domain (FD-OCT) and swept source (SS-OCT). The image is acquired rapidly - about 60 times faster than with TD-OCT. The image resolution in SD-OCT is 1 µm, as compared to 10 µm in TD-OCT. The practical impact of this improvement in resolution is the early detection of small cystic changes associated with the wet form of AMD. The great number of scans done per second allows SD-OCT systems to generate 3D reconstructions, which can be further manipulated. Visualization of these data in 3D demonstrates subtle pathology that are not evident with conventional 2D images. The most frequent application of OCT in retinal disease is the measurement and monitoring of the retinal thickness. The TD - OCT system (Stratus) gives a macular thickness map which is calculated from 6 radial B-scans crossing at the fovea. By interpolating data from these scans, the average macular thickness is calculated in 9 subfields centered on the fovea. Similarly, the total macular volume is obtained. The SD-OCT provides images with much higher resolution. Given the differences between the measurements with the two types of OCT (TD and SD), algorithms are necessary in order to establish correlations between them. Besides its contribution in the diagnosis of AMD, OCT examination is extremely useful in establishing the indication of the modern treatments in wet AMD (intravitreal injections with anti-VEGF agents) and in the monitoring of the response to treatment. Ideally, the OCT scan must be interpreted in correlation with the fundus photography, direction of scan and ideally, the angiography. Despite the obvious advantages offered by OCT at the present moment, there is still room for future developments and improvement.

4. Acknowledgment

This work has been financially supported by the Romanian Ministry of Education, Research and Youth, through The National University Research Council, Grant PN–II–ID–PCE–2007–1, code ID_459, 2007 - 2010.ID_459.

5. References

Brar, M.; Kozak, I. & Chang, L. (2009). Correlation between spectral-domain optical coherence tomography and fundus autofluorescence at the margins of geographic atrophy. *Am J Ophthalmol,*Vol. 148, No 3 (Sept. 2009), pp. 439-444, ISSN 0002-9394

Coscas, G. (2009). *Optical Coherence Tomography in Age-Related Macular Degeneration* (edition 2009), Springer Medizin Verlag, ISBN 978-3-642-01468-0, Heidelberg

Forte, R.; Cennamo, CL. & Finelli ML. (2009). Comparison of time domain Stratus OCT and spectral domain SLO/OCT for assessment of macular thickness and volume. *Eye,* Vol. 23, No 11 (September 2009), pp. 2071 – 2078, ISSN 1552 - 5783

Grover, S.; Murthy, RK & Brar VS (2010). Comparison of Retinal Thickness in Normal Eyes Using Stratus and Spectralis Optical Coherence Tomography. *Invest Ophthalmol Vis Sci,* Vol. 51, No 5 (May 2010), pp. 2644-2647, ISSN 0146-0404

Kakinoki, M.; Sawada, O. & Sawada, T. (2009). Comparison of Macular Thickness Between Cirrus HD-OCT ans Stratus OCT. *Ophthalmic Surg Lasers Imaging,* Vol. 40, No 2 (March/April 2009), pp 135-140, ISSN 1542-8877

Khaderi, K.; Ahmed, K.A. & Berry, G.L. (2011). Retinal Imaging Modalities: Advantages and Limitations for Clinical Practice. *Retinal Physician,* Vol. 8, No 3 (April 2011), pp. 44-48, ISSN 1552-812X

Luviano, D.; Benz, M.; & Kim, R. (2009). Selected Clinical Comparisons of Spectral Domain and Time Domain Optical Coherence Tomography. *Ophthalmic Surg Lasers Imaging,* Vol. 40, No 3 (May/June 2009), pp. 325-328, ISSN 1542-8877

Marschall, S.; Sander, B. & Mogensen, M. (2011). Optical coherence tomography - current technology and applications in clinical and biomedical research. *Anal Bioanal Chem,* Vol. 400, No 9 (May 2011), pp. 2699 - 2720, ISSN 1618 - 2650

Mylonas, G.; Ahlers, C. & Malamos, P. (2009). Comparison of retinal thickness measurements and segmentation performance of four different spectral and time domain OCT devices in neovascular age-related macular degeneration. *Brit J Ophthalmol,* Vol.93, No 11 (November 2009), pp. 1453 – 1460, ISSN 1468-2079

Osiac, E.; Saftoiu, A. & Gheonea, D.I. (2011). Optical coherence tomography and Doppler optical coherence tomography in the gastrointestinal tract. *World J Gastroenterol,* Vol. 17, No 1 (January 2011), pp. 15-20, ISSN 1007-9327

Sayanagi, K.; Sharma, S. & Yamamoto, T. (2009). Comparison of Spectral-Domain versus Time-Domain Optical Coherence Tomography in the Management of Age-Related Macular Degeneration with Ranibizumab, *Ophthalmology,* Vol. 116 No 5 (May 2009), pp. 947-955, ISSN 0161-6420

Schutze, C.; Ahlers, C. & Sacu, S. (2011). Performance of OCT segmentation procedures to assess morphology and extension in geographic atrophy, *Acta Ophthalmologica,* Vol. 89 No 3 (May 2011), pp. 235-240, ISSN 1755-3768

Talu, S.; Balta, F. & Talu, S.D. (2009). Fourier-Domain Optical Coherence Tomography in diagnosing and monitoring of retinal diseases. *IFMBE Proceedings,* Vol. 26, No 1 (September 2009), pp. 261-266, ISSN 1680-0737

Talu, S.; Demea, H. & Demea, S. (2010). Avastin in age-related macular degeneration, *Oftalmologia,* Vol.54, No 1 (January-March 2010), pp. 95 – 100, ISSN 1220-0875

Walther, J.; Gaertner, M. & Cimalla, P. (2011). Optical coherence tomography in biomedical research. *Anal Bioanal Chem,* Vol. 400, No 9 (May 2011), pp. 2721-2743, ISSN 1618-2650

Wenner, J.; Wismann, S. & Jäger, M. (2011) Interchangeability of macular thickness measurements between different volumetric protocols of Spectralis optical coherence tomography in normal eyes, *Graefes Arch Clin Exp Ophthalmol,* Vol. 249, No 8 (August 2011), pp. 1137-1145, ISSN 0721-832X

14

Treatments of Dry AMD

George C. Y. Chiou
Institute of Ocular Pharmacology
College of Medicine
Texas A&M Health Science Center
College Station, TX
USA

1. Introduction

Age-related macular degeneration (AMD) is the most common cause of legal blindness among those over 65 years of age in the United States (Mitchell et al., 1995; Klein et al., 1992). It is also a debilitating disease on central vision in patients over 50 years old (Ambati et al., 2003). As the baby boom generation ages, the incidence of AMD is expected to triple by the year 2025. It was first described in the medical literature as symmetrical central choroidoretinal disease occurring in senile persons (Hutchison 1875). It was not until 1980 that AMD was regenerated to be a significant cause of blindness in the United States (Leibowitz et al., 1980). Even though the prevalence of AMD is highest among Caucasians in western countries, Asians are as high as Caucasians in the development of AMD (Wang et al, 2010). In 2004, WHO estimated that there are 14 million persons worldwide suffering from blindness or severely impaired vision because of AMD. As the population in the Western World is growing older, the morbidity of losing the ability to read and drive resulting from AMD is becoming increasingly apparent (Klein, 1997). A 2004 analysis reported that among Americans over the age of 40, AMD and/or geographic atrophy were present in at least one eye in 1.47% of the population (Friedman et al., 2004). By the year 2020, there may be a 50% increase in the incidence of AMD. The study predicted that as a result of the rising prevalence of AMD, the number of blind people in the U.S. could increase by as much as 70% by 2020 (Congdon et al., 2004). Because of the enormous impact of AMD on the aging population, much public attention and research has been focused on this condition in the past decade.

The therapy that could treat patients at the dry AMD stage and prevent its progression have a huge impact in reducing the incidence of blindness, improving the quality of life and reducing the social costs of AMD, which equals to approximately $30 B in GDP annually in the year 2003.

AMD occurs initially in a "dry" form with pathological changes in the retinal pigment epithelium (RPE) and drusen accumulation and can progress to geographic atrophy (GA) (90%) and/or "wet" form of AMD (10%) with choroidal neovascularization (CNV) (Klein, 1997). The breakdown of Bruch's membrane under RPE serves as an entrance for new and immature choroid vessels to grow into the subretinal space that leads to the formation of

CNV (Klein, 1997; Lin and Chiou, 2008; Algveve and Seregard, 2002; Joussen, 2004). CNV can leak fluid as well as hemorrhage in the subretinal space resulting in blurry vision, visual distortion and sudden loss of vision (Nowak, 2006). If left untreated, these lesions progress to form an organized fibrous scar, termed diciform scar, which results in irreversible central vision loss.

The precise etiology is poorly understood despite intensive researches. Thus, we have limited choices of treatment for this kind of disease. Available treatment can be grouped into two major categories: physical and pharmacological (chemical) therapies. The former received extensive attention with little success whereas the latter attract new attention with great hope of success.

2. Etiology and pathogenesis of dry AMD

Drusen is a typical clinicopathologic entity in dry AMD, which causes the changes of retinal pigment epithelium (RPE) and Bruch's membrane (BRM). Drusen is deposited in between the basement membrane of RPE and BRM or external to BRM (Hope et al., 1992). The prevalence and severity of drusen formation in the eyes are linearly related to the progression of AMD. Oxydative stress has long been linked to age-related degenerative diseases and is implicated in the pathogenesis of AMD. The oxidative damage is likely to be the photo reactive pigments which accumulate progressively and constitute the lipofuscin of RPE cells (Imamura et al., 2006; Zhou et al, 2006).

The two major carotenoids in the human macula and retina are lutein and zeaxanthin. Lutein and zeaxanthin are deposited at an up to 5 fold higher content in the macular region of the retina as compared to the peripheral retina. Several functions of these pigments have been hypothesized and these include limitation of the damaging photo-oxidative effects of blue light through its absorption, reduction of the effects of light scatter and chromatic aberration on visual performance, and protection against the adverse effects of photochemical reactions because of the anti-oxidant properties of the carotenoids. So it has been further hypothesized that dietary supplementation with lutein and/or zeaxanthin might protect the retina and/or delay the progression of AMD (Mozaffarieh et al., 2003). Data from the Age-Related Eye Disease Study (AREDS) suggests that supplements that contain carotenoids, anti-oxidant vitamins A, C, and E, and minerals, such as zinc, showed a 25% decrease in the rate of progression to aggressive AMD among high risk patients (AREDS Report, 2001). The findings of the Lutein Anti-oxidant Supplementation Trial (LAST), a prospective, 12-month, randomized, double-masked, placebo-controlled trial, also support a possible therapeutic role of lutein in AMD (Richer et al., 2004). However, the controversial evidence also exists. The information available provides an indication that the carotenoids, lutein and zeaxanthin, may play a role in modulating the course of AMD, yet critical evidence of the beneficial effect has not been found, and crucial information for the most effective design of clinical trials is needed.

Similar to drusen, basal laminar deposit (BLD) is another typical sign of AMD development and led by extracellular deposit. BLD is located between the cell membrane of RPE and its basement membrane (Green and Enger, 1993; Kliffen et al., 1997). The pathogenesis of BLD could be enhanced by a high fat/cholesterol (HFC) diet. The accumulation of lipid particles in BRM is often associated with vascular endothelial growth factor (VEGF) expression and eventual development of CNV in wet AMD (Rudolf et al., 2005).

VEGF has a high degree of selectivity to endothelial cells, reciprocal oxygen regulation, diffusible to its target through extracellular secretion, and affecting multiple components of angiogenesis (endothelial cell proliferation, survival and migration) as well as vascular permeability (Ambati et al., 2003b). There is a lot of evidence showing a putative role of VEGF in CNV formation. Intravitreous injection of an anti-VEGF pegylated aptamer, a synthetic RNA compound specifically designed to bind to extracellular VEGF, stabilized or improved vision in 87.5% of patients with subfoveal CNV 3mo after treatment. However, elimination of VEGF threatens the normal survival of choriocapillaries, which is the trigger of the AMD to begin with. Thus, VEGF inhibitors are double blade swords, which make the control of VEGF levels during the treatment of AMD rather difficult. Inflammation and compromised immune systems are also implicated in the pathogenesis of dry AMD. As a result, anti-inflammatory agents, such as steroids, are frequently tried for the treatment of dry AMD. More specifically, complement components such as C3 and C5 are constituents of drusen in AMD patients (Ambati et al., 2003a). Others, such as interleukin-1, interleukin-6, and tumor necrosis factor (TNF) are implicated to develop dry AMD as well. Thus, interleukin-1 blockers have been tried in the dry AMD animal models as well.

The anti-angiogenic effect of corticosteroids has a dual mechanism. Not only do corticosteroids inhibit inflammation, but they also affect vascular endothelial cell extracellular matrix (ECM) turnover (Kaven, et al., 2001; Danis, et al., 2000). Similarly, corticosteroids decrease RPE cellular migration and proliferation by effecting a diminished enzymatic degradation of ECM components.

Invasion and migration of endothelial cells through the extracellular matrix during angiogenesis are orchestrated by the integrin family of cell adhesion molecules. They facilitate migration by interacting with adhesion proteins in the ECM, such as collagen, fibronectin, fibrinogen, laminin, vitronectin and von Willebrand factor. The process of interacting with adhesion proteins was potentiated by the secretion of matrix metalloproteinases (MMPs), a family of proteolytic enzymes that degrade basement membrane and extracellular matrix proteins, modulated by tissue inhibitors of metalloproteinases (TIMPs) (Ambati, et al., 2003b).

Drugs, which can change the construction of ECM or change the balance of MMPs and TIMPs, may have effects on angiogenesis process. Integrin alpha(v) beta3 is predominately expressed on endothelial cells in choroidal neovascularization (CNV). N-Biphenyl sulfonyl-phenylalanine hydroxamic acid (BPHA) is a synthetic, selective inhibitor of matrix metalloproteinase (MMP)-2, -9, -14. Oral administration of BPHA can reduce experimental laser-induced choroidal neovascularization (Kohri, et al., 2003). The binding of urokinase plasminogen activator (uPA) and its receptor (uPAR) triggers twin cascades of events during cancer research, the first of which is destruction of the extracellular matrix, and the second is intracellular signaling to program gene expression leading to cell migration, cell invasion, metasis, and angiogenesis. Overexpression of uPA/uPAR system has been shown in surgically excised CNV, and in laser-induced CNV. The octapeptide A6 is derived from the non-receptor-binding regulation of uPA. Subretinal injection of adenoviral or adeno-associated viral vectors have been used to transform the RPE into a factory for sustained local delivery of a drug or gene in experimental models of CNV. Angiostatin (act as a VEGF scavenger), TIMP-3. PEDF has been tested and showed inhibition of development of CNV in animal models (Ambati, et al., 2003b). An antiangiogenic activity that may last for several months after a single intravitreous injection of doses greater than 10(8) pu of AdPEDF. 11 have been reported. This study showed that adenoviral vector-mediated ocular gene transfer is a viable approval for the treatment of neovascular AMD (Rasmussen et.al., 2001; Campochiaro et al., 2006).

In addition to age, high fat diet, light oxidation, and inflammation, the factors of smoke, alcohol, and gene are frequently questioned. Cigarette smoke has been indicated by epidemiologic studies that it is the single greatest environmental risk factor for both dry and wet AMD (Evans, 2001). Mice experiments with inhaled cigarette smoke resulted in the formation of such-RPE deposits, thickening of BRM and accumulation of deposits, within BRM's membrane (Marin-Castano et al., 2006). On another experiment, mice were fed with nicotine in drinking water, the results showed nicotine increased the size and severity of experimental CNV formation (Suner, 2004).

The influence of alcohol on the development of CNV in wet AMD was studied by Bora et al (2006). The results showed that the activity of fatty acid ethyl ester synthase (FAEES) activity increased 4-fold in the choroid of alcohol treated rats as compared to controls. Further, the amount of ethylesters produced in the choroid was 10-fold higher in alcohol fed rats than the controls. The size of the CNV formation induced by laser treatment increased by 28% due to alcohol treatment.

In addition to environmental factors, gene also plays an important role in the development of dry AMD. Thus, some animal models used for AMD studies are transgenic mice treated with blue-green light (Espinosa-Heldmann et al., 2004).

There are some diseases which are similar to AMD. They include Stargardt macular dystrophy (STGD) and Sorsby's fundus dystrophy (SFD). STGD is characterized as dry AMD by accumulation of high level of lipofuscin in the RPE. It precedes to degeneration of photocells in the macular and atrophy of RPE (Karan et al., 2005; Raz-Prag et al., 2006). SFD is a rare autosomal dominant disorder that results in degeneration of the macular region, which leads to rapid loss of central vision like wet AMD (Li et al., 2005).

Most importantly, the choroidal blood flow of dry AMD and STGD is compromised and significantly lower than in normal eyes. (Grunwald et al., 2003, 2005) As a result, all metabolic wastes produced from oxidation, inflammation, aging, complement components, cytokines, cigarette smoke, nicotine, high lipid, alcohol and anything else are accumulated in RPE cells and BRM which trigger dry AMD and eventually wet AMD or GA. On the opposite direction, nutrient supply to BRM, RPE and photo cells at macula are markedly reduced which facilitate the worsening of dry AMD (Jiang and Chiou, 2007).

It is noteworthy that choroidal blood flow is found to be impaired by every method used to quantify it in the aging eye and in age-related macular degeneration: flourescein and indocyanine green angiography, color Doppler imaging, laser Doppler flowmetry, and pulsatile ocular blood flow (Freidman, 2000). The vascular model of AMD suggests that the elevation of intravascular pressure is the crucial hemodynamic factor in age-related macular degeneration. AMD is the result of the accumulation of lipids in the sclera and in Bruch's membrane, progressively increasing the stiffness of these tissues, and increasing the postcapillary resistance of the choroidal vasculature. In addition to decreasing choroidal blood flow, the increase in resistance tends to elevate the hydrostatic pressure of the choriocapillaries, enhancing leakage and deposition of extracellular proteins and lipids, particularly in the posterior pole. These deposits take the form of basal deposits within Bruch's membrane and of drusen, which can comprise the overlying retinal pigment epithelium and cause geographic atrophy of RPE. The progressive deposition of lipid in Bruch's membrane results in the degeneration of elastin and collagen, and ultimately calcification. The combination of elevated choriocapillary pressure, vascular endothelial growth factor, and a break in a calcified Bruch's membrane causes choroidal neovascularization in the neovascular form of AMD. Drusen, as well as the decrease in choroidal blood flow may be epiphenomena (Friedman, 2000; 2004). Vasoactive agents that selectively decrease postcapillary choroidal resistance may prevent the development of CNV. Drugs working in this field may provide a new way for AMD treatment.

3. Treatment of dry AMD with physical means

Treatment of AMD was initially focused in wet AMD and dry AMD was left untreated because no effective method was available then. Drusen is a marker for dry AMD as the size and number of drusen are proportionally related to the progression of the disease. However it was not clear whether it had a role in the pathogenesis of the disease until 2006 (CAPT) when laser therapy was applied to treat more than 1,000 patients in one eye and the other eye serving as the control. It was found that laser therapy had neither beneficial nor harmful effect for these patients, if any. The laser's energy can disrupt Bruch's membrane which loses the ability to prevent the growth of CNV under the retina, thus converting dry AMD to wet AMD (CAPT, 2006). On the other hand, laser therapy seems to delay the development of CNV by 6 months in studies, including patients with unilateral advanced AMD (Owen et al., 2006; Frikerg et al., 2006). In conclusion, presence and/or elimination of drusen with laser treatment did not affect the visual acuity, indicating that dry AMD cannot be treated with physical means at the present time.

4. Treatment of dry AMD with pharmacological agents

Most research and developments of dry AMD are focused on the prevention of metabolic wastes production with limited success. This is mainly because the production of metabolic wastes comes from numerous sources, including oxidation, aging, complement components, cytokines, inflammations, PEDF, VEGF, ECM turnover and the like. Thus, a complete inhibition of one branch of all pathogens can suppress the progression of dry AMD at only around 20% at best, which falls to the borderline efficacy only. Besides, metabolic wastes are normal products of physiological procedures of the body and complete inhibition of normal metabolism could result in other various pathological side effects. Further, visual acuity does NOT change significantly during the progression of dry AMD, thus, selection of proper end points to evaluate drug efficacy in the clinical trials are very difficult if not impossible.

4.1 Choroidal blood flow facilitators

Although fruitful progress has been made in the treatment of wet AMD, the treatment of dry AMD is still in the desert stage. There is no single drug available in the whole world for the treatment of dry AMD. Since 90% of AMD patient population is in the dry stage, there is active research carried out at the present time at different stages of research and development (Zou and Chiou, 2005).

A novel idea to solve the problem has been developed recently by Chiou in Texas A&M Health Science Center. He based on the risk factor of dry AMD as a reduction of choroidal blood flow (Friedman, 2000; Grundwald et al., 2003; 2005; Xu et al., 2010; Figueroa et al., 2006; Metelitsina et al., 2006), which lead to the accumulation of all waste products regardless of where they came from, including aging, oxidation, inflammation, complement components, VEGF, PEDF, cytokines and the like. Thus, instead of solving problems individually by using inhibiting/blocking agents of aging, oxidation, inflammation, complement components, VEGF, PEDF and cytokines, all waste products will be eliminated by improved choroidal circulation. Further, nutrients will be replenished to BRM, RPE, and photocells via improved choroidal circulation in macula to improve the vision.

In order to prove the concept that the disease severity of dry AMD is inversely proportional to choroidal blood flow (CBF), drugs that can facilitate CBF were identified with ocular hypertensive rabbits. The CBF was measured precisely with colored microsphere method. Drugs which can increase CBF were then administered to AMD rat models, including $NaIO_3$-induced and laser-induced AMD models. The former was used to prevent/reverse degeneration of RPE by drugs, representing the treatments of dry AMD. The latter was used to show the prevention of conversion of dry to wet AMD after the Bruch's membrane was broken down by laser treatment. It was interesting to note that those agents which can facilitate CBF can prevent/reverse AMD induced by $NaIO_3$ and/or laser beam. Those agents which did not improve CBF showed no effect on the AMD development. All drugs were administered with eye drops without preservatives in the ophthalmic solution. Phase I clinical trials and proof of the concept of MC1101 (MacuClear) in human patients had been carried out with encouraging results showing no major side effects observed and the drug can reach the back of the eye to facilitate CBF. If preclinical animal data are good indicators, it would most likely show drug efficacy in preventing/reversing the progression of dry AMD with these agents.

Numerous agents that can increase choroidal blood flow in rabbit eyes have been tested in dry AMD animal models. Among them, some were found to be quite efficacious in inhibiting the development of dry AMD. They include, but are not limited to, hydralazine (Jiang and Chiou, 2008; Jiang et al., 2008; Cheng and Chiou, 2008), tetramethylpyrazine (Zou et al., 2007; Shen et al., 2010a), flavone (Zhuang et al., 2010a; 2010b), naringenin (Lin and Chiou, 2008; Shen et al., 2010b), apigenin (Zou and Chiou, 2006), quercetin (Zhuang et al., 2011), guanabenz (Shen et al., 2011), interleukin-1 blockers (Zou et al., 2006) and D-timolol (Xu et al., 2005).

Reduction in choroidal blood flow causes deposition of extracellular proteins, lipids and metabolic wastes in the form of basal deposits within BRM and drusen in between BRM and RPE. The progressive deposition of lipid in BRM results in the degeneration of elastin and collagen, and ultimately calcification. The combination of elevated choriocapillary pressure, expansion of VEGF and break in the calcified BRM causes development of CNV and wet AMD. Vasoactive agents, which can facilitate choroidal blood flow are believed to prevent the progression of dry AMD and is the major focus of the research at the present time (Zou and Chiou, 2005).

4.2 Anti-oxidants

Antioxidants are the agents most extensively studied. Lutein and zeaxanthin are two major carotenoids in the human macula and retina. They are deposited at an up to 5-fold higher content in the macular region as compared to the peripheral retina. Because of antioxidant properties of carotenoids, lutein and zeaxanthin are considered to be able to protect and/or delay the progression of dry AMD (Mozaffarieh et al., 2003).

Age-related Eye Disease Study (AREDS, 2001) reported that food supplements that contain carotenoids, anti-oxidants vitamins A, C, and E, plus minerals, such as zinc, showed a 25% decrease in the rate of progression to aggressive AMD among high risk patients. The findings of Lutein Anti-oxidant Supplementation Trial (LAST) (Richer et al., 2004) also support a possible therapeutic role of Lutein in AMD treatment. However, the critical evidence of therapeutic efficacy has not been established.

In order to improve the initial success, AREDS-2 has been initiated with a new formulation for a six-year, multicenter, randomized trial. The new formula contains higher doses of lutein and zeaxanthin and/or Omega-3 fatty acids known as DHA and EPA. It also lowers the zinc from 80mg to 25mg and deletes β-carotene. Four thousand participants at ages 50 to 85 have been enrolled and the trial will last six years. The results should come out sometime in the near future (Karmel, 2011).

All agents, including hydralazine, tetramethylpyrazine, flavone, naringenin, apigenin, quercetin and guanabenz (Cheng and Chiou, 2008; Zou et al., 2006; 2007; Shen et al., 2010a; 2010b; 2011; Zhuang et al., 2010a; 2010b; 2011; Lin and Chiou, 2008) presented in section 4.1 as choroidal blood flow facilitators produce potent anti-oxidating actions as well. They can antagonize oxidation induced injuries on human RPE cells induced by H_2O_2, $NaIO_3$, t-BHP, and the like.

OT-551 is a piperidine derivative converted by ocular esterases to the actual metabolite, TEMPOL-H (TP-H) which serves as a potent free radical scavenger. It is a small molecule which can be administered as local eye drops (Tanito et al., 2007), OT-551 also possesses anti-inflammatory and antiangiogenic properties. OT-551 users are being investigated for the therapy of geographic atrophy in AMD. Unfortunately, the phase II trials failed to produce efficacy in preventing the enlargement rate of GA in AMD (OT-551, 2007).

4.3 Anti-inflammatory agents

Genetic association studies have shown that inflammation appears to be related to AMD (Patel and Chan, 2008). Further, complement factor H (CFH) was associated with an increased risk of developing AMD (Edwards et al., 2005; Hageman et al., 2005; Haines et al., 2005; Klein et al., 2005). Later studies linked AMD to even more complicated complement system. These studies indicated that inhibition of complement activation would be a reasonable strategy for the treatment of AMD. However, after a life-long damage on complement system, such a strategy might have little benefit on the AMD progression later in life (Arons, 2009).

Regardless, active investigation was carried out and numerous complement inhibitors were derived for clinical trials. Among them, POT-4 (Potentia Pharmaceuticals) was developed as a C3 inhibitor for wet AMD. Eculizumab (Soliris, Alexion Pharmaceuticals) was developed as a C5 antibody for the treatment of dry AMD. Since eculizumab is a monoclonal antibody, it has to be administered via intravenous infusion to patients with GA or high risk drusen. ARC-1905 (Ophthotech) is an anti-C5 aptamer administrated via intravitreal injection for dry and wet AMD. Another drug, anti-Complement Factor D antibody Fab (FCFD4514S) (Genetech/Roche) is in a phase II trial.

For preclinical R&D, JPE (Jerin: Ophthalmic) is developed with peptidomimetic molecular antagonist against C5a receptor. Interleukin-1 blockers (MacuClear) are also under investigation as eye drops for treatment of dry AMD.

For non-specific immune suppression for the treatment of dry AMD, subcutaneous glatiramer acetate (Copaxane, Teva Pharmaceuticals), intravitreal fluocinolone acetonide (Iluvein implant, Alimera Science) and subcutaneous sirolimus (Rapamycin, MacuSight) are under investigation (Arons, 2009).

4.4 Miscellaneous agents

Fenretinide (ST-602, Sirion Therapeutics) is an oral compound developed to slow down the progression of GA in AMD. It aims to reduce the accumulation of toxins which are end products of retinol (Vitamin A) related biochemical process. These toxins are accumulated in the form of lipofuscin when the elimination process is reduced such as in dry AMD and Stargardt's disease (Radu et al., 2005; Study of Fenretinide, 2007). Instead of slowing down the toxins productions, MC1101 (MacuClear) aims to facilitate the excretion of toxins by increasing the choroidal circulation (See Section 4.1).

Ciliary neurotrophic factors (CNTF, Neurotech Pharmaceuticals) have been developed to retard the progression of neurodegenerative diseases (A Phase II study, 2007). CNTF has been shown to reduce motor neuron loss in mouse and ciliary ganglion neurons in chick eyes. CNTF is delivered by genetically engineered cells that are housed in a patented delivery system called Encapsulated Cell Technology (ECT). They are surgically implanted through the pars plana into the vitreous and anchored to the sclera. It is designed to bypass the blood retinal barrier to reach the back of the eye (NTC201) (ECT Technology, 2007).

Drugs which can change the construction of extra cellular matrix (ECM) or change the balance of matrix metalloproteinases (MMPs) and tissue inhibitors of metalloproteinases (TIMPs) may have an effect on angiogenesis process as well (Berglin et al., 2003). These drugs are called ECM modifiers and are still in the experimental stage of development.

5. Clinical protocols for anti-dry AMD drug studies

There are at least two major obstacles which hinder the development of drugs for the treatment of dry AMD. First, the long time period that is required to observe progression of the disease (Csaky et al., 2008; AREDSRG, 2001), which discourages researchers as well as investors to get involved. Second, the clinical endpoints to show drug efficacy other than visual acuity are difficult to be determined. There are several promising methods under consideration and if approved by FDA, they can facilitate the drug evaluation and development in the future (FDA, 2008a; 2008b).

Dry AMD is an unique chronic disease whose visual acuity does not change much during the early stage of the progression of the disease. Its change does not parallel to the worsening of visual acuity until the late stage of the disease. Consequently, the efficacy of drug action to treat dry AMD is impossible to be assessed based on the changes in visual acuity. This is very different from the assessment of wet AMD drug actions, as the progression of wet AMD is parallel to the loss of visual acuity. Prolongation of dark adaptation is closely correlated to the severity of AMD (Jackson and Edward, 2008; Owsley et al., 2006; Jackson et al., 2002). Dark adaptation is strongly impacted in AMD long before there is any significant loss of visual acuity (Jackson and Edward, 2008). Thus, measurement of dark adaptation is one of the workable ways to measure the drug efficacy for the treatment of dry AMD. The commercially available prototype dark adaptometer (AdaptRx, Apeliotus Technologies Inc, Atlanta, GA) is now available.

It has been found that rod photoreceptor degeneration precedes cone degeneration in early AMD (Owsley et al., 2001; Curcio et al., 1996; Steinmetz et al., 1993; Chen et al., 2004; Jackson et al., 2004) and rod dysfunction may contribute to the later degeneration of cones because of their inter-dependence (Mohand-Said et al., 2001; 1998; Hicks and Sahel,1999). A ten-item night vision questionnaire (NVQ-10) has been developed by Ying et al (2008). Analysis of NVQ-10 implies that the wet AMD and GA may derive from two different disease physiological processes. Because of the ease of assessment, as compared to dark adaptation measurement with machine, assessing night vision symptoms may be useful in identifying patients with early or intermediate AMD at relatively high risk of progression (Ying et al., 2008).

Accumulation of the number and size of drusen is another parameter used to measure the progression of dry AMD. Since the change in drusen deposits is very slow and difficult to note subjectively, Matched Flicker (EyelC.com) has been developed to record the changes objectively and precisely. Basically, the precise high-tech use in the space science to record minute changes occurred in the sky at any time period has been applied to measure the changes of drusen occurred in the fundus of the same eye. Basically, two retinal images of the same eye from virtually any source can be loaded into Matched Flicker and the changes can be brought to life and observed as easy-to-detect motion. Since very minute change in drusen accumulation can be detected with the machine precisely and objectively, it allows to shorten the time to detect changes in drusen deposits as compared to inaccurate subjective observation with naked eyes in the past. As a result, clinical study of drug efficacy in slowing down the rate of drusen accumulation can be accomplished easily.

Optical Coherence Tomography (OCT) is an advanced technology that allows researchers to measure the increase in volume and area of drusen over time (Yehoshua et al., 2009; OCT, 2011). Information of detailed theory and selected application is available (OCT, 2011) and Spectral Domain OCT (SD-OCT) is particularly useful for monitoring drusen changes in volume and area which can be related to the progression of dry AMD (Yehoshua et al., 2009). This can be used as a novel clinical trial end point for investigation therapies of dry AMD.

RPE are critical cells to maintain healthy function of Bruch's membrane and photocells. The degeneration of RPE can be detected by measurement of the c-wave of ERG (Jiang and Chiou, 2007; Peachey et al., 2002). The suppression of c-wave is proportionally related to the deterioration of RPE in dry AMD.

A useful tool for determining patients' vision related function has been developed (Kokame, 2008) to allow the improved sensitivity for detection of even a slight change in visual activity in the stage of early and intermediate stages of dry AMD. The device is called NEI

VFQ-25 (National Eye Institute Visual Function Questionaire-25) which is responsive to changes in patients' visual activity and is able to differentiate between patients who are responders and those who are not.

Although NEI VFQ-25 measures patients' subjective evaluation of their visual function and how impairment in vision affects their lives, it is reliable, valid and responsive as compared to standard measure of vision used in clinical trials such as BCVA using standardized ETDRS (Early Treatment of diabetic retinopathy study) vision protocols (Kokame, 2008). The NEI VFQ-25 showed a large separation between the groups with improved BCVA (gained >15 letters) stable BCVA (gain or lost 15 < letters) and worse BCVA (lost ≥ 15 letters). It may also provide a more broad assessment of the visual function on life style and vision dependent activities than BCVA alone. On average, the 25-letter or better improvement in BCVA corresponds to an increase in the NEI VFQ-25 score of 8.2 in the MARINA Trial (Minimally Classic/Occult Trial of Anti-VEGF Antibody Ranibizumab in the Treatment of Neovascular AMD).

Although not all dry AMD would develop into wet AMD, 10-15% of dry AMD would eventually be converted into wet AMD. Thus, prevention of dry AMD to be converted into wet AMD is also a measurement of drug action to suppress the progression of dry to wet AMD. Since only 10-15% of dry AMD would be converted into wet AMD, a large number of patients are needed for this study to see the difference in drug treatment. In short, ideal clinical endpoints are urgently needed for the measurement of the efficacy of new drugs for the treatment of dry AMD. If approved by FDA, it can shorten the measurement of drug efficacy to save time, effort and funds.

6. Conclusions

Great deals of efforts have been poured in, in order to elucidate the etiology and pathogenesis of the dreadful disease, age-related macular degeneration, with a hope to develop an effective means of treatment and/or prevention of the disease. Although the etiology and pathogenesis have been largely revealed, its treatment with physical means has since failed and receded to the second line of treatment options. Fortunately, pharmacological agents are now available for the treatment of wet AMD. However, wet AMD is the very late stage of AMD and is too late to save the eyesight for normal daily function. Besides, wet AMD consists of only 10-15% of total AMD patients. Thus, developing efficacious drugs for dry AMD is most urgently needed. The key stage of the treatment of AMD is obviously at the early stage or dry phase of the disease. There are numerous groups of scientists working very hard to develop an efficacious drug yet none have succeeded as of yet.

The major obstacles for the development of ideal drugs for dry AMD are at least two folds. First, AMD is a long term chronic disease with little worsening of visual acuity until the very late stage of the disease. Thus, the clinical end point to measure improvement of visual acuity by drugs at early or even middle stages of the disease is very difficult. The agents for improving the choroidal circulation are under investigation. Alternative end points to measure visual functions have been developed including the measurement of dark adaptation for rod cell functions, the determination of c-wave of ERG for RPE cell functions and macular stress test for cone cell function in the macula. Secondly, the pathogenesis of the disease is closely related to numerous normal physiological functions, such as oxidation, aging, VEGF and PEDF expression, extracellular matrix modifications and the like. Thus, complete suppression of these normal functions is not only unrealistic and even detrimental to induce further devastating side effects. Since these factors are numerous, suppression of one of them can improve the disease only partially to bring it to the borderline, marginal improvement of the disease. The novel idea to solve the problem at the root of the disease is to improve the choroidal circulation which can eliminate all normal metabolic wastes from photocells, Bruch's membrane and RPE cells and to furnish nutrients to these critical tissues. This way, the macular function will go back to normal and the AMD would be reversed or suppressed without further development.

7. References

A phase II study of implants of encapsulated human NTC-201 cells releasing ciliary neurotrophic factor (CNTF) in participants with visual activity impairment associated with atrophic macular degeneration. ClinicalTrials.gov Web site. http://www.clinicaltrials.gov/ct/show/NCT00277134?order=2. Accessed on October 3, 2007.

AREDSRG (Age-related Eye Disease Study Research Group). A randomized, placebo-controlled, clinical trial of high-dose supplementation with vitamins C and E, beta carotene, and zinc for age-related macular degeneration and vision loss. *Archives of Ophthalmology*, 2001; 119:1417-1436

Algvere, P.V., Seregard, S. Age-related maculopathy: pathogenetic features and new treatment modalities. *Acta Ophthalmol Scand*, 2002; 80:136-143

Ambati, J., Ambati, B.K., Yoo, S.H., Ianchulev, S., Adamis, A.P. Age-related macular degeneration: etiology, pathogenesis, and therapeutic strategies. *Surv Ophthalmol*, 2003; 48:257-293

AREDS report No. 8. A randomized, placebo-controlled, clinical trial of high-dose supplementation with vitamins C and E, beta carotene, and zinc for age-related macular degeneration and vision loss. *Arch Ophthalmol*, 2001; 119:1417-1436

Arons, I. AMD update 6: An overview of new treatments for dry AMD. http://www.irvaronsjournal.blogspot.com/2009/12

Berglin, L., Sarman, S., van der Ploeg, I., Steen, B., Ming, Y., Itohara, S., Seregard, S., Kvanta, A. Reduced choroidal neovascular membrane formation in matrix metalloproteinase-2-deficient mice [J]. *Invest Ophthalmol Vis Sci*, 2003; 44:403-408

Bora, P.S., Kaliappan, S., Xu, Q., Kumar, S., Wang, Y., Kaplan, H.J., Bora, N.S. Alcohol linked to enhanced angiogenesis in rat model of choroidal neovascularization. *Fed Eur Biochem Soci J*, 2006; 273: 1403-1414

Campochiaro, P.A., Nguyen QD, Shah SM, Klein ML, Holz E, Frank RN, Saperstein DA, Gupta A, Stout JT, Macko J, DiBartolomeo R and Wei LL. Adenoviral vector-delivered pigment epithelium-deprived factor for neovascular age-related macular degeneration: results of phase I clinical trial. *Hum. Gene Ther*. 2006. 17:167-176

CAPT (Complications of Age-Related Macular Degeneration Prevention Trial Research Group) Laser treatment in patients with bilateral large drusen: the complications of age-related macular degeneration prevention trial. *Ophthalmology*. 2006;113:1974-1986.

Cheng, Y.W., Chiou, G.C.Y. Antioxidant effect of hydralazine on retinal pigment epithelial cells and its potential use in the therapy of age-related macular degeneration. *International J. Ophthalmol.* 2008; 8:1059-1064

Congdon, N., O'Colmain, B., Klaver, C.C., Klein, R., Munoz, B., Friedman, D.S., Kempen, J., Taylor, H.R., Mitchell, P. Causes and prevalence of visual impairment among adults in the United States. *Arch Ophthalmol* 2004; 122 (4) :477-485

Csaky, K.G., Richman, E.A., Ferris, F.L. 3rd. Report from the NEI/FDA Ophthalmic Clinical Trial Design and Endpoints Symposium. *Invest Ophthalmol Vis Sci.* Feb 2008; 49(2):479-489

Danis, R.P., Ciulla, T.A., Pratt, L.M. Intravitreal triamcinolone acetonide in exudative age-related macular degeneration [J]. R*etina*, 2000;20:244-250

ECT Technology. Neurotech Website. http://www.neurotechusa.com/product_tech.asp. Accessed on October 3, 2007

Edwards AO, Ritter R, 3rd, Abel KJ, et al. Complement factor H polymorphism and age-related macular degeneration. *Science.* 2005;308:421-424

Espinosa- Heidmann, D.G., Sall, J., Hernandez, E.P., Cousins, S.W. Basal Laminar deposit formation in APO B100 transgenic Mice: Complex interactions between dietary fat, blue light, and vitamin E. *Invest Opthalmol Vis Sci,* 2004; 45(1) :260-266

Evans, J.R. Risk factors for age-related macular degeneration. *Prog Retin Eye Res,* 2001; 20:227-253

Figueroa M, Schocket LS, DuPont J, Metelitsina TI, and Grunwald JE. Long-term effect of laser treatment for dry age-related macular degeneration on choroidal hemodynamics. *Am J Ophthalmol.* 2006, 141:863-867

Food and Drug Administration. Critical Path Initiative. http://www.fda.gov/oc/initiatives/criticalpath/. Accessed August 1, 2008a

Food and Drug Administration. Critical Path Opportunity Report. http://www.fda.gov/oc/initiatives/criticalpath/reports/opp_report.pdf. Accessed August 1, 2008b

Friberg TR, Musch DC, Lim JI, et al. Prophylactic treatment of age-related macular degeneration report number 1: 810-nanometer laser to eyes with drusen. Unilaterally eligible patients. *Ophthalmology.* 2006;113:612-622.

Friedman, D.S., O'Colmain, B.J., Munoz, B., Tomany, S.C., McCarty, C., de Jong P.T., Nemesure, B., Mitchell, P., Kempen, J. Prevalence of age-related macular degeneration in the United States. *Arch Ophthalmol* 2004; 122 (4):564-572

Friedman, E. The role of the atherosclerotic process in the pathogenesis of age-related macular degeneration [J]. *Am J Ophthalmol*, 2000 ;130:658-663

Green, W.R., Enger, C. Age-related macular degeneration histopathologic studies. The 1992 Lorenz E. Zimmerman Lecture. *Ophthalmology*, 1993; 100:1519-1535

Grunwald, J.E., Metelitsina, T.I., DuPont, J.C., Ying, G.S., Maguire, M.G. Reduced foveolar choroidal blood flow in eyes with increasing AMD severity. *Inv Ophthalmol Vis Sci* 2005; 46: 1033-1038

Grunwald, J.E., Metelitsina, T.I., Niknam, R.M. , DuPont, J.C. Foveolar choroidal blood flow in patients with AMD that have CNV in the fellow eye *Inv Ophthalmol Vis Sci.* 2003. 44: E-Abstract 4989

Hageman GS, Anderson DH, Johnson LV, et al. A common haplotype in the complement regulatory gene factor H (HF1/CFH) predisposes individuals to age-related macular degeneration. *Proc Natl Acad Sci USA.* 2005;102:7227-7232.

Haines JL, Hauser, MA, Schmidt S, et al. Complement factor H variant increases the risk of age-related macular degeneration. *Science.* 2005;308:419-421.

Hope, G.M., Dawson, W.W., Engel, H.M., Ulshafer, R.J., Kessler, M.J., Sherwood, M.B. A primate model for age related macular drusen. *Br J Ophthalmol,* 1992; 76 (1):11-16

Hutchison, W.T. Symmetrical central choroidretinal disease occurring in senile persons, R. Lond. Ophthal. Hosp. Rep. 1875; 8: 231-244

Imamura, Y., Noda, S., Hashizume, K., Shinoda, K., Yamaguchi, M., Uchiyama, S., Shimizu, T., Mizushima, Y., Shirasawa, T., Tsubota, K. Drusen, choroidal neovascularization, and retinal pigment epithelium dysfunction in SOD1-deficient Mice: A model of age-related macular degeneration. *Proc Natl Acad Sci,* 2006; 103 (30):11282-11287

Jackson, G.R., Edwards, J.G. A short-duration dark adaptation protocol for the assessment of age-related maculopathy. *J Occul Biol Dis Inform.* 2008. DOI 10. 1007/s12177-008-9002-6

Jackson G.R., Owsley, C., Curio, C.A. Photoreceptor degeneration and dysfunction in aging and age-related maculopathy. *Ageing Research Reviews.* 2002; 1:381-386

Jiang, W., Chiou, G.C.Y. Effects of hydralazine on ocular blood flow and laser-induced choroidal neovascularization in vivo and endothelial cells in vitro. *International J. Ophthalmol.* 2008;8: 2359-2363

Jiang, W., Chiou, G.C.Y. The development of AMD experimental models. *International J. Ophthalmol.* 2007; 7:585-589

Jiang, W., Zhang, W.Y., Chiou, G.C.Y. Effects of hydralazine on sodium iodate-induced rat retinal pigment epithelium degeneration. *International J. Ophthalmol,* 2008; 8:1504-1510

Joussen, A.M. Cell transplantation in age related macular degeneration: current concepts and future hopes. *Graefes Arch Clin Exp Ophthalmol,* 2004; 242: 1-2

Karan, G., Lillo, C., Yang, Z., Cameron, D.J., Locke, K.G., Zhao, Y. Thirumalaichary S, Li C, Birch DG, Vollmer- Snarr HR Williams DS, Zhang K. Lipofuscin accumulation, abnormal electrophysiology, and photoreceptor degeneration in mutant ELOVL4 transgenic mice: A model for macular degeneration. *Proc Natl Acad Sci,* 2005; 102(11) :4164-4169

Karmel M. The other AMD; Dry but drawing research attention *Eye Net. Amer. Academy Opthalmol.* 2011. www.aao.org/publications/eyenet/200702/retina.cfm.

Kaven, C., Spraul, C.W., Zavazava, N., Lang, G.K., Lang, G.E.. Thalidomide and prednisolone inhibt growth factor-induced human retinal pigment epithelium cell proliferation *in vitro*[J]. *Ophthalmologica* , 2001;215:284-289

Klein, R. The five-year incidence and progression of age-related maculopathy: The Beaver Dam Eye Study. *Ophthalmology* 1997; 104:7-21

Klein, R., Klein, B.E., Linton, K.L. Prevalence of age-related maculopathy. The Beaver Dam Eye Study. *Ophthalmology* 1992; 99:933-943

Klein RJ, Zeiss C, Chew EY, et al. Complement factor H polymorphism in age-related macular degeneration. *Science.* 2005;308:385-389

Kliffen, M., vd Schaft, T.L., Mooy, C.M., d Jong, P.T.V.M. Morphologic changes in age-related maculopathy. *Microsc Res Tech,* 1997; 36:106-122

Kohri, T., Moriwaki, M., Nakajima, M., Tabuchi, H., Shiraki, K. Reduction of experimental laser-induced choroidal neovascularization by orally administered BPHA, a selective metalloproteinase inhibitor [J]. *Graefes Arch Clin Exp Ophthalmol*, 2003;241(11):943-952

Kokame, G.T. NEI VFG-25, useful tool for determining patients vision-related function. *Retina Today* Nov/ Dec. 2008:27-29

Leibowitz, H.M., Krueger, D.A., Maunder, R.A. An ophthalmological study of cataract, glaucoma, diabetic retinopathy, macular degeneration and visual acuity in a general population of 2631 adults 1973-1975. *Surv Ophthalmol* 1980; 24 (Suppl):335-610

Li, Z., Clarke, M.P., Barker, M.D., McKie, N. TIMP3 mutation in Sorsby's fundus dystrophy: molecular insights. *Expert Rev Mol Med*, 2005; 31;7(24): 1-15

Lin, B.Q., Chiou, G.C.Y. Antioxidant activity of naringenin on various oxidants induced damages in ARPE-19 cells and HUVEC. *International J. Ophthalmol*, 2008; 10:1963-1967

Marin-Castaño, M.E., Striker, G.E., Alcazar, O., Catanuto, P., Espinosa-Heidmann, D.G., Cousins, S.W. Repetitive nonlethal oxidant injury to retinal pigment epithelium decreased extracellular matrix turnover in vitro and induced sub-RPE deposits in vivo. *Invest Ophthalmol Vis Sci*, 2006; 47(9):4098-4112

Metelitsina TI, Grunwald JE, DuPont JC, Ying GS. Effect of systemic hypertension on foveolar choroidal blood flow in age-related macular degeneration. *Br. J. Ophthalmol*. 2006,90:342-346

Mitchell, P., Smith, W., Attebo, K., Wang, J.J. Prevalence of age-related maculopathy in Australia. The Blue Mountains Eye Study. *Ophthalmology* 1995; 102:1450-1460

Mozaffarieh, M., Sacu, S., Wedrich, A. The role of the carotenoids, lutein and zeaxanthin, in protecting against age-related macular degeneration: a review based on controversial evidence [J]. *Nutr J*, 2003; 2:20

Nowak, J.Z. Age-related macular degeneration (AMD): pathogenesis and therapy. Pharmacol Rep 2006; 58: 353-363

OCT, Optical coherence tomography. en.wikipedia.org/wiki/optical_coherence_tomography , 2001

OT-551 antioxidant eye drops to treat geographic atrophy in age-related macular degeneration. ClinicalTrials.gov Web site. http://www.clinicaltrials.gov/ct/show/NCT00306488?order=1. Accessed on October 3, 2007.

Owen SL, Bunce C, Brannon AJ, et al. Prophylactic laser treatment hastens choroidal neovascularization in unilateral age-related maculopathy: final results of the drusen laser study. *Am J Ophthalmol*. 2006;141:276-281.

Owsley, C., McGwin, G., Jackson, G.R., et al. Effect of short-term, high-dose retinol on dark adaptation in aging and early age-related maculopathy. *Invest Ophthalmol Vis Sci*. Apr 2006; 47(4):1310-1318

Patel M and Chan C.C. Immunological aspects of age related macular degeneration. *Semi Immunopathol*. 2008,30:97-110

Peachey, NS., Staton, J.B. And Marmorstein, AD. Non-invasive recording and response characteristics of the rat dC-ERG. *Vis Nerosc*,. 2002;19:693-701.

Radu RA, Han Y, Bui TV, et al. Reductions in serum vitamin A arrest accumulation of toxic retinal flurophores: a potential therapy for treatment of lipofuscin based retinal diseases. *Invest Ophthalmol. Vis. Sci.* 2005;46:4393-4401

Rasmussen, H., Chu, K.W., Campochiaro, P., Gehlbach, P.L., Haller, J.A., Handa, J.T., Nguyen, Q.D., Sung, J.U. Clinical protocol. An open-label, phase I, single administration, dose-escalation study of ADGVPEDF.11D (ADPEDF) in neovascular age-related macular degeneration (AMD) [J]. *Hum Gene Ther,* 2001;12(16):2029-2032

Raz-Prag, D., Ayyagari, R., Fariss, R.N., Mandal, M.N.A, Vasireddy, V., Majchrzak, S., Webber, A.L., Bush, R.A., Salem, N. Jr, Petrukhin, K., Sieving, P.A. Haploinsufficiency is not the key mechanism of pathogenesis in a heterozygous Elov14 knockout mouse model of STGD3 disease. *Invest Ophthalmol Vis Sci,* 2006; 47(8): 3603-3611

Rechtman, E., Danis, R.P., Pratt, L.M., Harris, A. Intravitreal triamcinolone with photodynamic therapy for subfoveal choroidal neovascularization in age-related macular degeneration [J]. *Br J Ophthalmol,* 2004; 88:344-347

Richer, S., Stiles, W., Statkute, L., Pulido, J., Frankowski, J., Rudy, D., Pei, K., Tsipursky, M., Nyland, J. Double-masked, placebo-controlled, randomized trial of lutein and antioxidant supplementation in the intervention of atrophic age-related macular degeneration: the Veterans LAST Study (Lutein Antioxidant Supplementation Trial) [J]. *Optometry,* 2004; 75(4):216-230

Rudolf, M., Winkler, B., Aherrahou, Z., Doehring, L.C., Kaczmarek, P., Schmidt-Erfurth, U. Increased expression of vascular endothelial growth factor associated with accumulation of lipids in Bruch's membrane of LDL receptor knockout mice. *Br J Ophthalmol,* 2005; 89:1627-1630

Schachat, AP Safety issues related to the long-term use of VEGF inhibitors DSN SuperSite June, 2007

Shen, Y., Zhang W.Y., Chiou G.C.Y. Effects of naringenin on $NaIO_3$-induced retinal pigment epithelium degeneration and laser-induced choroidal neovascularization in rats. *International J. Ophthalmol,* 2010a; 10:1-4

Shen, Y., Zhuang, P., Zhang, W.Y., Chiou, G.C.Y. Effects of guanabenz on rat AMD models and rabbit choroidal blood flow. *The Open Ophthalmol. J.,* 2011; 5:27-31

Shen, Y., Zhuang, P., Zhang, W.Y., Chiou, G.C.Y. Effects of tetramethylpyrazine on RPE degeneration, choroidal blood flow and oxidative stress of RPE cells. *International J. Ophthalmol,* 2010b; 10:1843-1847

Study of Fenretinide in the treatment of geographic atrophy associated with age-related macular degeneration. ClinicalTrials.gov Website. http://www.clinicaltrials.gov/ct/show/NCT00429936?order=1. Accessed on October 3, 2007.

Suñer, I.J., Espinosa-Heidmann, D.G., Marin-Castaño, M.E., Hernandez, E.P., Pereira-Simon, S., Cousins, S.W. Nicotine increases size and severity of experimental choroidal neovascularization. *Invest Ophthalmol Vis Sci,* 2004;45 (1) :311-317

Tanito M, Li F, Elliott WH, et al. Protective effect of TEMPOL derivatives against light-induced retinal damage in rats. *Invest Ophthalmol. Vis. Sci.* 2007,48:1900-1905

Wang, T.Y, Loon, S-C, Saw, S-M. The epidemiology of age related eye diseases in Asia *Brit J. Ophthalmol,* 2006; 90:506-511

Xu, W, Grunwald JE, Metelitsina TI, DuPont JC, Ying GS, Martin ER, Dunaief JL and Brucker AJ. Association of risk factors for choroidal neovascularization in age-related macular degeneration with decreased foveolar choroidal circulation. *Amer J. Ophthalmol.* 2010, 150:40-47

Xu, X.R. Zhou, Y.H., Chiou, G.C.Y. The effect of D-timolol and L-timolol on rat experimental choroidal neovascularization (CNV) in vivo and endothelial cells culture in vitro. *International J. Ophthalmol,* 2005; 5:831-835

Yehoshua Z, Wang F, Rosenfield PJ, Penha FM, Feuer WJ and Gregori, G. Natural history of drusen morphology in age-related macular degeneration using spectral domain optical coherence tomography. www.ophsource.org/periodicals/article 2009.

Zhou, J.L., Gao, X.Q., Cai, B., Sparrow, J.R. Indirect antioxidant protection against photooxidative processes initiated in retinal pigment epithelial cells by a lipofuscin pigment. *Rejuvenation Res,* 2006; 9(2):256-263

Zhuang, P., Shen, Y., Chiou, G.C.Y. Effects of flavone on ocular blood flow and formation of choroidal neovascularization. *International J. Ophthalmol,* 2010a; 10:1455-58

Zhuang, P., Shen, Y., and Chiou, G.C.Y. Effects of flavone on oxidation-induced injury of retinal pigment epithelium cells. *International J. Ophthalmol,* 2010b; 10:1641-1644

Zhuang, P., Shen, Y., Lin, B.Q., Zhang, W.Y. and Chiou, G.C.Y. Effect of quercetin on formation of choroidal neovascularization (CNV) in age-related macular degeneration (AMD) *Eye Sci.* 2011,26:23-29

Zou, Y.H., Chiou, G.C.Y. Apigenin inhibits laser-induced choroidal neovascularization and regulates endothelial cell function. *J. Ocular Pharmacol.* Therap. 2006; 22:425-430

Zou, Y.H., Chiou, G.C.Y. Pharmacological therapy in AMD. *International J Ophthalmol,* 2005; 5:8-18

Zou, Y.H., Jiang, W., Chiou, G.C.Y. Affect of tetramethylpyrazine on rat experimental choroidal neovascularization in vivo and endothelial cell culture in vitro. *Current Eye Res,* 2007; 32:71-75

Zou, Y.H., Xu X.R., Chiou, G.C.Y. Effort of interleukin-1 blockers, CK112 and CK116 on rat experimental choroidal neovascularization (CNV) in vivo and endothelial cells culture in vitro. *J. Ocular Pharmacol. Therap.* 2006; 22:19-25

15

Promising Treatment Strategies for Neovascular AMD: Anti-VEGF Therapy

Young Gun Park, Hyun Wook Ryu,
Seungbum Kang and Young Jung Roh
*Department of Ophthalmology, Yeouido St. Mary's Hospital,
College of Medicine, The Catholic University of Korea, Seoul,
Korea*

1. Introduction

Age-related macular degeneration (AMD) is one of the leading causes of substantial and irreversible vision loss. The prevalence of AMD can be expected to increase along with life expectancy, which has risen steadily [1, 2]. Without treatment, the neovascular form of AMD leads to severe quality-of-life loss within a short time period and considerable economic burden.

Vascular endothelial growth factor (VEGF) is a key mediator involved in the control of angiogenesis and vascular permeability and has been shown to be induced by hypoxia in cultured human retinal pigment epithelium (RPE) [3]. VEGF-A is the most potent promoter of angiogenesis and vascular permeability within the VEGF family and its role in the pathogenesis of neovascular AMD is well recognized [4, 5]. The advent of intravitreous VEGF inhibitors has revolutionized the management of neovascular AMD. Yet, frequently, indefinite injections of VEGF blocking agents introduce a significant treatment burden for patients with neovascular AMD, and may potentially put patients in the risk of developing ocular and systemic adverse effects from injections. Many studies on modified treatment regimens have been performed in an attempt to mitigate this burden without compromise to visual acuity outcomes. Meanwhile, various randomized clinical trials on combination therapies and efforts to develop new pharmacologic agents are ongoing.

2. Therapeutic monoclonal antibodies and fragments

2.1 Intravitreal ranibizumab and bevacizumab monotherapy

2.1.1 Vascular endothelial growth factor

VEGF plays an important role in a variety of in vitro processes, including angiogenesis, microvascular permeability, and endothelial cell survival. On the other hand, these activities are all essential to survival, VEGF has been linked to a number of pathogenic conditions, including neovascular AMD, diabetic retinopathy, and cancer.

Three VEGF therapies are currently used for the treatment of patients with neovascular AMD: pegaptanib (Macugen, OSI Pharmaceuticals, USA), ranibizumab (Lucentis, Genentech, USA), and bevacizumab (Avastin, Genentech, USA).

Pegaptanib is an oligonucleotide aptamer and was the first VEGF antagonist to be approved by the US Food and Drug Administration (FDA) for use in wet AMD. However, wet AMD patients treated with pegaptanib still experience visual decline. [2, 6] The first monoclonal antibody developed to target VEGF was bevacizumab, a humanized murine monoclonal antibody. Bevacizumab was initially developed for applications in oncology, and received approval as a first-line therapy for widespread colorectal cancer from the US FDA in 2004. Bevacizumab has subsequently been approved for use in non-small cell lung cancer and breast cancer.

The successful development of VEGF as an oncology target led to interest in the potential of anti-VEGF treatment for other therapeutic indications, including ocular neovascular disorders. VEGF-A has been identified as the primary angiogenesis mediator in the eye. It is implicated in ocular neovascularization through its promotion of blood vessel formation and permeability. A role for VEGF-A in neovascular AMD is suggested by immunohistochemistry localization in human choroidal neovascular (CNV) lesions and extrapolation from other disease models [5, 7-9].

New blood vessel formation and leakage play important roles in the development of the neovascular form of AMD, and clinical trials of agents that block VEGF-A activity have produced more evidence that VEGF-A is important in development of this disease.

Ranibizumab is a humanized antibody fragment against VEGF which was specifically designed for intraocular use as a smaller antibody fragment to penetrate through the retina better. The Food and Drug Administration (FDA) approved ranibizumab for treatment of subfoveal neovascular AMD in June, 2006. It was the first drug for AMD treatment shown to improve visual acuity in a substantial percentage of patients.

Bevacizumab is a recombinant humanized monoclonal immunoglobulin antibody that inhibits the activity of VEGF. It has a similar action and is related to the ranibizumab compound with respect to its structure. Bevacizumab was approved by the FDA for the treatment of metastatic colorectal cancer in 2004, but it has not been licensed for the treatment of wet AMD or any other ocular conditions. However, it is recently used off-label worldwide not only for wet AMD but also for other ocular disease entities associated with macular edema and abnormal vessel growth.

Intraocular pharmacokinetic data derived from studies in monkeys demonstrated that through intravitreal administration, ranibizumab distributed rapidly to the retina and had a vitreous half-life of 3 days. Studies in rabbits have demonstrated that ranibizumab can rapidly penetrate through the retina to reach the choroid, just 1 hr after intravitreal admidistration [10]. In primates, serum ranibizumab levels were found to be more than 1000-fold lower than in the vitreous and aquous humor following a single intravitreal injection [11]. These were negligible and tissue concentrations were undetectable.

2.1.2 Safety

Systemic VEGF inhibition is suspected to be associated with an increased risk of hypertension and arterial thromboembolic events. Given the average age of patients requiring treatment for AMD, it is important that their treatment does not significantly increase the risk of these events. The rate of arterial thromboembolic events and hypertension was low. Over the 24 months trial period, the rates in the ranibizumab 0.5 mg treatment group of the ANCHOR, MARINA, and PIER trials was 5.0 %, 4.6 %, and 0 %, respectively, compared with 4.2 %, 3.8 %, and 0 % in the control group.

2.1.3 Efficacy

The pivotal phase III Minimally Classic/Occult Trial of the Anti-VEGF Antibody Ranibizumab in the Treatment of Neovascular AMD (MARINA) [12] and the Anti-VEGF Antibody for the Treatment of Predominantly Classic CNV in AMD (ANCHOR) trial [13, 14] demonstrated best-corrected visual acuity (BCVA) outcomes were far superior to any previously published study in the treatment of this disease. At the end of 24 months in the MARINA trial, significantly more ranibizumab-treated patients had maintained [lost <15 Early Treatment Diabetic Retinopathy Study (ETDRS) letters] or improved vision than sham-injected patients. Indeed, 90–95% of patients treated with 0.3 and 0.5 mg ranibizumab maintained vision compared with 53–64% of control patients. Over the same period, vision improved in 25–34% of treated eyes, compared with 4–5% of sham-injected patients.

In the ANCHOR trial, ranibizumab was compared with verteporfin photodynamic therapy (PDT) and demonstrated similar findings: 90–96% of the ranibizumab-treated versus 64–66% of the PDT-treated patients maintained vision, whereas 34–41% versus 6% of each group, respectively, gained more than 15 letters.

These outcomes were significantly better than those achieved by the control groups.

In both trials, a biphasic treatment effect was observed, with the majority of the visual gain achieved in the first 3 months of treatment (the loading phase) followed by stabilization of the gain (the maintenance phase).

Patient-reported outcomes were also assessed in the ANCHOR and MARINA trials to measure the influence of the ranibizumab-mediated improvement in visual acuity (VA) on quality of life. The data demonstrated that patients treated with ranibizumab were more likely to report improvements in near activities, distance activities, and vision specific dependency which were maintained over the 2 year duration of the trial [15, 16]. These data demonstrate that the clinical improvements seen with ranibizumab treatment translate into meaningful benefits for the patient.

More recently, the anatomical benefit of ranibizumab treatment in both the MARINA and ANCHOR studies with regard to angiographic and optical coherence tomography (OCT) characteristics has also been demonstrated. [12, 15, 16] Both functional and anatomical improvements were maintained over the 24 month study period with monthly injections.

Bevacizumab, the predecessor of ranibizumab, is a full-length monoclonal antibody that binds to and blocks the action of all VEGF isoforms. Numerous retrospective [17-20] and prospective studies [21-23] of intravitreal bevacizumab have reported its efficacy for neovascular AMD and low rates of treatment related complications [24]. Although a number of these studies were uncontrolled, relatively small in sample size, of limited follow-up, and varied with regard to outcome measures and retreatment criteria, the reported efficacy of bevacizumab coupled with its low cost when utilized as an intraocular agent has propelled its adoption worldwide.

A recent, large, multicenter, randomized prospective study (Bevacizumab for Neovascular Age-Related Macular Degeneration [ABC] trial) that demonstrated MARINA/ANCHOR-like results lends further support for its use in neovascular AMD [25, 26]. On the basis of results from the pivotal phase III clinical trials, ranibizumab dosed monthly represents the gold standard to which all other therapeutics and regimens are to be compared. In clinical practice, many retinal physicians have extrapolated the data and continued using bevacizumab. A formal head-to-head comparison of bevacizumab and ranibizumab is being conducted by the National Eye Institute of the National Institute of Health in the Comparisons of Age-Related Macular Degeneration Treatment Trials (CATTs) [27, 28]. The CATT study design includes four treatment arms: either bevacizumab or ranibizumab on a variable schedule means that monthly follow-up and evaluation of fluid based on OCT, and anti-VEGF injection when CNV becomes active and either bevacizumab or ranibizumab on a fixed monthly schedule for 1 year followed by random assignment to either continued monthly injections or a variable schedule based on the treatment response. The primary outcome measure is mean change in BCVA; secondary outcome measures include number of treatments, anatomical changes in the retina, adverse events, and cost. Preliminary results are reported in 2011 and will provide insight into how ranibizumab and bevacizumab compare with each other within the context of either a fixed monthly or traditional pro re nata (PRN) approach. At 1 year, bevacizumab and ranibizumab had equivalent effects on VA when administered according to the same schedule. Bevacizumab administered monthly was equivalent to ranibizumab administered monthly, with 8.0 and 8.5 letters gained, respectively. Bevacizumab administered as needed was equivalent to ranibizumab as needed, with 5.9 and 6.8 letters gained, respectively. Ranibizumab given as needed with monthly evaluation had effects on vision that were equivalent to those of ranibizumab administered monthly, although the comparison between bevacizumab as needed and monthly bevacizumab was inclusive. Differences in rate of serious adverse events require further study.

3. Modified treatment regimens

The prospect of indefinitely adhering to the monthly treatment schedules of MARINA and ANCHOR has raised ocular and systemic safety concerns as well as convenience and cost issues for patient and physician alike. The identification of alternative dosing strategies capable of reducing the number of required anti-VEGF injections while still achieving VA outcomes similar to those reached in the pivotal trials has since been a subject of great interest.

The observed biphasic treatment effect raised the possibility that, after the initial 3-months loading phase, maintenance of VA gain may be achieved with less frequent treatments. A PIER trial evaluated ranibizumab administered monthly for 3 months, followed by quarterly injections, and compared this with sham treatment. Under this schedule, ranibizumab did provide a significant VA benefit; a significantly greater number of patients achieved VA stabilization at 24 months compared with patients receiving sham treatment. However, subgroup analysis revealed that VA gains observed during the first 3 months of treatment were only maintained in 40% of patients over the duration of the trial, and for the remaining 60% quarterly dosing was not suitable [29, 30]. Results for both ranibizumab doses in the PIER trial (0.3 and 0.5mg) showed an initial mean improvement in BCVA during the initiation phase with monthly dosing, but after month 3 in the maintenance phase with quarterly dosing, there was a gradual decline in mean BCVA to below the pretreatment baseline (2.2 letters) at 12 months, which remained unchanged at 24 months [30].

More recently, the Efficacy and Safety of Ranibizumab in Patients with Subfoveal Choroidal Neovascularization Secondary to Age-Related Macular Degeneration (EXCITE) study directly compared the PIER regimen with a fixed monthly treatment arm (0.3 mg ranibizumab) [31]. Although BCVA outcomes in the two quarterly treatment arms fared better than those in the PIER study at 12 months (2.2 and 3.1 letters gain with 0.3 and 0.5 mg ranibizumab, respectively), neither was as good as monthly dosing (0.9 letters gain). These suboptimal results demonstrate that, on average, quarterly treatment is inferior to monthly treatment; thus, it has never been adopted in practice.

Subsequently to the PIER trial, further investigation of a flexible dosing approach was carried out. The EXCITE trial directly compared a maintenance phase of quarterly injections against the monthly regimen. Consistent with previous observations, an initial gain was made in the first 3 months, after which patients receiving monthly injections contributed to gain VA, whilst those receiving quarterly injections showed a decrease from their 3 months VA levels. **(Table 1.)**

Study design	MARINA	ANCHOR	PIER	EXCITE
Study duration	24 months	24 months	24 months	12 months
Number of patients	716	423	184	353
Visit regimen in maintenance phase	Monthly	Monthly	Quarterly	Monthly for control Quarterly for study
Ranibizumab regimen in maintenance phase	Monthly	Monthly	Quarterly	Monthly for control Quarterly for study
No. of injections in maintenance phase	9	9	3	9 for control 3 for study

Table 1. Summary table of many different treatment regimen.

The current norm in clinical practice with ranibizumab or bevacizumab is to implement an initiation/induction phase followed by an individualized maintenance phase that is modeled after one of two basic approaches: traditional PRN [32] or 'treat and extend' [33, 34]. Traditional PRN involves both regular follow-up and treatment until the macula is more or less free of exudation, with treatment thereafter during the maintenance phase only in the presence of recurrent exudation. The original prospective studies that evaluated a PRN approach to the maintenance phase were the Prospective Optical Coherence Tomography Imaging of Patients with Neovascular AMD Treated with Intra-Ocular Lucentis (PrONTO) study [35] and the Secondary to Age-Related Macular Degeneration (SAILOR) study [36]. More recently, the Study of Ranibizumab in Patients with Subfoveal Choroidal Neovascularization Secondary to Age-Related Macular Degeneration (SUSTAIN) study has contributed additional data [37]. In each of these trials, patients received three consecutive, monthly intravitreal injections of ranibizumab for induction, followed by monthly office visits. Thereafter, a PRN maintenance phase adhered to the following retreatment criteria: loss of at least five ETDRS letters, increase in central macular thickness on OCT of at least 100μm, or new hemorrhage.

Of the three studies, the PrONTO study demonstrated the best VA results. The PrONTO study evaluated an OCT guided, variable-dosing regimen with ranibizumab (0.5 mg) and showed that mean VA improved by 9.3 ETDRS letters at 12 months. Over a 2-year period, mean BCVA outcomes were similar to MARINA and ANCHOR with a mean of 9.9 injections (5.6 in the first year and 4.3 in the second). In comparison, results from the SAILOR study were not as good. In this study, the mean change in BCVA at 12 months from baseline was 0.5 and 1.7 letters in the treatment-naive and previously treated groups, respectively, at the 0.3 mg dose and 2.3 letters in both groups at 0.5 mg. It is worth noting that participants were not monitored as closely in SAILOR as compared with PrONTO, averaging nine visits through 1 year and a mean of 4.9 injections.

The 12-month results from SUSTAIN were slightly better than those from SAILOR (mean BCVA from baseline of 3.6 letters), yet still not as good as the monthly treatment trials. In contrast to SAILOR, participants in the SUSTAIN trial were followed monthly (more like PrONTO) and the mean number of injections over the first year was higher at 5.6.

Other relatively large studies using a traditional PRN approach have recently been published [38-40]. An analysis of these reports highlights an important trend: the best visual acuity results come from the study with the greatest mean number of treatments and closest follow-up, whereas the poorest outcomes were observed in the study with the lowest mean number of treatments and office visits. Unlike traditional PRN, a treat and extend approach initially involves regular and frequent treatment until the macula is dry, followed by a gradual extension of the treatment interval and corresponding follow-up visit. Treatment interval extension continues until there are signs of recurrence, at which point the treatment interval is then reduced.

Kang et al. [41, 42] recently published a retrospective analysis that monthly injections were not given in contrast to the three injections during the initial treatment period in the PIER and PrONTO trials. This study showed that visual acuity improved by 0.078 logMAR units and minimized the number of injections given during 12 months of follow-up (a mean of 4.07 injections were given over the 12 months). The decreased need for retreatment is of great benefit to both patients and clinicians. These results may raise doubts about the need for the three initial loading injections. They reported another study [42], the mean number of injections given in the 12 months period was 4.2 (range, 1-6). Patients were also offered reinjection with ranibizumab on an "as needed" basis. Data showed that the percentage of patients (71.9%) with no visual loss or improved visual acuity was comparable to the percentages in the monthly injection-based studies.

In addition, Gupta et al. evaluated a treat and extend approach with bevacizumab and found nearly identical results at 12 months following a mean of 7.3 injections in the first year [40]. Although various methods for individualizing maintenance therapy have been proposed, the optimal non-monthly dosing regimen still remains unclear.

4. Combination therapy: Photodynamic therapy and antivascular endothelial growth factor therapy

The development and propagation of CNV membranes involve pro-angiogenic factors, vascular permeability molecules, and inflammatory proteins. Current standard treatment with monthly intravitreal injections of anti-VEGF monotherapy can be limited to the angiogenic component of CNV development and burdensome for both the physician and patient. Patients are subjected to increased risk of adverse effects from monthly treatments that may be lessened with treatment options given with less frequency [43]. While current monotherapy with anti-VEGF agents are effective therapy for CNV, their benefits are short-lived as they are unable to regress the lesions completely. Combination therapy with PDT proven to be effective in CNV regression may have a role not only in the treatment of CNV development but also may provide synergy through blocking adverse effects.

PDT was approved in 2000 by the FDA for the treatment of CNV secondary to AMD. Treatment involves intravenous administration of a light-sensitive dye called verteporfin followed by laser-guided, location-specific activation within the CNV membrane. Activation of the verteporfin molecules incite a phototoxic event within blood vessels, induce endothelial cell damage, platelet aggregation, and eventually lead to thrombosis of vascular channels. Treatment size is limited by the greatest linear diameter of the CNV lesion being treated [44, 45].

Variable factors within PDT treatment regimens include time of laser application and laser fluence. Standard fluence PDT (sfPDT) was commonly employed in the early studies. The Treatment of AMD with PDT (TAP) study showed stabilization but no improvement in vision with this protocol. In addition, other studies have reported that PDT may inadvertently perturb the normal choriocapillaris bordering a pathologic CNV lesion, resulting in up-regulation and expression of VEGF [46, 47]. This collateral damage may potentially be minimized with reduced-fluence PDT (rfPDT) [46]. rfPDT protocols have gained popularity because of its potential for increased CNV membrane selectivity and propensity to cause less surrounding retinal inflammation. The Verteporfin in Minimally Classic (VIM) trial employed both a standard and reduced fluence PDT protocol and showed stability of vision with either treatment over placebo, but it showed a clear trend toward a better visual outcome with rfPDT. In another comparative study, patients treated with rfPDT tended to have lower rates of severe visual loss and an overall better visual prognosis [46].

While PDT is intended to specifically target CNV vessels, collateral damage to surrounding blood vessels may lead to ischemia of healthy tissue. Following PDT of a CNV membrane, induced ischemia can lead to production of pro-angiogenic factors, especially VEGF. Therefore, combining verteporfin PDT and anti-VEGF therapy may be beneficial compared with either modality alone, yielding longer treatment-free intervals and requiring fewer intravitreal injections [44].

The RhuFab V2 Ocular Treatment Combining the Use of Visudyne to Evaluate Safety (FOCUS) study is a multicenter, randomized, single-blind study designed to evaluate the safety and efficacy of sfPDT in combination with intravitreal ranibizumab [48, 49]. It compared sfPDT to combination sfPDT and intravitreal ranibizumab in the treatment of predominantly classic CNV secondary to AMD. One-year data showed greater visual stability in the patients treated with combination therapy and 23.8% of patients experienced improvement in visual acuity, compared with 5% of patients treated with PDT monotherapy alone. The number of re-treatments with sfPDT were decreased as well with 91% of patients treated with sfPDT monotherapy requiring repeat treatment while only 28% of patients treated with combination therapy requiring re-treatment within one year. Two-year data showed similar results with 88% of combination treated patients losing less than 15 lines of vision versus 75% of sfPDT alone treated patients. Combination therapy required an average of 0.4 repeat PDT treatments compared with an average of 3.0 in the sfPDT group [49].

5. Vascular endothelial growth factor Trap-Eye

The most effective dosing regimen and monitoring program for anti-VEGF therapy has yet to be firmly established but new treatments are aimed at extending and improving on the efficacy of ranibizumab. VEGF Trap-Eye (aflibercept, Regeneron Pharmaceuticals, USA) is a promising new anti-VEGF drug. Structurally, VEGF Trap-Eye is a fusion protein of key binding domains of human VEGF receptor 1 and 2 combined with a human IgG Fc fragment. Functionally, VEGF Trap-Eye acts as a receptor decoy with high affinity for all VEGF isoforms, binding more tightly. VEGF Trap-Eye differs from established anti-VEGF therapies in its higher binding affinity for VEGF-A and its blockage of placental growth factors-1 and -2 [50, 51].

Recently, the 1 year results of two parallel randomized, double-masked phase 3 clinical trials (VIEW 1 and VIEW 2) on the efficacy and safety of VEGF Trap-Eye for the treatment of neovascular AMD were reported [51]. Phase I data demonstrated acceptable safety and tolerability of VEGF Trap-Eye in the treatment of neovascular AMD. In Phase II study data, patients dosed in a similar fashion to the PrONTO trial demonstrated stabilization of their vision that was similar to previous studies of ranibizumab at 1 year. All dosing regimens of VEGF Trap-Eye, including 2 mg bimonthly met the primary endpoint of non inferiority compared with monthly 0.5 mg ranibizumab with regard to the percentage of patients with maintenance (loss of <15 ETDRS letters) or improvement in vision. The all treatment groups showed a mean gain of 5.3 letters at 1 year. A greater mean improvement in VA compared with monthly 0.5 mg ranibizumab at 1 year versus baseline represented the secondary endpoint of the study. In both the North American study (VIEW 1) and international study (VIEW 2), more than 95% of patients in each of the following VEGF Trap-Eye dosing groups achieved maintenance of vision compared with 94% of patients on monthly ranibizumab: 0.5 mg monthly, 2 mg monthly, and 2 mg every 2 months. In VIEW 1, patients on 2 mg monthly dosing achieved the secondary endpoint with a mean gain of 10.9 ETDRS letters compared with 8.1 for monthly ranibizumab [51].

The results of the VIEW studies come at a critical time, when clinical evidence suggests that less frequent dosing of existing anti-VEGF therapy, particularly in the first year, may yield inconsistent visual acuity outcome. In particular, the ability to achieve maintenance or improvement in VA with a more convenient every-other-month injection without need for intervening office visits may potentiate a shift in the current management of neovascular AMD. Continuation of the VIEW studies through the second year will assess the various VEGF Trap-Eye doses administered every 3 months, or more often in the case of worsening disease, as per protocol-defined 'quarterly capped PRN' schedule. Based on phase II data, VEGF Trap-Eye seems to be generally well tolerated with no serious drug-related adverse events. In the 157 patients enrolled in phase II trial, there were two deaths (one from pre-existing pulmonary hypertension and one from pancreatic carcinoma) and one arterial thromboembolic events (patient with a history of previous stroke), but no serious systemic events occurred related to VEGF Trap-Eye [51].

In contrast to current anti-VEGF antibodies, which are rapidly cleared, the VEGF Trap-Eye is relatively degraded more slowly. Due to its high binding affinity and the ability to safely inject high doses into the eye, VEGF Trap-Eye may have longer duration of effect in the eye. Its adoption into clinical practice will depend on efficacy at 4 and 8 week intervals. If effective at 4 and 8 week intervals, VEGF Trap-Eye may offer a competitive price advantage over ranibizumab and the opportunity to significantly reduce treatment burden on patients and physicians.

6. Conclusion

Blindness secondary to AMD is common across the world and the pathogenesis of this severe condition is not fully understood. However, the advent of anti-VEGF therapy has revolutionized therapy in the management of neovascular AMD. The appropriate method, dose, regimen, types of combination therapy, and the safety of anti-VEGF remain to be investigated but randomized trials are pending and may provide a clearer answer, which hopefully can help in the treatment of resistant CNV with longer time between treatments.

7. References

[1] Bressler, N.M., *Age-related macular degeneration is the leading cause of blindness.* JAMA, 2004. 291(15): p. 1900-1.

[2] Emerson, M.V. and A.K. Lauer, *Current and emerging therapies for the treatment of age-related macular degeneration.* Clin Ophthalmol, 2008. 2(2): p. 377-88.

[3] Shima, D.T., et al., *Hypoxic induction of endothelial cell growth factors in retinal cells: identification and characterization of vascular endothelial growth factor (VEGF) as the mitogen.* Mol Med, 1995. 1(2): p. 182-93.

[4] Ferrara, N., H.P. Gerber, and J. LeCouter, *The biology of VEGF and its receptors.* Nat Med, 2003. 9(6): p. 669-76.

[5] Kliffen, M., et al., *Increased expression of angiogenic growth factors in age-related maculopathy.* Br J Ophthalmol, 1997. 81(2): p. 154-62.

[6] Gragoudas, E.S., et al., *Pegaptanib for neovascular age-related macular degeneration.* N Engl J Med, 2004. 351(27): p. 2805-16.

[7] Aiello, L.P., et al., *Vascular endothelial growth factor in ocular fluid of patients with diabetic retinopathy and other retinal disorders.* N Engl J Med, 1994. 331(22): p. 1480-7.

[8] Boyd, S.R., et al., *Correlation of increased vascular endothelial growth factor with neovascularization and permeability in ischemic central vein occlusion.* Arch Ophthalmol, 2002. 120(12): p. 1644-50.

[9] Kvanta, A., et al., *Subfoveal fibrovascular membranes in age-related macular degeneration express vascular endothelial growth factor.* Invest Ophthalmol Vis Sci, 1996. 37(9): p. 1929-34.
[10] Gaudreault, J., et al., *Pharmacokinetics and retinal distribution of ranibizumab, a humanized antibody fragment directed against VEGF-A, following intravitreal administration in rabbits.* Retina, 2007. 27(9): p. 1260-6.
[11] Gaudreault, J., et al., *Preclinical pharmacokinetics of Ranibizumab (rhuFabV2) after a single intravitreal administration.* Invest Ophthalmol Vis Sci, 2005. 46(2): p. 726-33.
[12] Brown, D.M., et al., *Ranibizumab versus verteporfin for neovascular age-related macular degeneration.* N Engl J Med, 2006. 355(14): p. 1432-44.
[13] Brown, D.M., et al., *Ranibizumab versus verteporfin photodynamic therapy for neovascular age-related macular degeneration: Two-year results of the ANCHOR study.* Ophthalmology, 2009. 116(1): p. 57-65 e5.
[14] Rosenfeld, P.J., et al., *Ranibizumab for neovascular age-related macular degeneration.* N Engl J Med, 2006. 355(14): p. 1419-31.
[15] Kaiser, P.K., et al., *Angiographic and optical coherence tomographic results of the MARINA study of ranibizumab in neovascular age-related macular degeneration.* Ophthalmology, 2007. 114(10): p. 1868-75.
[16] Sadda, S.R., et al., *Anatomical benefit from ranibizumab treatment of predominantly classic neovascular age-related macular degeneration in the 2-year anchor study.* Retina, 2010. 30(9): p. 1390-9.
[17] Spaide, R.F., et al., *Intravitreal bevacizumab treatment of choroidal neovascularization secondary to age-related macular degeneration.* Retina, 2006. 26(4): p. 383-90.
[18] Emerson, M.V., et al., *Intravitreal bevacizumab (Avastin) treatment of neovascular age-related macular degeneration.* Retina, 2007. 27(4): p. 439-44.
[19] Cleary, C.A., et al., *Intravitreal bevacizumab in the treatment of neovascular age-related macular degeneration, 6- and 9-month results.* Eye (Lond), 2008. 22(1): p. 82-6.
[20] Yoganathan, P., et al., *Visual improvement following intravitreal bevacizumab (Avastin) in exudative age-related macular degeneration.* Retina, 2006. 26(9): p. 994-8.
[21] Avery, R.L., et al., *Intravitreal bevacizumab (Avastin) for neovascular age-related macular degeneration.* Ophthalmology, 2006. 113(3): p. 363-372 e5.
[22] Bashshur, Z.F., et al., *Intravitreal bevacizumab for treatment of neovascular age-related macular degeneration: a one-year prospective study.* Am J Ophthalmol, 2008. 145(2): p. 249-256.
[23] Algvere, P.V., et al., *A prospective study on intravitreal bevacizumab (Avastin) for neovascular age-related macular degeneration of different durations.* Acta Ophthalmol, 2008. 86(5): p. 482-9.
[24] Wu, L., et al., *Twelve-month safety of intravitreal injections of bevacizumab (Avastin): results of the Pan-American Collaborative Retina Study Group (PACORES).* Graefes Arch Clin Exp Ophthalmol, 2008. 246(1): p. 81-7.
[25] Arevalo, J.F., et al., *Intravitreal bevacizumab for subfoveal choroidal neovascularization in age-related macular degeneration at twenty-four months: the Pan-American Collaborative Retina Study.* Ophthalmology, 2010. 117(10): p. 1974-81, 1981 e1.
[26] Tufail, A., et al., *Bevacizumab for neovascular age related macular degeneration (ABC Trial): multicentre randomised double masked study.* BMJ, 2010. 340: p. c2459.
[27] Martin, D.F., et al., *Ranibizumab and bevacizumab for neovascular age-related macular degeneration.* N Engl J Med, 2011. 364(20): p. 1897-908.
[28] Rosenfeld, P.J., *Bevacizumab versus ranibizumab for AMD.* N Engl J Med, 2011. 364(20): p. 1966-7.
[29] Regillo, C.D., et al., *Randomized, double-masked, sham-controlled trial of ranibizumab for neovascular age-related macular degeneration: PIER Study year 1.* Am J Ophthalmol, 2008. 145(2): p. 239-248.

[30] Abraham, P., H. Yue, and L. Wilson, *Randomized, double-masked, sham-controlled trial of ranibizumab for neovascular age-related macular degeneration: PIER study year 2.* Am J Ophthalmol, 2010. 150(3): p. 315-324 e1.
[31] Schmidt-Erfurth, U., et al., *Efficacy and safety of monthly versus quarterly ranibizumab treatment in neovascular age-related macular degeneration: the EXCITE study.* Ophthalmology, 2011. 118(5): p. 831-9.
[32] Spaide, R., *Ranibizumab according to need: a treatment for age-related macular degeneration.* Am J Ophthalmol, 2007. 143(4): p. 679-80.
[33] Brown, D.M. and C.D. Regillo, *Anti-VEGF agents in the treatment of neovascular age-related macular degeneration: applying clinical trial results to the treatment of everyday patients.* Am J Ophthalmol, 2007. 144(4): p. 627-37.
[34] Chiang, A. and C.D. Regillo, *Preferred therapies for neovascular age-related macular degeneration.* Curr Opin Ophthalmol, 2011. 22(3): p. 199-204.
[35] Lalwani, G.A., et al., *A variable-dosing regimen with intravitreal ranibizumab for neovascular age-related macular degeneration: year 2 of the PrONTO Study.* Am J Ophthalmol, 2009. 148(1): p. 43-58 e1.
[36] Boyer, D.S., et al., *A Phase IIIb study to evaluate the safety of ranibizumab in subjects with neovascular age-related macular degeneration.* Ophthalmology, 2009. 116(9): p. 1731-9.
[37] Tano, Y. and M. Ohji, *EXTEND-I: safety and efficacy of ranibizumab in Japanese patients with subfoveal choroidal neovascularization secondary to age-related macular degeneration.* Acta Ophthalmol, 2010. 88(3): p. 309-16.
[38] Dadgostar, H., et al., *Evaluation of injection frequency and visual acuity outcomes for ranibizumab monotherapy in exudative age-related macular degeneration.* Ophthalmology, 2009. 116(9): p. 1740-7.
[39] Rothenbuehler, S.P., et al., *Effects of ranibizumab in patients with subfoveal choroidal neovascularization attributable to age-related macular degeneration.* Am J Ophthalmol, 2009. 147(5): p. 831-7.
[40] Gupta, O.P., et al., *A treat and extend regimen using ranibizumab for neovascular age-related macular degeneration clinical and economic impact.* Ophthalmology, 2010. 117(11): p. 2134-40.
[41] Kang, S. and Y.J. Roh, *Ranibizumab treatment administered as needed for occult and minimally classic neovascular membranes in age-related macular degeneration.* Jpn J Ophthalmol, 2011. 55(2): p. 123-7.
[42] Kang, S. and Y.J. Roh, *One-year results of intravitreal ranibizumab for neovascular age-related macular degeneration and clinical responses of various subgroups.* Jpn J Ophthalmol, 2009. 53(4): p. 389-95.
[43] Beer, P.M., et al., *Intraocular concentration and pharmacokinetics of triamcinolone acetonide after a single intravitreal injection.* Ophthalmology, 2003. 110(4): p. 681-6.
[44] Cruess, A.F., et al., *Photodynamic therapy with verteporfin in age-related macular degeneration: a systematic review of efficacy, safety, treatment modifications and pharmacoeconomic properties.* Acta Ophthalmol, 2009. 87(2): p. 118-32.
[45] *Verteporfin therapy of subfoveal choroidal neovascularization in age-related macular degeneration: two-year results of a randomized clinical trial including lesions with occult with no classic choroidal neovascularization--verteporfin in photodynamic therapy report 2.* Am J Ophthalmol, 2001. 131(5): p. 541-60.
[46] Azab, M., et al., *Verteporfin therapy of subfoveal minimally classic choroidal neovascularization in age-related macular degeneration: 2-year results of a randomized clinical trial.* Arch Ophthalmol, 2005. 123(4): p. 448-57.

[47] Azab, M., et al., *Verteporfin therapy of subfoveal choroidal neovascularization in age-related macular degeneration: meta-analysis of 2-year safety results in three randomized clinical trials: Treatment Of Age-Related Macular Degeneration With Photodynamic Therapy and Verteporfin In Photodynamic Therapy Study Report no. 4.* Retina, 2004. 24(1): p. 1-12.
[48] Antoszyk, A.N., et al., *Ranibizumab combined with verteporfin photodynamic therapy in neovascular age-related macular degeneration (FOCUS): year 2 results.* Am J Ophthalmol, 2008. 145(5): p. 862-74.
[49] Heier, J.S., et al., *Ranibizumab combined with verteporfin photodynamic therapy in neovascular age-related macular degeneration: year 1 results of the FOCUS Study.* Arch Ophthalmol, 2006. 124(11): p. 1532-42.
[50] *Aflibercept: AVE 0005, AVE 005, AVE0005, VEGF Trap - Regeneron, VEGF Trap (R1R2), VEGF Trap-Eye.* Drugs R D, 2008. 9(4): p. 261-9.
[51] Dixon, J.A., et al., *VEGF Trap-Eye for the treatment of neovascular age-related macular degeneration.* Expert Opin Investig Drugs, 2009. 18(10): p. 1573-80.